The Shape of Things to Come

DRUIN BURCH is a physician who practises at the John Radcliffe Hospital in Oxford. He is the author of *Digging Up the Dead* and *Taking the Medicine*.

The Shape of Things to Come

Future Lives, Future Bodies

Druin Burch

HEAD of ZEUS

An Apollo Book

This is an Apollo book, first published in the UK in 2019 by
Head of Zeus Ltd

9 7 5 3 1 2 4 6 8

A catalogue record for this book is available from
the British Library.

ISBN (HB): 9781788543385
ISBN (E): 9781788543378

Typeset by Adrian McLaughlin

Printed and bound in Great Britain by
CPI Group (UK) Ltd, Croydon CR0 4YY

Head of Zeus Ltd
First Floor East
5–8 Hardwick Street
London EC1R 4RG

WWW.HEADOFZEUS.COM

To Rachel Eleanor Burch,
whose spring helps make my summer

Contents

The shape of
things to come

Speculating on what changes lie ahead for human lives, and human bodies, is relatively new. Science fiction has been fondly enthusiastic, as likely to attach tentacles as facts. But the serious exercise of imagination has not been possible for long, and not solely because we lacked the power to change very much. Before the late 1700s even the concept of change was unavailable. In a few dizzying decades at the end of the eighteenth and beginning of the nineteenth centuries, everything altered. You cannot look to the future without a feel for the past, and during those decades we first properly acquired it. Before that our knowledge told us our world had been largely unchanged in the 6,000 years since Creation. Explore the Holy Land and you would find that the Bible spoke accurately of its geography. Dig up mummified people and animals from beneath great pyramids and it was plain they were our fellow creatures. The only difference that was palpable was that the spirit of the age could always be compared unfavourably against that which was fading – but that impulse, too, showed its own constancy over the years. 'What times, what manners', complained Cicero in 63 BC. 'My dear old friend, you and I shall never see such days again! The peaches are not so big now as they were', wrote the painter Benjamin Robert Haydon to Wordsworth in 1842. 'Happiness', said Spike Milligan, more than a hundred years later, 'is a yesterday thing.'*

Only slightly more than two centuries ago did we become able to see further back. Humans had not always been around, it turned out, nor mountains, nor seas, nor earth. Geologists, realising how old and strange the world was, complained of being deafened by the terrifying drip, drip, drip of time. Everything is in flux, Heraclitus had said, but he hadn't realised quite how true that was. A gentle meandering trickle had slowly carved out valleys and mountains and epochs. Tennyson wrote in melancholy amazement of nature as being too huge to treasure us. Gone was the sense of life on a scale such that not a sparrow fell without notice. Tennyson called nature indifferent to individuals and caring only to preserve species – but even species, as life's record became more readable, were expendable, even legions of them.

Astronomers wrote of looking to the heavens and feeling vertigo, their sense of self spinning out into the chilling hugeness. 'The days of our years are threescore years and ten; and if by reason of strength they be fourscore years, yet is their strength labour and sorrow; for it is soon cut off, and we fly away.' Thus spoke the psalm, confident and precise. As the vast stretch of the world swam into view, framed by what came to be called Deep Time and Deep Space, the Bible ceased to seem an easy and obvious guide to non-spiritual knowledge. Medicine became excitingly unmoored – the assumption that the Greeks and Romans had known all there was to know, that it was the job of modern practitioners solely to guard and preserve their

---

* Santayana believed we began to think less of the world as we grew old enough to sense that it was more than willing to carry on without us.

wisdom, evaporated into the cold gap between the stars, split apart with the relentless tapping of the geologist's hammer. When the past turned out to have been so unfathomably strange, what might the future bring? Who knew now what was possible? While he was developing vaccination, Edward Jenner wrote excitedly to John Hunter, asking his old mentor whether he thought an idea would work. 'Why think?' Hunter replied scornfully, 'why not try the experiment?' Our physiques, our lifespans and our vitality were no longer set in the stone frame of constancy. In them, as in all else, lay a boundless potential for experiment, change and discovery. The past no longer belonged to us. As a consequence, the future did. The sense that its form was not fixed meant it was ours to mould.

Life reshapes itself. Plants take in carbon dioxide but breathe out oxygen. Their expirations allowed the inspiration giving life to a million others. Many creatures became enrolled, usually to mutual benefit, as sex aids to the plants. Reshaping goes on within species too. An old joke has two weary fellows bathing their feet in an African stream. They see a group of hungry lions approach, and one man dries his feet and starts putting on his socks and his shoes. 'What's the point?' asks the other, 'we can't outrun lions.' 'True,' the first replies, with a touch of manly regret, 'but I can outrun you.' Competition fuels survival, and survival is the engine of change. As the biologist J. B. S. Haldane pointed out, even the origins of altruism can be explained by genetic self-interest – he would sacrifice himself, he said, to save eight first cousins or two brothers. It was Darwin who noticed that natural selection did not merely pick out traits of direct advantage but did other, subtler things too. Stephen Jay Gould, late in the twentieth century, described some as

3

'ineluctable consequences of structural design'. Male humans, like male lions, became faster and stronger and larger than their female counterparts because males compete by fighting with each other. Women with a taste for pace, strength and size in their men were more likely to have successful offspring. Qualities that began as practical became aesthetic. The same applies outside the limited boundaries of physicality. Truth and honour emerge as characteristics that aid survival and reproductive success, but they win their place in our genes by winning a place in our hearts. Our sense of morality and beauty is not a false overlay on our real desires but the structure that supports them. 'I could not love thee, dear, so much, / Loved I not honour more' has a spine of truth.[1]

Sexual taste, not solely for an isolated physical act but for a relationship and a shared family life, literally blends everything together. Within an alpha male system, where males fight to the death and females take the winner, males are larger in order to give themselves the outside chance of bloody success. But the pressures remain when the race is no longer to the swiftest, nor the battle to the strong. To live is to choose. Selecting on the basis of wit, honeyed voice, sound judgement or upright morality is still to select. Your choices shape the future just as, over generations, tastes shape success, and success shapes taste. It says something about different human cultures and shared evolution that one can no longer become American president without being tall; it says something else that this is not so vital for a British prime minister. Linking specifics too glibly to evolution is hazardous, a guarantee of superficiality, but some relationship exists, however indirect and hard to trace. We strive to suit our own tastes and those of others. When you see a wildflower you see a bee's sense of beauty. We develop to match the tastes of those we seek to please, to make hungry where most we satisfy. There is a reason peacocks and birds of paradise come easily to mind when contemplating human preening. Beauty might be skin deep but similarities are not.

There is no choice over whether we compete, unless it dissolves into a sad choice over whether to half-live or to live at all,* but the spirit in which we strive is a different matter. To run a race for the pleasure of beating others is different from running for the delight in the stretch and power of one's legs. As a young man I boxed, and I vividly recall a fight's audience being divided into those who had come to see bloodshed – to see someone beaten up and someone doing the beating – and those wanting to see a contest drawing out the skill and spirit of the fighters. It was heartening that those with some experience of boxing were in the second group. It is hard not to believe that songbirds have full-throated joy in their song, whatever their territorial intentions. The judgement is an aesthetic one. In the nineteenth century some masters of mills and factories pioneered health care for the working classes. We admire or deplore them depending on what we think of their motivation.

Human lives continue to change. We wish to do better, look better, beat others and better ourselves. Physical capacities vary and so does the capacity for making an effort. We grow faster and taller, fatter and lazier, stronger and fitter – better able to read but less well read, more educated and more spoon fed, better medicated and more given to cranks and fads. We alter our stresses and our recreations, our sleeping patterns and our childhoods. We make new joints from metal and grow new cartilage in laboratories. We transplant kidneys and hearts, bone and hands and faces, and we breed and alter pigs with the hope

---

* 'I would prefer not to', says Melville's Bartleby, in the haunting story – and he doesn't.

of harvesting not bacon but organs. We innovate and explore, reshaping viruses to alter our genes and eliminate disease. We scan fetuses and abort some to spare them pain, and others to spare ourselves tragedy or inconvenience or daughters. We make ourselves more or less fertile, storing our eggs and sperm and deciding which fertilised embryos to reject and which to accept. We inject fat into our lips and buttocks and suck it from our bellies. We ink and stain and pierce ourselves, bathe in the sunshine and block it out, stuff ourselves with drugs and potions and remedies, alter our looks and change our height and shape. We want drugs to change our mood and our sexual potency so badly that we have a long tradition of seeing them where they don't exist. A good portion of our life is spent consciously trying to reshape ourselves. The rest of the time the shaping continues all the same. We are thoroughly normal in all of this, save that we have become more effective and more deliberate at it than any species or any generation that has gone before.

In 1860 infant mortality rates were higher in the richest countries in the world – the richest the world had ever known – than they now are *anywhere*. Modern Afghanistan offers newborns a better hope of life than the wealthiest nation on earth did a century and a half ago. In science and human health there really is the possibility for progression, for history to be the story of improvement, however stuttering and unevenly spread. But neither science nor science fiction predicted the decline of infant mortality any more than the rise of diabetes. Malthusian population projections have tended to underestimate our growth and wildly (and often with a curious relish) overestimate the catastrophe, chaos and starvation it would bring. We cannot look into the future without being wrong – but we can look, and learn from doing so. Plans are worthless, Eisenhower was fond of saying, but planning is indispensable, and there is progress even in predicting progress. Overall, medicine did more harm than good up until the 1930s: except for the simplest of interventions, we had not figured out how to measure the impact of what we did, and most of our favourite cures turned out, in retrospect, to be noxious and mistaken. The leech that has become such a standing joke was wholeheartedly believed in by the most thoughtful and observant. We are now approaching almost a century's experience of being able to do better. Today no newspaper is complete without some dismal story about a new aspect of our daily lives alleged to be bad for us, or some miracle breakthrough just around the corner. It is also true that no sober discussion of a drug is free of cautiously weighing its benefits against its harms. The drugs and the interventions mount up, as does our understanding of how they affect our bodies and our lives. Not that it is complete. In my twenty-five years of medicine I have seen some conditions grow rare, and others common, without either myself or my profession always fully understanding why. Over those years the frailties and strengths and trajectories of life have changed. Mostly, they have changed for the better.

The pace is intimidating, and fear of what lies ahead periodically convulses us. It isn't only in science fiction that worries have emerged. The fantasies may be fictions, but their effects have been real. *Brave New World* and *1984* speculated about how human societies might stratify, how power might be so misused that class differences would solidify into impenetrable physical and social and evolutionary barriers. Malthusian terrors have given rise to the plot lines of novels and also to actual forced sterilisations and slaughter. Fertility rates are higher in lower social classes, a phenomenon whose consequences have often been questioned. 'Genocide' was a term first used in 1943. It 'does not necessarily mean the immediate destruction of a

7

nation' or a group, wrote Raphael Lemkin, who coined it, but can also be 'a co-ordinated plan of different actions aiming at the destruction of [their] essential foundations'.[2] In a limited sense we still seek some genocide: there are diseases, defects, abnormalities we mean to wipe out. With artificial ears and eyes growing ever more capable, some groups have expressed unease at being viewed as so completely undesirable. Eliminate deafness and you eliminate the deaf community and deaf culture. Few people worry that the use of growth hormone will eliminate the community and culture of the short, but what will be the effect of us getting ever taller? Will we at some stage seek to rein it in? And if sexuality can be influenced, would that be of interest? Yes, of course: it already is, even without any scientific warrant – think of those claiming to cure homosexuality or concerned with how liberalism provokes it or conservatism stops it flowering. Our interest means we become so concerned about our powers we easily overestimate them. Not that these things are always easy to know. Even in areas free of the immeasurables of psychology and culture, the effects of our interventions are hard to judge. Part of the concern over the metal blades of Oscar Pistorius was that it was so hard to be certain where the line was between eliminating handicap and frank enhancement. Deciding what is fair and what actually works can both be difficult. Early Tour de France cyclists attempted to cheat by drinking alcohol, not something many sports scientists would these days believe in. The athletes who inject themselves with erythropoietin or blood may be just as mistaken.

It is not just the adornments and baroque exceptions of human lives that alter but the basics too. In 1991 two hikers in the Alps found a corpse. Ötzi, as he came to be called, had been shot dead – some 5,000 years before, by an arrow. Frozen in glacial ice, his body had been preserved down to its stomach contents.

He was of average height and a good age. Both parameters have changed over the millennia and now we would think of him as short and relatively young. He was skinny and wiry with a gap between his upper incisors. Modern life would have made him fatter – his lack was not entirely healthy – and, had he kept his habit of exercise, given him more upper body strength. A brace would have eliminated that gap between his front teeth. What else might it have done for him and what more may it still do, for us and our children's children? The tools and clothes Ötzi possessed, like the knowledge in his mind, added to his naked capacities. What changes have we undergone between Ötzi's death and now, and what stands ready tomorrow?

There is a contemporary tendency to start every piece of non-fiction with a preface explaining why the time to write it is *now*. It has become something of a bad cultural habit. Most issues in science and history and human life can be spoken of at any time, without fear of somehow hitting a moment, like a sudden silence at a party, when it is better to be quiet. In this case, however, the story could not have been told much earlier. It will be capable of being retold in the years to come, as knowledge and experience accumulate. But we live now at a point where we can look backwards far enough to turn and peer ahead. We have a track record not only of what we have achieved, but also of our guesses, our expectations and our presumptions. 'The activity of science being necessarily performed with the passion of Hope,' observed Samuel Taylor Coleridge, 'it is poetical.'[3] There is a certain style of science writing, particularly when evolution and social sciences are invoked, which breezily explains too much, more than it has the warrant for. Passion, hope and poetry – meaning science – is better served by attending as closely to uncertainty as to confidence, as much to misapprehension as to insight. The errors we have made in trying to guess the future have often inadvertently flaunted our often half-examined points of view. Yet our tastes, our habits and our technology, our lifestyles and our ambitions, our weaknesses and foibles: we have some idea what they have done and what they will do to our bodies and our lives in the near future. Humans are not special in reshaping themselves or the world around them, only unique in being able to make predictions, and to learn from and even enjoy our errors. We are unique in being able to think consciously about where tomorrow might take us, and how. We are unique in being able to think about what the lives of the people of the future – and what the people themselves – might look like.

Death

'Begin at the beginning,' advised the King in Alice in Wonderland gravely, 'and go on till you come to the end: then stop.'[1] Death is a grave place to start with instead but doing so comes naturally. For a quarter of a century death has been my day job.

I started in hospitals in the 1990s. For a long time that date seemed almost embarrassingly close at hand. Subtly it has moved away until now it seems almost from another age. That's what happens as we get older – we notice that the most profound changes happen slowly. Or at least we partly notice. Even in my first year of work I spotted that when you matched people's stories to their written notes, the discrepancy veered in one direction. If a patient recalled they'd been taking a pill for three years it was probably five. The freshness of our memory betrays us. For most of us, the gift of recall inspires a mild but persistent state of overoptimism. It's what we react to when we're reminded of our error and exclaim over how long ago something turns out to have been. Most of the time it still seems like yesterday. I am still perplexed that I am not more often still mistaken for a junior doctor. In truth, it hasn't happened for five years – which, regrettably, probably means ten.

The first time I was called in an emergency, because someone had become catastrophically unwell, I remember running from the hospital accommodation where I was sleeping, across a wide lawn by a car park, and seeing the daisies in the summer night make the grass look full of stars. The memory was fixed in my head by the terror that followed, of rushing into a side room and seeing something hard to make sense of. In a bed an old woman was sitting up, her eyes open but unfocused, taking deep, odd breaths. A nurse was there, trying to put an oxygen mask on the woman's face, but the woman's bony hands were moving about and pushing it away. Then she stopped pushing but carried on with her deep, odd, gasping breaths. I don't remember much about what happened or what I did in the short space of time before a more experienced doctor arrived, I only remember the deep relief when he came and how exceedingly, unmistakably and disturbingly wrong the woman looked. 'Well,' said my senior to the nurse and to me, taking a glance and shrugging, 'she's dying, isn't she?'

At the time I heard his words as having a question mark. I was wrong. Having seen it before, many times, the situation was obvious to him. My panic did not totally resolve, and as we walked away I kept wondering if, despite the other doctor's assurance, there was something we should have been doing. It took the experience of many more deaths – until almost the end of that first month – to understand what the other doctor had seen. Once you recognise death you can, to a huge extent, relax. Much of the terror comes from the uncertainty over whether there is some desperate action it would be calamitous to miss. Explain to a panicking family that their relative is dying and their reaction can sometimes be relief. Death is often expected; panic comes from anxiety over whether something needs to be done. Making sure someone is comfortable as they die is important but usually straightforward. Another recent book about the future of mankind, Yuval Noah Harari's *Homo Deus*, wrote about the extent to which we 'have become used to thinking about death as a technical problem' rather than as our natural end. 'When a woman goes to her physician and asks, "Doctor, what is wrong with me?" the doctor is likely to say, "Well, you have the flu," or "You have tuberculosis," or "You have cancer." But the doctor will never say, "You have death.""[2] I can report that not only do they often say just that, but it is something people can be relieved to hear. To know the dissolution is real, to give it a name, to know that there is nothing one needs to be frantically doing to ward it off, these things matter. They are normally done well. See them done badly once and you never forget.

I speak of death that comes towards the end of life, towards the end of a long life, because most of the time that is when it happens. It's what modernity has given us. Death, for most people, is a fading out, with no last words and little awareness (often none at all) of the final experience. One breaks the news of it to the family; the person themselves may not be interested. Their interest has already faded – read Tolstoy's account in *War and Peace* of the death of Prince Andrei. (Not many people die with Andrei's lucidity but then not many live with it.) I say it took only weeks to recognise the final approach of death; I should add that it took years to sense its looming shadow. Sometime around 2007 I remember we bought Christmas presents for our patients. It was straightforward: being Christmas the hospital was so quiet we had few people to buy for and time to send a member of the team shopping. One old man liked whisky and we got him a bottle of malt. He was obviously pleased, despite being mostly withdrawn and absent. Over the following week he drank a couple of thimblefuls. The bottle remained by his bed while he spent his time sitting, or lying, without books and without complaint. He was waiting while his family (who did not visit him) made plans and our social workers made theirs. The plans were never completed. One morning someone else was in his bed and the bottle was gone.

Death in old age is predictably unpredictable. Frailty, the profound frailty of age, was there in his lack of impatience. It was unmistakeable except I had not learnt that yet. Most of my patients – the vast, vast majority – fade and are gone. Sometimes an infection gives warning of the final event, sometimes not. To be able to recognise where someone is in life's trajectory is essential. The world's oldest medical textbook, the Egyptian Ebers papyrus, which dates back to around 1,600 years before Christ but is almost certainly based on Sumerian teachings of millennia before, divides up the conditions that a doctor sees. It divides them into those of which he says 'I shall treat' and 'I shall not treat'. Managing expectations and not overselling yourself mattered then as now, and so did knowing your power and acting appropriately. When someone is dying, treatments whose only impact can be to give them a less pleasant death are not good medicine. They are not medicine at all.

Only very rarely have I had patients dying with full, bright consciousness. I remember two, both brilliant. One was a woman whose lungs were filling with fluid as her heart failed. She remained alert not because we were unwilling or unable to treat her sensation of drowning but because she chose alertness over comfort. There was nothing masochistic about her bravery, it was simply her choice. Another I cared for because his own team (not on duty that weekend) had asked me to check on him. Knocking on his door and entering, I was startled by his immediate enquiry of 'Am I dying?' His enquiry was not panicked, merely imperious. If he had had any time for fools before, he had none now. I replied that I understood that he was and he seemed satisfied. The next day he died, surrounded by his family.

Most of my patients fade out. They have begun fading years before. A friend noted his own decline. He reported finding himself of less interest, to himself and others, than he had before. In his ninth decade he told me he did not want to die too slowly nor too quickly. So many of those he had loved, he pointed out, had already died. He did not want his death to be drawn out but he wanted time to see what it was like.

My patients are usually old. The hospices, which have done so much good for so many, are not for them. Hospices provide privacy and peace and relative luxury. They tend to be for the middle-aged, for those dying before their time of diseases discrete enough to be predictable. The old and the frail, those for whom the precise timing and events of their decline and fall can be less well prophesied, do not get to hospices. Most of us, when elderly, die in acute hospital beds like the ones I tend, where wards are noisy and lacking in privacy, dignity or space.[3] My partisan resentment of the hospice movement is eased by how seldom my patients notice what they lack, or complain of dying on chaotic wards packed with open bays of the sick and demented. This is not the same as saying that they do not deserve better.

While most of my patients are old, I am not a geriatrician. I am a general physician. If you arrive at hospital with a complaint which cannot be sorted out by the emergency department, and particularly if you have problems with more than one organ system, I am likely to be looking after you. I see young people but almost invariably I can get them rapidly home. The ones who stay are those who are frail, those in whom there is more than one problem afflicting them. Medicine is so good – the state of normal human life has become so good – that, by and large, these people are all elderly. Even including rare diseases, or common diseases that have taken an unusually bad turn, most people who are young or middle-aged can be turned around at pace and discharged. It is worth celebrating that the majority of hospital inpatients are now the elderly.

This book is about what has changed and what will change in human lives. Some things, though, remain the same. We are born, we live, we die. It is my experience that those in old age who are terrified to die are those who sense they never properly lived. The people who were waiting for something to start, which never did, can find their death unbearable. 'Older people who are reasonable, good-tempered and gracious bear ageing well', wrote Cicero. 'Those who are mean-spirited and irritable will be unhappy at every stage of their lives.'[4] My friend told me he regretted the thought of not seeing his wife's face again, but that he did not resent dying. This was the man who had noted that the decline of his mind with age had made his thoughts and conversation less interesting. He was right, but these had been at such a level that even the remnants sparkled. 'There is something pleasant', he said towards the end, 'about handing back your badge.'

'Due to an uncompromising humanist belief in the sanctity of human life,' wrote Harari, 'we keep people alive till they reach such a pitiful state that we are forced to ask, "What exactly is so sacred here?"'[5] In fact what we offer is kindness, intelligently applied, and neither doctors nor their patients are usually so frightened by death as to become phobic about it. The rise in senescence has not happened through fear of mortality. The extension of old age, and the continued survival of those in the greatest states of frailty, is a side effect, an ineluctable consequence of preventing people from dying young. In recent wars casualties have survived with injuries that would have been fatal in any conflict before. They have not survived chiefly because of specific efforts to help those with the most extreme injuries. They have survived because combat care of the wounded has improved in every way, and when the outcomes improve for the average they also get better at the extremes.

An eminent twentieth-century physician and epidemiologist named Richard Doll remarked that death in the old was inevitable but death before old age was not. Old age has grown more common because we have been so successful in stopping the premature deaths that pinch us off before we reach it.

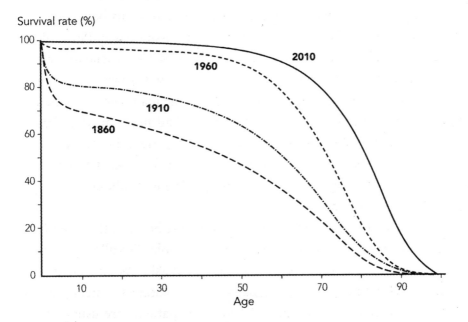

Fig. 1. Percentage survival at period rates for males in England and Wales. Reproduced by permission of the Clinical Trial Service Unit, University of Oxford. Data taken from the reports of the Registrar-General for England and Wales and the Human Mortality Database.

In Fig. 1 the area under the curve represents life and the area above it holds more than death. The area above the curve – so dominant in 1860, so slimmed down today – is the domain of heartbreak, grief and lost opportunity, agonisingly palpable to the survivors. Anyone wishing to bemoan modernity would be right to say that the graph is made of numbers. They would be lost to reason if they forgot what those numbers meant. The coffins on the upper left side of the graph are small ones. The fact we need so few of them today is part of the reason so many of us will experience decay.

Age

Growing up in cities, and on a bike, I missed out on any early interest in cars. The only flash of fascination came from studying evolution, and a story about Henry Ford visiting scrapyards. What piece of his Model Ts, he wanted to know, was most often in good working order? He went back to the factory and instructed those responsible to make it cheaper.

The story held a frisson of the evil capitalist; of cloven hooves under the boardroom table. I understood that the anecdote was about evolution – don't make anything stronger than it needs to be – but failed to spot that Ford's attempt to make his product cheaper by not overengineering any components was no betrayal of his customers. It was in their interest.

For many years, until the impracticality of commuting by bicycle while living in the countryside overcame my idiocy – it had been no moral choice so much as moronic incompetence at attaining essential life skills – I had no concern with cars. Then they were a vehicle in which to commute. They still are, although I can see why others become more interested. That I can see such a basic thing is down to my son. At the age of seven, when his television diet had consisted only of children's programmes and natural history, he came into the kitchen. A friend had visited and they had watched some TV; we had overheard scraps but only some of David Attenborough. 'Mummy, Daddy,' our son said, 'what's female sexual appetite and what has it got to do with handbrake turns?'

It was the start of a *Top Gear* obsession of his that we were helpless to escape. Initially we were helpless because we wanted to keep an eye on what a seven-year-old was watching. Soon it was because we were laughing as much as he was. Watching grown men deliberately make fools out of themselves was a distinct step up from most children's programmes and funnier than Attenborough. As a primer on some forms of male behaviour it was a fine textbook. In the episode my son first watched the late-middle-aged presenters recalled their youthful conviction that if only they could perform dramatic handbrake turns, women would not be able to contain their sexual fervour. Cue scenes in which their attempts met with the lofty scorn and cold indifference they merited. The trinity of risk-taking, wit and bullshit was funny and that was its lesson. Fail with sufficient style and you become a memorable success.

Evolutionary point number 1: men, particularly adolescent men, take risks. It's a generalisation to say that they take more than women because generally speaking it's true. There are more deaths among adolescent men than women, and violence and accidents account for the difference.[1] It's part of the reason men have shorter lives. Men do so well in so many other ways that society's sympathy has been limited – campaigns to bring life expectancy into balance by preferentially spending healthcare resources on men have sold no wristbands. But we have been actively interested in modifying young men's risk-taking. Might we find the genes that control this behaviour and switch them off? As it happens we can do this already, as plenty of people have wanted to do to the *Top Gear* presenters. Castrate someone, physically or chemically or by knocking out the one gene that flicks an embryo over from being female to being male, and you feminise them. The earlier in life you do it, the more effective it is. Will we ever be able to be more precise, to eliminate individual aspects of masculinity without affecting the whole? No. There's no more a single gene or neurotransmitter or neural nucleus for recklessness or daring than there is for making handbrake turns.

Evolutionary point number 2: the risk-taking of young men is often not impressive to young women. Lots of the risk-taking that men engage in, even when they believe it impresses women, is not attractive at all. But it does not necessarily need to be. Human males exist in a hierarchy. The more sophisticated the society, the more multifactorial the hierarchy, and the greater the room for something more grown up than a single pecking order, but hierarchies remain: and for adolescents, sophistication is not at a lifetime high. Young women distinctly unimpressed with handbrake turns or fast driving may nevertheless be very aware of which young men around them are treated by the others as being leaders of their pack.

Evolutionary point number 3 is that it's not only capitalists who are concerned about reducing wasteful expenditure. To muddle famous phrases from evolutionary biology, a chicken is just an egg's way of making another egg, genes are selfish and flesh is disposable. We are designed to promote the survival of the genes we carry but we are not overengineered. With this in mind, here are four observations about our species:

1. We are sexually dimorphic. That is, men and women look different.
2. Our longevity and physical frailties are sexually dimorphic too. Young men die more often than young women do from

risk-taking behaviour. Later, men die more often than women from cardiovascular disease. Women live longer.

3. We often survive for a long period after we have stopped having children and after our children are physically independent. This is not new: life expectancy at birth was in the low to mid-twenties in many historical societies but that was because so many died before the age of five. Those who got through those first years had a decent chance of being around when their children had children of their own.

4. There is a female menopause.

Exaggerated sexual dimorphism does not fit with monogamy. Think of lions, deer, walruses, gorillas, sparrows or other animals with alpha-males and harems. The males have extra size and strength and power and they have it in order to fight other males. Animals such as swans or turtle doves look more similar, lead more similar lives and mate more as lasting pairs.

It is straightforward to summarise the implications of these observations for whether we should be sexually faithful: they have none whatever. Evolutionary history cannot be extrapolated to moral advice. Many birds, previously thought monogamous, can, by DNA fingerprinting, be proven to cheat,[2] but converting that to conclusions about acceptable behaviour within a marriage is a non sequitur. Natural selection provides rich metaphors for describing human behaviour but metaphors are not excuses. The survival of the fittest is a law of population genetics but apply it to the behaviour of people in society and it is not a law but a comparison. There is a sorry history of taking biological metaphors as social rules – and often then of presuming each to have its own gene. Such thinking has been a part of human life for long enough that we can be confident it will unhelpfully persist.

Male menopause is another metaphor, a description by analogy for vague changes in late middle life that include an irregular and variable reduction in fertility. It acquires a false sense of reality by sharing a name with something real. Female menopause is a highly consistent and discrete set of biological changes. At about the age of fifty ovulation and menstruation cease. Menopause does not exist in other primates, it is peculiar to women.[3] Why?

The evolutionary biologist Stephen Jay Gould referred to responses to these sorts of 'why?' question as 'Just So stories', after Kipling's fiction. He was not trying to denigrate them but attempting to point out they cannot be tested, so their truthfulness cannot be judged by the direct testing of science. Our assessment of their truth rests on how persuasive we find them as stories.

Menopause stops women having more children. The accepted explanation notes that having children is physically risky and that children take a long time, and a lot of parental investment, before they are independent. The risks of childbirth rise with age. Menopause seems to be a consequence of women doing better by their genes if, after a certain age, they concentrate on aiding the survival of existing relatives rather than chancing themselves on making more.

We benefit from relatives. We benefit not only when we are infants or young adults, but also late into our life and perhaps throughout it. Aunts, uncles, grandparents and even great-grandparents count. We are a species in which social groups and culture matter. We are not unique in this but we are unique in its extent. Menopause is the result of natural selection reflecting the fact older women have value in themselves, a value too precious to risk on the increasing hazards of childbirth and raising infants.

Fertility and menopause have hormonal control systems that are relatively simple (relative, say, to the workings of the mind) and which we have learnt to manipulate. We will undoubtedly get better at this, but already our main limitations in extending fertility relate to what feels right and desirable rather than what is technically feasible; the techniques of in vitro fertilisation have led to successful pregnancies for women in their seventies. More straightforwardly, research will continue to yield results in reducing the number of younger women stuck with infertility. The future is always easiest to predict when it consists of more of the same.

Cars that are designed for power and performance are unlikely to last as long as those built to cover many miles. If you want to judge what models are reliable, you pay attention to those the taxi-drivers choose, not those the boy racers rev late at night. Male success in primates has been driven by power and performance. Creatures whose sexual success is lavish but brief and violently won tend to have large testicles relative to their body size. (The pomp of this image is defused for me by memories of my son's pet rats. The pendulous weight of their testicles made their bodies wobble ludicrously as they walked. It was also plain they could not be judged by their balls. They illustrated the diversity powering evolutionary success. One was bold and fearless, permanently on the verge of catastrophe, the other nervous, conservative, too fearful of risk to leap from the sofa to the floor. One small step for his brother, too giant a leap for him.) Monogamous creatures whose sexual success lies in steady domestic effort have relatively small testicles. They have no requirement to widely spread their seed when brief opportunity presents her many selves. Humans, on this continuum, are not designed in expectation of monogamy – but they are closer to it than many creatures and significantly closer to it than chimps.* Human males average out as being faster, stronger and more physically powerful than females. For the same reason, they do not live as long. In terms of where evolution put her energy, human men are designed to burn more brightly at the price of more quickly burning out. As with adolescent risk-taking, we could adjust this immediately if we wished, but we cannot do it without adjusting all that goes along with it. Gene therapy is not required, only castration.

Our increasing lifespans have not, so far, been the result of efforts to make the span of human life longer, to stretch out the life expectancy of someone free from illness or trauma. The improvements we have seen have been the result of efforts to prevent premature death, not to postpone the date at which death seems mature.

Years ago I admitted the chief executive of a large, global car company. He had had a heart attack, and he received the appropriate treatment. A powerful clot-busting drug, some morphine to take the pain away,† a range of drugs to thin his blood in the short and long term, a pocketful of others to take home to lower his risk of another heart attack. The evidence was clear that this line of approach worked. It is still clear today, and it shows the benefits are not restricted to reducing the future risk of your heart. They reduce the chance of strokes

---

* The research for my master's degree consisted of watching wild chimps. Their lack of manners and wholesale distaste for privacy are boons to the notebook-wielding academic.

† Actually it was Heroin. I use the capital letter here because it is a trade name. Bayer called it that after their volunteers who tried it said it made them feel heroic. Heroin is a more concentrated version of morphine: there's no added extra evil, just half the volume.

and other conditions too. They have these benefits because they reduce the risk of ongoing problems – over months and over the following few years – with the circulatory system overall.

This patient was a cheerful man, even in the crisis of his heart attack. I asked him whether he enjoyed his job and he answered with persuasive enthusiasm. He didn't enjoy it, he said, he loved it. Having finally learnt to drive, I asked him how long cars were designed to last. At the back of my mind was the thought of devilish corporations making sure of built-in obsolescence to encourage future orders. He gave me an answer for the longevity of cars. Ten years, he said: they were designed to last ten years or a 100,000 miles, give or take. I didn't ask about built-in obsolescence – I could see the notion made no sense, economically or in engineering terms or psychologically. I had got on well with the man, made an emotional connection, something which is not only easiest to do in a crisis, but also part of the job. I had also put an intravenous line into the back of the man's foot. I had seen his sole: five toes, no cloven hoof. The answer he gave me, however, was not true.

In the last third of the twentieth century, cars were lasting longer. At the beginning of that period the odometer was typically five digits – past 99,999 miles and it rolled back to zero – but by the end, it was always six. Part of the improvement came spurred by competition: more reliable Japanese cars put others to shame and designers on their mettle. Manufacturing processes and materials improved. Where it had hardly mattered before if a car had rusted to bits after a decade, now, when much of the rest of the car was lasting better, the rust stuck out more. Environmental regulations acted as another prod. Anticorrosion and antipollution regulations came in. The state of California required catalytic converters to operate at a high level of efficiency even when a car reached high mileages, and California is a big market. 'The California Air Resources Board and the EPA have been very focused on making sure that catalytic converters perform within 96 per cent of their original capability at 100,000 miles', a Ford engine designer said in 2012, and

> because of this, we needed to reduce the amount of oil being used by the engine to reduce the oil reaching the catalysts... Fifteen years ago, piston rings would show perhaps 50 microns of wear over the useful life of a vehicle, today, it is less than 10 microns. As a benchmark, a human hair is 200 microns thick. Materials are much better. We can use very durable, diamondlike carbon finishes to prevent wear. We have tested our newest breed of EcoBoost engines, in our F-150 pickup, for 250,000 miles. When we tear the engines down, we cannot see any evidence of wear.'[4]

The summed effect of efforts individually targeted at particular signs of premature ageing in cars meant the overall life expectancy of vehicles rose. The executive wasn't lying with his notion of ten years and 100,000 miles, he was out of date without realising it. When I told him I was treating him for his heart attack, so was I.

In 1858 the Harvard physician Oliver Wendell Holmes wrote a poem called 'The Wonderful "One-hoss Shay"'. This shay, a one-horse carriage, was designed so superbly that no part wore out before any other. After a century of faultless running, the carriage shuddered and – in its entirety – dissolved.

> You see, of course, if you're not a dunce,
> How it went to pieces all at once, –

All at once, and nothing first, –
Just as bubbles do when they burst.

The weak points in humans, the bits that wear out first, cause disease. More than half of all deaths are caused by problems with the circulatory system, problems resulting in a loss of blood to the heart or the brain.* Years of damage to smaller blood vessels underlie the development of leg ulcers, dementia and a host of other problems.

The drugs we have developed to ward off the atherosclerosis that furs up our circulatory system work, but each one works only a little. Young people or those at low risk stand a very small chance in any year of seeing benefit, even if they take all these drugs combined, because the events the drugs are warding off are so unlikely to begin with. We are not intervening early, to stop the first signs of ageing, because the benefits per year are too small (and the side effects of the drugs too real) and because we see our treatments still as ones that treat disease. It was Alexander Pope who asked 'to help me through this long disease, my life',[5] but that was a simile; young people have no disease, not in any normal sense. Our knowledge of what drugs would do if given early and over the long term is lacking; treatment decisions are made on the basis of trials looking at effects over a few years in those who are older and at higher risk of disease, since that is the setting in which we have done

---

* This is true not only for high-income countries, but also for the world as a whole and for lower-middle-income countries. Low-income countries are the exception, with stroke and heart attacks being the third and fourth most common causes of death behind respiratory infections and diarrhoea. See https://www.who.int/en/news-room/fact-sheets/detail/the-top-10-causes-of-death and http://www.who.int/mediacentre/factsheets/fs310/en/index1.html [accessed 7th March 2019].

our trials. We can estimate what would happen if we used the drugs earlier, based partly on studies of those whose genes mimic the effects of lifelong medication, but we do not know for certain.

New agents will be added, old ones refined; people will continue to take them from an earlier age. Drugs to treat our raised sugar and lipid levels and our raised blood pressure treat the effects of modern life but it is also true to say that the main effect they treat is life itself: they treat the entropy and decay of age. As they accumulate, their effect on life expectancy will build. They will become not a way of staving off premature death but a means of slowing death's approach. They already have become that, but we have been slow to realise. Just as with cars, a suite of interventions aimed at preventing early breakdowns and promoting health in late middle age have resulted, inadvertently, in wholesale increases in longevity. Medicine thinks of itself as being in the business of disease treatment and disease prevention. Actually, it is most often now devoted to life prolongation, specifically the extension of healthy life.

'To many,' wrote a thoughtful physician in 2017, 'it sounds absurd that there is no such thing as healthy ageing and that everyone eventually will need some medication.'[6] In truth healthy ageing is an oxymoron and 'need' is the wrong term. There is never any need to take any medicine. The question is always whether you prefer the likely consequences of taking it to those of abstaining.

Pressures and opportunities for medicalisation will grow ever greater. Whether they are experienced as progress or oppression will depend on how well we understand them and how we are encouraged and informed to decide for ourselves on how much health promotion we will tolerate for any given gain. Compromises over how vigorously medicine should intrude into the quest for health promotion will be essential and imperfect. An additional problem will be how to stop our increasing medical power from widening the gap in health that wealth makes.

Genes for ageing will be constantly discovered and just as constantly discovered to be something else. There will never be a gene for ageing since ageing is not a single process. Understanding the host of genetic variants that influence ageing will continue to help us find ways of extending healthy lives. We have evolved to face a host of challenges that are no longer so frequent or so pressing. The suites of adaptations we possess to fight off infections and trauma come at a cost. The treatments for many middle- and late-life conditions are treatments aimed not at augmenting the body's natural responses but at suppressing them. They differ from the antibiotics that support the immune system. Anti-inflammatories for arthritis, drugs for heart failure, antihypertensives and antidiabetic drugs, drugs thinning the blood after a heart attack or a stroke, all of these and a host of others stop or modulate the body's natural (and unhelpful) responses to a world where early death from disease or trauma is no longer the greatest risk. We will continue to get better at intervening in this way. Genes have been discovered that raise cardiovascular risk in middle and late life. It may be that for our ancestors they offered survival advantages in a world beset by early death. Now they may provide tools for altering the scars of time. Genetic variants in how we process cholesterol opened windows onto treating it.[7] Other mutations published as being genes for ageing are also often modifiers of cardiovascular risk.[8] We are optimally adapted to a life we no longer lead, and the production of drugs and the alteration of genes are likely to be most fruitful when exploring this mismatch. In other respects we will have to do better than evolution (not impossible, given we have different tools) but here we merely need to spot the ways in which we have wrong-footed her by changing so swiftly. Squinting towards the horizon and muttering about genetic redesign in order that humans do not age at all will remain a different thing, a way of dissolving real prospects into mists of fantasy.

'Our grand business undoubtedly is', wrote Thomas Carlyle in 1829, 'not to see what lies dimly at a distance, but to *do* what lies clearly at hand.'[9] Life expectancy will continue to grow as we get better and better at reducing premature deaths. The corollary will be that our efforts gradually alter what we think of as prematurity. 'The cardinal principle of all science [is] that the profession, as an art, dedicates itself above all to fruitful doing, not clever thinking; to claims that can be tested by actual research, not to exciting thoughts that inspire no activity.'[10] Rejuvenation machines, telomere alteration and the other favourites of bad journalism will remain alluring and misleading. In the meantime my current car is approaching 200,000 miles without problems and I will be disappointed if it doesn't make it, just as I would be to be told that my grandchild would not live a longer and healthier life than me.

'Recent studies have shown that life expectancy at birth has, since the 1970s, steadily increased by 3 months per year in high-income countries and there are no signs that the trend is slowing'.[11] A pessimist would note that unless that improvement quadruples, we're all doomed. A realist could comment that the steady increase began long ago, and while human activities like war can make it dip, it is cheerful and encouraging that there is nothing sudden about it. No abrupt lifts follow from the breakthroughs of genius, not even after the development of antibiotics, the closest we have ever come to miracle drugs. There is only a general trend towards improvement, cut back now and again by calamitous war. It is the steady accumulation of progress, summed over generations, that makes the miracle. If we can avoid global conflict and catastrophic global warming, it will continue to do so.

Early childhood

The first five years

In 1890 Luke Fildes painted *The Doctor* (Fig. 2). A pale child lies collapsed across a makeshift bed. A jug and bowl of water nearby have been used to ease the child's fever; on a table is a half-full medicine bottle. The mother sits despairing, her head in her hands. The father stands next to her, watching the face of the doctor who is seated by the child. The doctor gazes at the child intently. Morning light begins to show at the window – 'the dawn that is the critical time of all deadly illnesses',[1] wrote the artist – shining with the possibility of hope or of the child's departure from this earthly world.

It was a picture portraying the best that medicine could offer. The physician's power was limited but his compassion was not, nor his patience in watching, waiting, and willing for a recovery, despite having been awake through the night (with a family, the picture makes clear, too poor to pay well). It was a picture painted from life, a memory of the childhood illness of the artist's own son. Aged just one year the child had fallen ill. The devotion of the doctor who attended stayed with Fildes. Thirteen years later, when he was commissioned to paint but left free to choose his subject, he painted from experience.

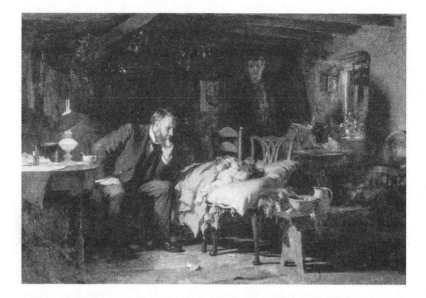

Fig. 2. *The Doctor*, Luke Fildes.

The painting is of its own time, not ours. Not only have the trappings of technology changed, but so too has the experience of childhood infection. Measles, mumps, rubella, chickenpox, whooping cough, scarlet fever, smallpox, streptococcal and staphylococcal and most other infections of childhood – their outbreaks and epidemics were the common stuff of tragedy. Now they are rare, gone, or mild. Infections take their toll when we are old but rarely before. Childhood death has been reduced beyond the dreams of our ancestors.

Fildes' painting remembers his own domestic tragedy. Despite the care received by his son, despite the best and most serious attempts of the doctor, the one-year-old boy died. That early deaths were once so common did not make them easier. We are not so attached to our children now because they live. Hence the painting that became a memory and hence the success of the painting. Back then the adults who looked at the picture would have recognised the scene and most would have recalled the times – more than once – when it ended with the death of their own child.

To say that early deaths were common obscures the fact it is today's experience that is unusual. Throughout history, from before history began, childhood mortality was common. It was common in all societies as it is common in all other animals. No part of life is as perilous as its beginning. Those saddened at living with the barbarism of the modern world can take heart from how much barbarism has gone. For the first time since parental love arose, the fraught anxiety of every parent will not end for most in heartbreak.

In 1800 more than four in ten children born in the world died without reaching the age of five. Death's dominion over infancy fell steadily over the course of that century,[2] all without significant medical advances. Economic and social development were responsible. A hundred years later only a quarter of British children were dying before the age of five.[3] Elsewhere the figure was worse, but also better than it had been, the global average having fallen to just over a third. Halfway through the twentieth century, the situation improved to the extent that the world in 1950 had caught up with Britain in 1900. By 1960 global infant mortality fell below one in five. It has continued to fall – below 15 per cent a decade later, below 10 by the mid-1980s, under 8 by 2000 and reaching 4 per cent in 2015. This is not all the effect of high- and middle-income countries pulling up the average – mortality in even the poorest countries has fallen.

'There is a danger that people will lose faith in progress when they hear so little that would support their faith in it,' wrote the physician and Nobel peace laureate Albert Schweitzer, 'and real progress is closely linked to the faith of a society who considers this progress possible.' The quote sits on the website www.ourworldindata.org, which exists to point the progress out. 'On no day in the last five decades', notes the founder of the site, 'was there ever the headline "Global Child Mortality Fell by 0.00719% Since Yesterday".' It did, and it will continue to, and it is remaking our world beyond recognition.

Youth

From five to thirty-four

For all its formative power, the dramas of youth are mostly personal. Within those years lie excess deaths for males as a result of their tendency to violence and risk-taking. The tendency is slight, but against the backdrop of little else happening it acquires importance. It is easy to come up with frightening figures showing that horse-riding or trampolining or knife fights are leading causes of death for the young. They are, but it's principally because little else can touch them. Society's job can be seen as that of a designer of a playground. The goal is to keep the interest and adventure while making sure the falls are safer. Society has been more than helpful. It has not eliminated our impulses but it has tamed them. Duels are no longer a requirement of masculine honour. Wars are still fought but they are fought less, which is to say that, for decades, the number of lives claimed by battle has been falling not only relative to the number of people alive, but, more impressively, in absolute numbers too.[1] The effects of global media have been important in increasing the value of the lives of the lowest ranked, but so have the declines in infant and youthful mortality. To lose a young man in war was no less catastrophic for the parents of previous generations but the loss to society was not as noticeable.

So many were lost each day anyway. The best thing we can do for the young is to let them grow old – a reminder that we do not just want them to avoid an early death, we want them to grow up. The point of youth is to waste it and the point of being able to do that is to learn from experience how to stop.

Events do occur in youth, however, with important effects on health. The obvious ones are those responsible for the few lives lost during these years. Trauma, in the absence of other problems, looms large, with violence and road traffic injury the most reducible parts. The latter is modifiable in the immediate future by spending on road safety and, to a far more exciting degree, by the automation of cars. Those changes have a chapter of their own later, and the aim of the chapter is to persuade you that it merits being one. Violence is a harder part of human ecology to deal with but it remains modifiable. Causes of death and ill health remain just that when the interventions required to deal with them are not medicines but changes in culture. Women are more likely to be victims of violence where they are less educated and marry younger.[2] Interventions to improve the situation need to consist of cultural change, of better education, greater sexual equality and later marriage. That these interventions are not drugs or vaccines makes them no less relevant or powerful.

Vaccinations continue to offer new benefits: vaccinating against human papillomavirus (HPV), it has been conservatively estimated,[3] could prevent half a million deaths each year. The estimate is conservative because it looks only at the reduction in deaths of cervical cancer, a disease now known to be almost entirely sexually spread through transmission of the virus. The benefits are undoubtedly greater and more varied.

The notion that a virus could cause cancer was incredible for most of the twentieth century: Peyton Rous suggested it in 1910[4] but was not believed. Only from the 1960s onwards did its existence seem real, and then only in non-human settings (the first cancer-causing virus identified affected only chickens; the second, rabbits). When Rous received his Nobel Prize in 1966 it was not for his clinical or his veterinary impact but because he had changed our ideas of what viruses could do. The main benefit of Rous's discovery was understood as being the better comprehension that cancer cells operated under the same physiological rules as others. It took until the 1970s for the role of a virus in a human cancer to be demonstrated. The demonstration was of HPV in the neck of the uterus* and the Nobel Prize for that came only in 2008. The true extent of HPV in human cancers is still uncertain but appears broad. Spread by close contact† the virus causes benign tumours, warts, which can progress to malignant ones, cancers. It accounts for most cervical, anal and rectal cancers, as well as the majority of vaginal, vulval, penile, oral and pharyngeal ones.[5] At the moment the strategy in most high-income countries is to vaccinate girls and men who have sex with men. The vaccine is timed to be given before sexual lives start but, because its effects are thought to wane, not too long before. A more rational (and cost-effective[6]) strategy would be to vaccinate everyone, thereby increasing herd immunity, removing any requirement to pry into sexual choices, and not incidentally giving wholly heterosexual men the reassurance that they were not killing their lovers. An Australian study showed that even a limited vaccination strategy was already

* Cervix means neck in Latin and the underlying image is of the uterus as an upside down flask, its opening and neck at its base.

† The relative contributions of sex, kissing, oral sex and other close contact are not certain. Unless one is going to allow intimate behaviour to be more determined by hygiene than desire, they probably don't matter, and they certainly don't if you have a vaccine.

having much greater effects than merely the protection against cervical cancer – the occurrence of genital warts was plunging and, in young women who had been vaccinated, had entirely disappeared.[7] Improvements in the appearance of Australian genitals herald deeper improvements to come in later life and its vulnerability to cancer.

The eventual number of deaths that could be preventable by HPV vaccination is immense but unknown. In the meantime childhood cancer trends, affecting far fewer than are struck down by HPV-associated diseases, are an established success. Survival rates have climbed steadily and progressively: whereas a century ago cancers of childhood were overwhelmingly likely to kill those who got them, survival rates are now of the order of 90 per cent. The way cancer care and cancer research for children have been organised has been partly responsible. Cancer in children attracts our attention because of its horror but also because it is rare. Its rarity means its treatment has tended to be concentrated in specialist centres. The proportion of children entering clinical trials has, as a result, always been extremely high,[8] which is not true of adults. Progress has not come from miracle breakthroughs but the accumulation of steady benefits, each minor or moderate, but each adding to the sum (a recurring story in this book, but a formulation that bears repeating.) There is also something physiologically different about childhood cancers. As one editorial put it, 'for reasons that are still obscure, many childhood cancers are very responsive to treatment, and cure has long been both a feasible objective for treatment and a powerful motivator of physicians' behaviour'.[9] Tumours in adults, the combination of decades of mutations, are fantastically varied in the genetic changes that underwrite their escape from the body's normal control of cell division. Those that emerge in childhood and youth often involve a smaller number of molecular pathways. The fewer of those there are, the more able we are to attack them.

For these reasons – reasons of physiology and genetics, and also of culture – improvements in the treatment of childhood cancers have proven particularly achievable. Here too, where progress has been most rapid, the story is of steady improvement, not great leaps forward. Half the trials report no benefits at all while those that do show benefits adding a few percentage points to a good outcome here, an extension of life by a fraction there.[10] There have been so many trials that these small steps combined have taken us a very long way.

That cultural traits apply so powerfully to what at first glance seems a purely technical problem – how do you stop the rapidly dividing cells of childhood cancer? – is a reminder that the problem of human health is never a strictly scientific one. Or more accurately a reminder that science itself cannot be separated from our wider culture. Neither the questions asked nor the answers we come up with nor the tools available to us are impartial, drawn simply from objective calculations.

Émile Durkheim, struggling to argue that there was such a thing as sociology, chose suicide as a major example. There was, he argued, such a thing as society: a level of organisation that gave rise to phenomena which could only properly be understood at that level. Suicide was a good example partly because it was such a personal act, a test case to see whether considering it at the level of a society would reveal qualities invisible at the level of individuals.

Suicide can be explained as a chain of levels, some explanations being more proximate to the event and others more distant. The distance does not alter an explanation's truth quotient, only the level of organisation they address and the sorts of insight they give. Suicide from paracetamol overdose can be explained in a very proximate manner as a result of the toxicity of the drug: the liver breaks it down into a substance that destroys glutathione, an antioxidant the liver uses to protect itself against certain cellular reactions. Take enough paracetamol and the liver dies.

For any individual suicide from paracetamol, this explains their death. So do the reasons behind the person taking the overdose. Answers emerge from psychology that are just as true as, but different in nature from, answers from pharmacology and hepatic physiology. At a societal level, Durkheim argued, new insights appeared that could no more have been reliably predicted from psychology than the psychology could have been understood by peering at the liver. Emergent or irreducible properties needed to be approached differently from resultant properties, those that could be understood by extrapolating from simpler levels of understanding. 'Human beings in society have no properties but those which are derived from, and may be resolved into, the laws of the nature of individual man,' John Stuart Mill had declared.[11] Sociology and Durkheim said otherwise. The phenomena of society could not be wholly resolved into the properties of individuals. Conglomeration was not accumulation. New properties emerged, new phenomena requiring new explanations.

The idea that we should be seeking to understand the underlying reasons for events, not just their proximate causes, lay behind the rebranding, in the UK, of hospital emergency departments. Previously, they were known as 'accident and emergency'. When a person trips over their cat, it's an accident. National figures for these injuries, however, show trends and show links with other properties of society; these figures represent a collection of random events which, taken together, have non-random properties. In America the Centers for Disease

Control and Prevention record pet-related injuries. They record injuries separately for cats and for dogs and for owners tripping over the pets themselves or a pet-related item.* Medicine meets sociology and the upshots were recommendations for reducing such injuries.[12,13] It may not seem a terrific step forward for human welfare to raise awareness of the potential to trip over your hound, or the extent to which it can be reduced by taking them for obedience training, but its triviality makes it a fine example of how medicine works and how it has come about that we live longer and healthier lives than our ancestors. In the last year reported, 80,000 Americans sought emergency treatment after falls related to pets. Some were bumps and bruises people should never have sought attention for but 10 per cent of individuals – 8,000 – had serious enough injuries to require admission to hospital. In the pursuit of better human health, small differences matter. Whether they matter enough to warrant the fuss they involve is a different matter, but the answer is, at least potentially, that they do.

In Britain, reductions in emergency department attendances were noted in particular weeks scattered through the early 2000s. Investigations revealed that each one followed, and appeared to be explained by, the release of the latest Harry Potter book.[14] The authors of the study considered 'a committee of safety conscious, talented writers who could produce high-quality books for the purpose of injury prevention' but noted the potential problems of an 'increase in childhood obesity, rickets, and loss of cardiovascular fitness'. The study was a deliberate

---

* And separately still if the pet was in no way responsible. 'Patient jumped off a fence and fell onto a doghouse,' was the example given. The medical journals publish this stuff partly because it matters and partly to brighten up the lives of those of us who have to read them. Aware of what else they print, they know we need it.

joke but the sort of relationship it demonstrated between societal and apparently entirely individual events was real.

Durkheim identified cultural traits he thought contributed to some societies having higher suicide rates than others. He was trying to prove a point rather than alter practice, but the point is that practice followed. Durkheim noted a rise in suicide when economies boomed and when they bust. It was the disruption to normality, he thought, that was dangerous. A modern study of economic hardship in Greece found suicide to be linked not to the 2008 recession, but to the policies of economic austerity it inspired.[15] Durkheim thought prosperity harmful (reducing the ties that bound societies together in harder times) but the Greek study concluded prosperity's effects on suicide rates had been absent or actively helpful. What matters is not so much which of them is correct, as that Durkheim won his argument. We can disagree with the conclusions of his sociology but we do so by challenging them with alternative sociological evidence. Arguing that sociology can be done badly only strengthens the notion that it matters when done well.

How one could make society less alienating and more encouraging is a question medical science cannot answer – answers have to come from social psychology and politics, culture and religion – but it can suggest methods by which proposals can be tested rather than argued over. Randomised controlled trials have allowed us to test interventions that change the odds of events to a degree that unstructured observation could never safely distinguish from the background noise of human variety. These techniques are used in agriculture and medicine and veterinary science but rarely elsewhere. They have the transforming power to replace belief with knowledge. Many questions in politics, economics, criminology, education and other fields that are currently decided by ideology and argument would be better settled by experiment. The experiments are often possible, we just lack the culture of doing them, and as a result we suffer by their absence. Even in medicine, where the majority of interventions are based on reliable interventions in a way they were not a few decades ago,[16] the use of trials has not extended far enough. Opinions are fiercest, it has been dryly observed, when the evidence to support or refute them is weakest.

Medicine has shown itself capable of proposing smaller scale interventions that make a substantial difference even to individual choices like suicide. One example, and a good one for illustrating where evidence can be good but should have been better, comes from changes made to the size of packets of paracetamol.

In both the UK and the USA, paracetamol poisoning is the top cause of liver failure. In 1998, UK law limited the amount of paracetamol people could buy at any one time. The aim was to make it harder, however slightly, to kill oneself. At the cost of making life slightly more irritating for those with pain or fevers, the hope was that numbers of impulsive suicide attempts would be thwarted. We think the measure worked but we are not sure. A before and after study showed that rates of suicide by paracetamol overdose went down, but suicide rates in general were falling so it was impossible to be sure why that happened.[17] We could have trialled the intervention properly. The changes could have been rolled out in a randomised fashion, with different geographical locations allocated the new limits or the old. Such an approach would have had benefits beyond the satisfaction of revealing the truth. The irritation of limiting sales of paracetamol to those with pain or a fever is minor but real. The minor irritations of ever-increasing bureaucracy and risk-averse policies accumulate, just like the benefits they aim to bring. Since some of the benefits are real, and add up, the whole business deserves to be taken seriously enough to remember that the same can be said for the harms. A cluster-randomised test of the effect of limiting paracetamol pack size (where different geographical locations were randomised to different strategies) would not only have determined its effects, but would also have set a powerful precedent for testing well-meaning interventions that may or may not work.

Childhood cancer rates have dropped partly because of a consistent culture of subjecting every well-meaning and well-designed intervention to a proper test. Interventions for childhood cancer are, in the scheme of things, relatively predictable – certainly more so than societal interventions aimed at altering human behaviour. Despite that, when subjected to proper trials, interventions for childhood cancer are as likely to harm as to help. Taken overall, when the history of childhood cancer research was explored, each trial was shown only to have a fifty–fifty chance of working.[18] Progress does not come from expert opinion which, even in a field so highly reducible to physiological theory, is no better than a coin toss. Progress comes from structured experiments that reliably test those theories and opinions and identify which are right. We are wrong to assume that it is better to do something than nothing, or that wisdom and compassion act first and worry later.

The history of medicine, and its increasingly explosive success over the past century, makes a powerful argument for the limited ability of wisdom when it comes to predicting outcomes. 'It is a layman's illusion that in science we caper from pinnacle to pinnacle of achievement,' wrote the immunologist and Nobel laureate Peter Medawar,

and that we exercise a Method which preserves us from error.

Indeed we do not; our way of going about things takes it for granted that we guess less often right than wrong, but at the same time ensures that we need not persist if we earnestly and honestly endeavour not to do so.[19]

The mistake medicine historically made was to use science to generate guesses about interventions and then put the guesses into practice. Only over the past ninety years has medicine developed ways (and noticed the need) to test whether the guesses are correct.

The amino acid methionine acts as an antidote to the toxic effects of paracetamol. It may be that combining it with paracetamol in tablets would eliminate all remaining deaths from deliberate or accidental overdose of the drug and at the same time abolish any need to limit pack size. We are unsure to what extent methionine might cause mild irritations, both physical ones like headache and nausea and more certain commercial ones like the cost of building it in. Hence we are uncertain whether the combination is worth introducing.[20] What holds us back is cultural as much as scientific – the partial penetration of scientific method into culture. Lacking the tradition of testing our hypotheses, we overlook the need to and the answers go begging. People die today from paracetamol overdose who we might have saved. If all paracetamol packets contained their own antidote to an overdose, no sales limits would be needed. Similar issues plague the question of whether putting barriers on bridges, to make it harder to jump, reduces suicide rates. Before and after studies show confidently they reduce suicides at those bridges, but leave uncertain whether people simply find somewhere else.[21,22] The difference matters. We are left unsure whether we have wasted resources and inappropriately intruded into society by erecting barriers that do not work, or whether we are causing harm and needless death by not intervening more.

Most people survive the years between their fifth birthday and the start of middle age three decades later. Habits and predispositions are learnt, adopted and cemented with implications for future health. But the immediate hazards remain small. For those between the ages of five and nineteen, the most likely thing to kill you is a road traffic accident, followed by suicide or accidental poisoning. Between the ages of twenty and thirty-four those two causes of death remain pre-eminent but their order is reversed. Suicide will rise in importance in the years to come. It will do so because roads will get safer. 'Drive safely', said a memorable Ugandan road sign; 'bloodless roads look good.' Haphazard deaths by car are common. They will soon be rare.

In Jane Austen's novels a cough and cold are enough to convulse her characters with fear. They gather in hushed tones by bedsides or make anxious enquiries from a distance. As a teenage boy I recognised how ridiculous this was. With the warm and generous heart of youth, I pitied the sentimental melodrama of the author.

Not the first adolescent male to be too stupid to understand Austen, it took years for me to realise the full extent of my error. To force teenage boys to study *Mansfield Park*, as my syllabus did, was to guarantee a bad result, and the moment I discovered Austen's other books my doltish adolescence began to recede a little. Admiring delight in her work was quick; what took longer was a proper understanding of history. Austen was a tough and realistic woman. Writing to a brother in the navy, she wholeheartedly wished him warm luck, urging him to remain good humoured even in the likely event he realised his death was upon him. The hazards of the navy were known to her. So were those of life on land. She lived in a time when mild infections were often fatal, and with little warning. Well on Monday, a fever on Tuesday, dead by the weekend. Her books, and books of her period and in all the periods of human life before antibiotics, are littered with the accidents of premature death. They were the stuff of novels because they were what shaped and determined lives. People gathered anxiously at bedsides or sent nervously for news because they feared the worst. They were right to do so.

Middle age

From thirty-five to sixty-nine

In 1907 three men gathered in Oxford. William Osler was the host. Regius Professor of Medicine, he was a world-leading doctor, his success largely due to personal charisma. Osler was on the university's governing council and hence partly responsible for the academic year's recent closing ceremony and the presentation there of honorary degrees to his two guests.[1] Osler's title declared that he held one of the few academic positions in the Empire where appointments were made directly by the monarch. Rudyard Kipling, who regretted his lack of university education and whose parents had lacked the money to send him to Oxford, had received an honorary doctorate. So too had Samuel Langhorne Clemens, Mark Twain, for whom the award was the brightest point of his public career.[2] 'Oxford is healing an old sore of mine, which has been causing me sharp anguish once a year for many, many years,' wrote Twain in his private diary, continuing with characteristic relish:

Privately, I am quite well aware that for a generation I have been as widely celebrated a literary person as America has ever produced... and so it has been an annual pain to me to see our universities confer an aggregate of 250 honorary degrees on persons of small and temporary consequences – persons of local and evanescent notoriety, persons who drift into obscurity and are forgotten inside of ten years – and never a degree offered to me! In these past thirty-five or forty years I have seen our universities distribute nine or ten thousand honorary degrees and overlook me every time... This neglect would have killed a less robust person than I am, but it has not killed me; it has only shortened my life and weakened my constitution; but I shall get my strength back now.[3]

All three men had married American women: Twain's wife was born in 1845, Osler's in 1854 and Kipling's in 1862. In the accounts of the day, and in the accounts of the lives of the three men, their wives are shaded in the background, in a way they would not be today. One part of women's lives that was recorded was their experience of childbirth and of loss. Women in America in 1845 gave birth to an average of six children, of whom half died before the age of five. By 1862 the average number born had dropped to five, of whom three might survive infancy.[4] The world was already improving but death in childhood remained common. To lose a child now is not only heart-breaking, it is also extraordinary bad luck. To lose a child then was normal; most lost more than one. Its normality made it no less heart-breaking.

That July, the three men enjoyed the sun in a beautiful garden backing onto the University Parks in Oxford. They enjoyed their success and each other's company among the flourishing roses and sweet peas. 'Mark Twain was most enthusiastic about Kipling', wrote Osler. 'It was delightful to hear them joking together.'[5] All three ended their days bereaved and broken-hearted. Of Kipling's three children, Josephine died aged six from pneumonia and John at the Battle of Loos in 1915.

Osler's first son died in 1893, within a week of his birth, while his second, Revere, died of wounds at Passchendaele in 1917. That was despite the connection with his father meaning he received a degree of medical attention other soldiers could not dream of: Harvey Cushing, one of the world's finest surgeons and Osler's future biographer, opened Revere's belly to try and remove the shell fragments and fix the damage they had done.[6] Of Twain's four children, his son Langdon died of diphtheria in 1872, Susy of meningitis in 1896 at twenty-four and Jane of drowning brought on by a seizure in 1909. By that stage she was twenty-nine but had suffered ill health most of her life – the consequence of a head injury aged eight and the epilepsy that followed. At least Twain and Kipling each had one who survived: Clara Clemens who died in 1962 aged eighty-eight, and Elsie Bambridge (nee Kipling) who was eighty when she died in 1976. Exceptional then and normal now.

Part of Osler's charm was his famously sunny humour. He inspired a generation of doctors (he inspires many today) through his infectious optimism. The reason the scene of him in the garden on a summer's afternoon in Oxford sticks in the mind, surrounded by flowers and good company, was that his life seemed made of such days. After Revere's death he was still observed to walk through his hospital wards whistling with his customary cheerfulness, raising the spirits of those around him, but he was seen sometimes to dive into cupboards or behind doors when he could keep it up no longer and the whistling broke into weeping. Osler wrote a note echoing Herodotus: 'The Fates do not allow the good fortune that has followed me to go with me to the grave – call no man happy until he dies.'[7] He died grieving for his son and when you read Cushing's Pulitzer prize-winning biography it is hard to escape the conviction that it was the heartbreak that killed him.

The effect of loss on Clemens was similarly severe. 'Some of those who in later years wondered at Mark Twain's occasional attitude of pessimism and bitterness towards all creation, when his natural instinct lay all the other way', wrote his biographer, 'may find here some reason in his logic of gloom.'[8] Ditto for Kipling. The death of his child defined his life, as it defined so many. The difference was only that, being Kipling, his sorrow is there for us to read.

> 'Have you news of my boy Jack?'
> *Not this tide.*
> 'When d'you think that he'll come back?'
> *Not with this wind blowing, and this tide.*
>
> 'Has any one else had word of him?'
> *Not this tide.*
> *For what is sunk will hardly swim,*
> *Not with this wind blowing, and this tide.*
>
> 'Oh, dear, what comfort can I find?'
> *None this tide,*
> *Nor any tide,*
> *Except he did not shame his kind—*
> *Not even with that wind blowing, and that tide.*
>
> *Then hold your head up all the more,*
> *This tide,*
> *And every tide;*
> *Because he was the son you bore,*
> *And gave to that wind blowing and that tide!*

There neither are nor ever will be guarantees, but most of us will progress through the prime of our lives safe from having to bury our children. Our kids will grow up confidently expecting their own health and ours. Just as two generations ago it was normal to grow up and have friends who died in childhood, in another generation it will be abnormal to grow up and have friends who, as children, lost a parent. Global mortality statistics are concatenations of bereavement and those bereavements have declined beyond belief. Fewer orphans, fewer broken hearts, fewer lost lives and fewer blighted lives. What was unimaginable a hundred years ago has become so ordinary we don't see it.

Fig. 3 is a plot of the uses of two terms in books and journals over the period in which life expectancy has exploded and infant mortality collapsed.

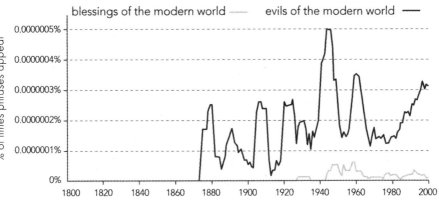

Fig. 3. Use of the terms 'evils of the modern world' and 'blessings of the modern world'.

There's something to be said for worrying about the problems we have rather than dwelling on those that are largely solved, but we can take it too far. Middle age has changed from being good fortune to almost a birthright. And we get to enjoy it without witnessing the death of our children.

*

The biggest reason for recent improvements in the lives and life expectancy of the middle-aged is not a particularly interesting one. It's not technologically sophisticated or intellectually challenging, and it is straightforward to say how it will extend into the future and what we can do to affect it. But neither intellectual challenge nor technological sophistication are necessarily guides to importance. The biggest reason for the transformation of middle-aged life is that the world, at least the richest part of it, has been giving up smoking.

In giving the data here from Britain, I am not merely being parochial. Britain was one of the first countries to take up smoking, using industrially produced cigarettes, seriously. In the 1960s, with enough decades of the habit under our belts and inside our chests to manifest its full effects, a greater proportion of us were dying from smoking than in any other country – almost half of all British men died from tobacco.[9] British women had taken up smoking later, and initially at a lesser rate; only 15 per cent were then dying from their habit. That figure rose but will never now reach the same peak.

The early evidence that smoking caused cancer brought little change. Richard Doll and Austin Bradford Hill showed the dominance of smoking among those with lung cancer in 1950,[10] with little impact. More effective was a study they published in 1954, under the title 'The mortality of doctors in relation to their smoking habits'.[11] The first of a series of papers drawn from an observational study – the fifty-year follow-up was published in 2004[12] – the paper had the effect of making its results palpable to one key group of the British public, the doctors themselves. One of the immediate consequences of the 1950 paper had been that Doll, recognising his own results, stopped smoking. After the 1954 paper, many others did the same. As doctors began to quit smoking and to argue for public recognition of its hazards; and the fact they did the former made the latter more persuasive. British smoking rates began to drop. The result, partly due to the popularity of the habit to begin with, was that Britain went from experiencing the greatest proportion of tobacco-related deaths to seeing the greatest reduction in them.

In Britain in the 1960s, 42 per cent of men who reached middle age, thirty-five to sixty-nine years old, died before it finished. Of that 42 per cent, almost half were dying from tobacco. By 2010 that figure had dropped to a tenth. Overall health had improved – the chance of dying in middle age had fallen by half – and the biggest contribution to that improvement was that smoking-related deaths had plummeted.[13] The improvement in mid-life survival in Britain between 1970 and 2010 consisted of twenty-two more of every 100 middle-aged people surviving into old age; the vast bulk of the improvement – in fifteen of the twenty-two, equating to 68 per cent of the improvement achieved over forty years – was due to the fall in smoking. That impact dwarfs the benefit achieved over the same period by all medical advances and all health improvements combined. Smoking does more to make people die early than all of medicine put together does to prevent them. Smoking was responsible for more deaths in the twentieth century than both world wars combined. At current rates it will kill more than a billion in the century now begun.[14] If you got rid of every hospital and every doctor and every medicine in the world, and got rid of smoking at the same time, you would do more good than harm.

What's true for the world, however, as a whole is not true everywhere. The more developed countries now smoke less and have better medical care. Both these things have contributed, as have other factors, to the most important trend in human life over past decades and what will be most important over the century to come – the reduction in cardiovascular disease. As with smoking, its importance is a function not of its glitz but of its impact.

In Britain suicide is the biggest killer of men between the ages of thirty-five and forty-nine.[15] Not many people now die of anything in that part of life, so its pre-eminence comes from the lack of competition. For all that, suicide remains a non-trivial problem: not the occasional act of a few tortured romantics but a reasonably frequent hazard. For women between thirty-five and forty-nine, the biggest killer is not suicide but cancer. Charities and pressure groups warn of the growing modern risk of cancer. They are right to do so but their attempt to frighten is inappropriate. Cancer's growing frequency means it merits growing attention, but its growing frequency is mostly a cause for celebration. As smoking rates have gone down, and pollutants have been better identified and controlled, the risk of getting cancer at any particular age has declined. The risks of dying from infection, trauma or other forms of early death, though, have plummeted. So cancer has climbed in relative importance for younger people as young lives have grown safer – and it has climbed in absolute importance for older people because cancer overall is a disease of age. As long as we keep living longer, more of us will get it. Cancer in middle-aged women is a major problem relative to the other threats to them but those other threats are small. Their cancer risk is minor compared with cancer risk later in life.

Between thirty-five and forty-nine, women die most often of cancer, while men die most often of suicide.[16] The second most common causes of death also differ. Women are killed by their livers and men by their hearts. The emergence of heart disease hits men first and hardest but men are hit first and hardest by many things: at this age, liver disease is only their third most common fatal frailty but still kills more of them than it does women. From conception to near the very end, men die young more often than women. At conception there are around a quarter more boys than girls, by birth only 5 per cent more and within a short space of time they are in the minority. Altogether the differential death rates mean women have about four extra years of life expectancy at birth. It also means many more women than men spend their final years alone.

While lung, bowel and other cancers affect women, breast cancer does the most damage. The same is not true for men, even though they get breast cancer too.

Men get breast cancer because they have breasts. Being male or female is determined by a single gene on the Y chromosome, which men possess and women generally do not. If the gene is missing or its function is faulty, a person develops normally as female despite possessing a Y chromosome. The single gene – testis-determining factor – produces a protein that turns on a hormonal cascade which results in masculinity. In the absence of that cascade the default is female.* There's precious little else on the Y chromosome; it's relatively blank. If the Y chromosome contained multiple genes designed for all the 'bits' of maleness – a male hand, a male foot, and every other piece, as Juliet mused, belonging to a man – there would be problems. There would be huge genetic duplication, with the two sexes designed from different blueprints, and the result would be

---

* There is no moral implication to female being the default. In some other creatures it's male.

endless errors. Selection has produced genes and chromosomes that muddle up and produce variation. Natural selection has also been superbly efficient in making sure that this muddle almost never gives rise to someone intersex, neither quite male nor quite female. Such people are usually infertile. The virtue of a single genetic switch, with all embryos possessing everything they need to be either sex, is simplicity: there is less to go wrong.

Since men have all the genes needed to be women, though, and women virtually all those needed to be men, there are consequences. Men, for example, have nipples they do not need. The cost of these bits of the body is small, smaller than the costs of the genetic tinkering needed to delete their redundancy.

Identical genetic design of the breasts explains why men get breast cancer. What it does not explain is why men get so little of it, of the order of 1 per cent. The switch controlled by testis-determining factor, left in its default female pathway, gives rise to a different hormonal environment for the cells of the body. Organs and tissues respond to these differences. And the hormonal environment they develop in is shaped by more than genetics. In 1700 an Italian Professor of Medicine in Padua, Bernardino Ramazzini, published a book called *De morbis artificum diatriba* – on the diseases of workers. He noted that women in one profession, a long-standing one in which the women led extreme variants of normal sexual lives, had peculiarly high rates of breast cancer.

Links between sexual activity and disease had long been made, and have continued to be made ever since, but most were, as many remain, entirely fictional. Hysteria was the disease caused by the uterus, unhappy at not being filled with a gestating fetus, wandering around the body and making trouble. Chlorosis, caused by young women being romantically and sexually unsatisfied, tinged their skin green. Masturbation caused blindness, fellatio produced halitosis, and homosexuality was a disease like any other: some notions linger on. One can predict with certainty that new ones, equally mistaken and equally harmful, will be invented and believed in. Ramazzini, although he thought the problem to be caused by a straightforward lack of sex, noted something that was otherwise entirely true. Breast cancer rates were higher in nuns.

Another of Ramazzini's insights – less original but more widespread and more important – had been published two years earlier. '*Quando longe praestantius est praeservare, quam curare, licuti satius est tempestatem praevidere, ac illam effugere, quam ab ipsa evader*' ('It is far better to anticipate, rather than cure, just as it is better to foresee a storm, and avoid it, rather than to escape from it').[17] More briefly, prevention is better than cure.

Many of the occupational hazards Ramazzini wrote about in *De morbis artificum diatriba* were avoidable, preventable or at least reducible: he studied jobs exposed to harm through poor sanitation and ventilation, hazardous chemicals or constricted environments. For nuns, however, there was nothing to be done by way of prevention; all that was possible was to be aware of the higher risk and to focus on detection and treatment. Breast cancer turns out not to be the only physical danger of their sexual abstinence. 'Today', wrote *The Lancet* in 2012, 'the world's 94,790 nuns still pay a terrible price for their chastity because they have a greatly increased risk of breast, ovarian, and uterine cancers: the hazards of their nulliparity.'[18] To be nulliparous is to have never given birth.

Cancer is a condition in which cells of the body break normal bonds of regulatory control and multiply. No single error is enough to cause cancer, the safeguards being so great; a series is needed. The more a cell divides, the greater the chance of a mutation. Cancer is a disease of age since more cell divisions have then taken place. It arises in some tissues more than others because not all cells divide to the same extent. Nerve and muscle cells divide very little so their cancers are rare. Skin, gut, breast and prostate cells divide frequently.

Cell division in reproductive organs is not only a function of time. Breast tissue is profoundly affected by lactation. So are the ovaries and the uterus, as they all are by pregnancy and by menstrual cycles. Each cycle prompts the cell division that creates a state of reproductive readiness. The greater the number of cycles, the higher the risk of reproductive cancers. In developed societies, women reach puberty earlier and menopause later, the result of being healthier. They are older when they have their first child, they have far fewer children overall, and for each child they breastfeed, if at all, for far shorter a time. Historically, as in poorer countries today, breastfeeding continued for years. Falling pregnant is not impossible while breastfeeding but it's less likely: the hormones involved in lactation have a contraceptive effect, a mechanism for reducing the chance of a woman having a baby while still suckling a fully dependent infant. The name of kwashiorkor, a severe form of infant malnutrition, means 'the disease of the deposed baby when the next one is born'.[19]

Women have evolved in the setting of undergoing far fewer menstrual cycles than modern life involves. Nuns have the most of all, and have the added risk of never undergoing pregnancy and lactation, but the risk for all women has risen and not just because other dangers have diminished. Below the age of sixty, women in developed societies have more than a hundred times the chance of getting breast cancer than their preagricultural ancestors.[20]

We cannot engineer a society in which the pursuit of health determines too strongly how we live. What, then, can be done to avoid the storm of raised cancer risk, 'to improve the health of breasts that do not need to lactate, ovaries that need not ovulate, and a uterus that does not need to menstruate'?[21]

Something, certainly. Perhaps a very great deal. Not always an enthusiast for change, the Catholic Church under Pope Paul VI nevertheless said that it 'in no way regards as unlawful therapeutic means considered necessary to cure organic diseases, even though they also have a contraceptive effect'.[22] Oral contraceptives consist of hormones designed to fool the body into believing it is already pregnant. They suppress those normal hormonal changes which raise the risk of reproductive cancers. If nuns took the pill, as it is normally taken for contraception, they would cut their chance of suffering ovarian and uterine cancers by more than half.[23] And oral contraceptives do not need to be taken in such a way as to preserve a monthly menstrual cycle; it might be that if taken in other ways, reducing the number of cycles further, the reduction in cancer they confer would be even greater.

Might we develop regimens of hormones specifically to reduce a woman's risk, to return it as much as possible to that of her ancient ancestors? Could similar pills fool ovaries, uterus and breasts into thinking pregnancy had taken place? The difference between male and female breast cancer risk is entirely hormonal. It cannot be totally abolished except by giving women a male hormonal environment, which would be to make them men. But oral contraceptives show our power to make changes without such costs. Hormones taken around the time of puberty could make the body believe a pregnancy had come to term at the earliest possible point. Such a strategy would likely be impossible without serious side effects such as breast swelling and brief lactation, and perhaps the small rise in blood clots seen with oral contraceptives. Given the cost of breast cancer, though, significant harms and intrusions would be potentially worthwhile if they reduced the risk of women dying from cancers that such treatments made largely preventable.

There is massive scope to reduce the risk of breast cancer in women through faking the hormonal changes of pregnancy. Lying so plainly in the realm of the possible, it is likely to lie near in the future. Other changes, too, stand close by. Genetic assessment of breast cancer risk and prophylactic mastectomy (as well as removal of ovaries and uterus on completion of reproductive life) are already used. Some of the same drugs that treat breast cancer have been shown to have effects in preventing it, but are not yet widely used for that purpose. Then there are the normal risk factors – smoking, alcohol, diet, exercise, weight – which also play a part and are modifiable. There is much that can be done in the near future to reduce the burden of breast and reproductive cancers on human lives.

Old age

Seventy to death

Old age is not what it was. Gone is the brief descent into retirement or senescence, the glint of a passing moment of late golden afternoon before the night draws in.

These days, old age is lengthy and healthy. Less like an equatorial dusk, gone as soon as noticed, more like a summer evening in England, stretching into the fade. For most of us, that is: for we many, we happy many, as Shakespeare might have put it if infection had not hurried him away at the age of fifty-two. Such infections are not conquered, for few victories in medicine are absolute. They can strike down those whose immune systems were born odd, or achieved oddness by virtue of some misfortune or medical intervention. But we no longer live in general fear of sudden infection. Not until old age is advanced enough to have properly got its teeth into us. By then, even its worst outcome has lost much of its horror. Osler, the medical professor we met in his garden with Twain and Kipling, called pneumonia the old man's friend. When it came for him he welcomed it.

As we weaken, as dusk thickens, the ground we live on once more becomes the battlefield of infectious illness that so recently made up all of human life. Antibiotics get less effective;

their power only ever being to support the response our bodies mustered. The infections happen more because we weaken, eventually because our mechanism for swallowing becomes so poor that what should be going from mouth to stomach finds its way to lungs instead. For most of old age such infections are troublesome and treatable. When we are very elderly they are troublesome still, but eventually all troubles end and pneumonia is often what does it. The art is determining where a patient is in their life. Not to rescue someone from pneumonia, when intervening might grant some span of happy days, is a failure. So is not recognising the soft footsteps of death and mistaking it for a medical problem.

Osler reached seventy. Any seventy-year-old on my ward would be prefaced, whenever anyone spoke of them, by the adjective 'young'. The average age of my patients is in the mid-eighties. Is it now the case that medicine has achieved the appalling trick of prolonging our decline in ever more awful ways? In 1616 Shakespeare went from full health to gone in a blink – 'We wondered, Shakespeare, that thou went'st so soon,' wrote a contemporary, 'From the world's stage to the grave's tiring room'.[1] In 1920 Osler declined more slowly but in a manner still swift by modern standards.

Decay has undoubtedly been stretched out, but this has happened neither deliberately nor exclusively. We spend more of our lives old and frail and dependent on others. But we have longer lives and, as a proportion, the amount of our lives we spend in senescence has actually gone down. We are more likely to reach old age alive and in good health and we are more likely to stay that way. The independent time we have gained in old age is still increasing at double the rate of the time when we need the most basic help.[2] The drawbacks are real, but to enjoy extended good health in old age is now the norm and never was before.

Doing an autumn afternoon outpatient clinic for the elderly, I saw a standard referral letter for a man in his early eighties: the problem, it said, was a shortness of breath on exercise. I asked the gentleman concerned, who looked notably sprightly. He admitted that it was, explaining that things he had once been able to do with ease he now noticed himself labouring at, needing to stop and rest frequently. How many yards, I asked, could he now walk before needing to rest? It's a standard question, and the answer is often half a mile or ten or twenty yards. This gentleman explained he never used to have any problems, but had grown concerned that summer at needing to stop occasionally on his annual ascent of Scafell Pike.

Drugs developed to treat disease have extended health. All drugs have side effects, meaning impacts beside the one intended, and not all side effects are bad. By aiming at treating disease we have extended frailty and altered expectations. We have developed the capacity to medicalise ourselves, to treat the natural process of ageing as though it were a disease to be fended off. The virtue of doing so is that we have grown powerful in our success. Prevention is better than cure? Taken seriously, it means reckoning what can be done by medicalising the normal progress of life.

Delaying cardiovascular disease buys time, and good quality time. 'Eighty is not without its pleasures', wrote the American essayist Joseph Epstein, commemorating his arrival.[3]

> One sees the trajectory of others' lives and careers—'the trajectory from life to death, with the final vertical plunge not far away', Proust called it in *Time Regained*. One thinks here of those prodigies who came whirring out of the gate but lost

ground on the second turn, with nothing left for the home stretch. Or those who were good at school but, as it turned out, nothing else. Or those who made all the predictably correct career and personal moves and yet ended up with supremely boring lives. Or those whose success, given their utter absence of talent and paucity of charm, remind one that the world is not an entirely just place.

Though much is taken, much abides, of mental as well as physical vivacity. So long as the pleasure in our capacities outweighs the burden of their limitations, relish remains.

'Santayana wrote that whatever one's age, one should always assume that one still has a decade left to live', Epstein continued.

In one of his letters he noted that, in his early 80s, his physician wanted him to lose 15 pounds, adding that he apparently desired him in perfect health just in time for his death. (He lived to 88.) In his 80s my friend Edward Shils still bought dishes and other new household items: 'It gives one a sense of futurity,' he explained.

In old age, people are willing to look old – to be old. 'In the late nineteenth and early twentieth centuries, old people in America had prayed, "Please, God, don't let me look poor." In the year 2000,' wrote Tom Wolfe, 'they prayed, "Please, God, don't let me look old." Sexiness was equated with youth, and youth ruled. The most widespread age-related disease was not senility but juvenility.'[4] People talk of having a wasted youth. Not wasting our maturity should be our chief concern and one of our modern blessings is that we have more of it to play with.

★

Eventually the end comes. Most of us do not die from one thing, no matter how much a death certificate demands that such a single cause be named. Frailty is always varied. Lungs lose capacity, muscles weaken, the brain and the heart subside, the liver shuts down its synthesis of albumin. Egg whites are made of the stuff and it is essential to human life. When the body is busy with an inflammatory process – an infection, a cancer, a ruptured plaque within a blood vessel – the liver reduces its production. The lack of albumin means fluid leaks from the bits of the body where it is meant to be to those where it is not. The swollen ankles that in a minor way are a common part of many lives, particularly for women, become something quite different. The swelling can get everywhere, as fluid leaks from blood vessels into the tissues, but it starts in the ankles, and spreads upward as it worsens, since it obeys the pull of gravity. More leaking fluid enters the lungs and makes us breathless. The process can be swift but is normally slow and superimposed on our other weaknesses. In a stuttering and unpredictable manner, frailty makes us halt and trip and fall and eventually fail.

Life expectancy in the UK at age seventy has gone from nine years in 1922 to sixteen in 2010.[5] Perhaps the change is more apparent if we note our double-take at the notion of sixty-five or seventy being described as marking the onset of old age. What felt true in 1922 feels wrong today and the difference is progress. It has not stopped. Between 2010 and 2015 healthy life expectancy at age sixty-five increased for the twenty-eight EU countries by 0.6 of a year.[6] Many have worried that medicine tends only to prolong our decay – in fact it means that we spend fewer years than ever before disabled by ill health.[7,8,9] Neither pessimism nor scepticism challenges the fact that we enjoy a greater percentage of life in good health, and that our good health extends over more years than ever before.

★

Our health buys us illness. Because we dodge bullets and cars and heart attacks we make it, eventually, to old age. The arms of old age may be frail and trembling but they are open wide, if only because the person they belong to is often falling. When they get old enough they are sometimes falling backwards. Even older and their arms don't go out at all. In early old age we fall forward and break our wrists, later we collapse more clumsily and smash our hips. When we react too slowly to break our falls voluntarily we break them all the same, but with our heads. Wrist fractures, pelvic fractures, head injuries: the sequence makes a steady pattern in how we present to hospital as our years go by. When *The King's Speech* hit the cinemas a number of its audience hit the floor – people not given to leaving the house made the journey in order to see a film about a monarch and a flurry of them arrived in hospital to have their broken hips replaced.

As muscle strength declines and reaction speeds drop we change from being the same person slowed down to being a different, slower person. The line between increasing forget-fulness and early dementia scares us so much because we understand it's not a line at all but a shadow, and by the time our sun is low on the horizon the edges of the shadows are never crisp. That so many more of us than ever before will become demented is not a failure but a success. We will live to become demented whereas before we would not have got so far. The change seems less miserable when you remember that it is not a matter of having swapped a past when a heart attack pinched us off the day before dementia came fumbling for the doorbell. That heart attack would just as likely have stopped us seeing our children finish school and stopped them from growing up and remembering who we were. Dementia robs us of our memories but it comes in place of being robbed of the chance of making them.

Our assault on dementia – an explicit and expensive one, quite as deliberate and almost as well funded as our war on cancer – has yielded little. Its most abiding lesson is of failure, no less valuable a lesson for not being the one we hoped for. Drugs to treat dementia have performed so poorly that even the greatest successes make a dubious difference. We can put Alzheimer's back by a few months, in certain limited circumstances, and in a way that does nothing to stop the pace of its progression. Drug company after drug company has withdrawn from the field, believing the value of the lesson is that they should study different problems. The future of specific anti-dementia agents seems bleak and unpromising. Its hopes were based on the notion that these conditions were discrete diseases, single-pathway problems, a notion that now seems mistaken. Alzheimer's has no infective agent to be fought off and no genetic switch to be reset. The very best drugs we have managed are less helpful than Zimmer frames but similar in effect – crutches that extend our independence a little but do nothing to stop its decline. Which is not to say that treating dementia is hopeless, only that the hope appears more and more to lie in fending it off for longer, not in dissolving it once it arrives. Dementia means ageing as it affects our brains. It is a category, not a pathway. It also seems to be a disease longer in the making than cardiovascular disease. High blood pressure in late life causes strokes but it appears to be high blood pressure in middle age that most predicts dementia. 'Not only underground are the brains of men / Eaten by maggots,' wrote Edna Vincent Millay.[10] Dementia is the final result of many years of time's munching.

Statins and antihypertensives and the anti-inflammatories

being introduced to treat cardiovascular disease[11] will all, I predict, be shown to reduce and retard dementia when given early enough. The armamentarium that reduces the ageing of our blood vessels will reduce age-related damage to the brain. The chance of getting dementia at any given age will continue to fall. The number of people with dementia, and the lifetime chance of developing it, will go up. Single-pathway attempts to treat it will continue to disappoint, while single-pathway attempts to reduce its progression and slow its initial onset will yield a series of mild to moderate successes.

These will combine and old age will not merely be deferred and extended but reshaped. Throughout history we have imagined that as societies and technology grow more efficient we will have more leisure time. We tend to think this hasn't happened. We overlook the extent to which it has already occurred, the leisure time not being spread throughout our lives but added at their end. To labour hard and then have decades of retirement suits many, but so does having a profession one enjoys – and that one does not wish to be forced into renouncing on reaching an arbitrary age. Less skilled jobs are often those which people are more pleased to give up. They are certainly those more subject to being eliminated through technological innovation. The jobs that are likely to expand in the future are the skilled ones. A British political drama portrayed a newly elected left-wing prime minister, travelling by train, being asked if he intended to abolish the privilege of first-class carriages. 'No,' he replies, 'I'll abolish second.'[12] Divided societies can hope to take the same approach, and such hopes are more likely to be fulfilled if they are conscious aims. Inequality is unavoidable – and efforts to delete it by executive order have had monstrous consequences – but attacking privilege can be helpfully replaced by expanding it and opening it up. The number of people capable of living first-class lives, in whatever way you wish to measure them, is not limited by our genes. We may end up working longer not because we have to, nor because it is the only reasonable response to living longer, but because it pleases and satisfies and interests us, and because we choose to do so. To be able to work longer at what we enjoy seems an inordinately attractive consequence of progress. 'The lyf so short, the craft so long to lerne', wrote Chaucer.[13] Hippocrates, with his famous *ars longa, vita brevis* – the art is long, the life is short – had opened one of his books with the same.

We can work while we still have light, and we can glory in our expectation of having more of it and bequeathing still more again. Some of the improvements came inadvertently but none happened by accident.

The UK Office for National Statistics reported in 2015 that:

> Dementia and Alzheimer's disease was the leading cause of death for women over 80 accounting for 17% of deaths and was the second leading cause for men causing 11% of deaths in this age group. Deaths from dementia and Alzheimer's disease are increasing as people live longer, and are more common in women as women live longer than men. The leading cause of death for men in this age group was ischaemic heart disease accounting for 15% of deaths, this was the second leading cause for women causing 11% of deaths.[14]

Dementia almost never occurs in isolation. Dementia and ischaemic heart disease are manifestations of ageing, both heavily mediated by deteriorations in our vascular tree. Which ailment happens to have its nose in front on the day life crosses its finish line is not what matters most. The goal is to put together effective responses to slow, retard, regress and fight against the dying of the light. Dylan Thomas's 'Do not go gentle into that good night' is usually misremembered as being about old age facing death. It's not, it's about the experience of the middle-aged man faced with the death of his father. It is the business of fierce middle age to improve the ways of fending off death. Those at the end of their lives have no obligation to feel the same way.

The way in which single diagnoses can hide complex reality is apparent in old age. The changes seen at autopsy in the brains of those with Alzheimer's are seen in 40 per cent of those without it: it is unclear whether these changes, the clumps of proteins called amyloid plaques that build up in our brains over the years, are cause or consequence. We have focused on them as the cause for Alzheimer's because the possibility that they were gave us a target for our investigations and our drugs. Neither has yielded benefits and the plaques may not be the cause of the disease at all. Brain scans of elderly individuals are similarly uninformative, with the vast majority of mentally intact elderly people showing changes on their scans that could be seen as firm evidence for dementia – if they had had any. A recent review noted these problems:

> A hypothesis that remains unproven yet catches the collective imagination can become, with the passage of time, so seductive that it dominates... [medical] opinion and arrests the development of alternative ideas. Such is the case for the amyloid hypothesis of [Alzheimer's disease].[15]

Waging war on cancer has proven hard enough, and that was a disease where the cause – the cancerous cells – was straightforward to identify. With dementia, nothing is so clear.

Never before have diseases of decay been so overwhelmingly those which affect us; in the past they never had the chance. Decay tends to be more multifarious in its causes than infections or trauma. The human body is packed with overlapping safety features. Single parts of it rarely fail by themselves. With Alzheimer's our focus on amyloid deposition, on the misfolded proteins that accumulate with age, was driven partly by noting that this amyloid seemed responsible for an odd, minor variant of the disease, a rare type that strikes people when young. It is yielding to genetic analysis and it is known to be connected to genes giving rise to amyloid deposition when faulty. We have extrapolated from such rare variants of the disease to the much more common form, a disease whose genetics are not understood and which does not appear to operate as a genetic disorder. Normal amyloid plaques in the brain are not a manifestation of a genetic disease and may not be the cause of a disease at all. They may be the evidence of our body fighting one off or they may be nothing more than the traces of time passing.

This is not to suggest that there can be no useful insights from comparing the rare forms of dementia with the common ones – to do so was a sensible strategy – but when dealing with diseases of old age we often need to approach them differently from others. In 1854 Thomas Snow removed the handle of the Broad Street pump in London, simultaneously ending the local cholera outbreak and proving that the disease was a waterborne infection.* Diseases not transmitted by a particular

---

* Actually, not quite, although it makes a neat story and is close to the truth. The pump handle was removed because Snow had won the fight to establish cholera as water-borne – and the outbreak may have already been dying out. The intellectual appeal of medical science is not that it is clean and precise. It has all the muddled complexity of history and art, being made of both.

infective organism or caused by single-gene defects are not so straightforward. Their causes are multifarious. When you have been asking a question for a long period without finding an answer, the explanation is sometimes that the answer is hard to find – but often that the question itself is wrong. Dementia, like depression, cardiovascular disease, cancer, arthritis, sexual dysfunction and many of our other afflictions, is not a single entity caused by a single problem. The hazard of reducing a phenomenon to a single cause (like amyloid deposition) is that the simplification can move you further away from reality.

'It matters not how a man dies,' said Johnson, 'but how he lives. The act of dying is not of importance, it lasts so short a time.'[16] Another great quotable disagreed: 'In judging another's life,' wrote Montaigne, 'I always see how its end was borne: and one of my main concerns for my own is that it be borne well.'[17] How one died mattered partly because it was the reflection, the culmination, of how one lived. Johnson would have allowed for that had he not been so devoted to expressions that flattened all opposition – in other words, if he had not been Johnson.

How we bear our deaths is not recorded on the certificates with which civil authorities mark them. Nor is the need to bear death bravely so demanding as it once was. We are better at eliminating the pain and physical suffering that dying can entail and effective at ensuring that death comes in old age, which also makes it easier to bear. 'There is a great difference between going off in warm blood like Romeo', wrote Keats, 'and making one's exit like a frog in a frost.'[18] We mostly do the latter, and only when our long year is so mature that it does not seem unnatural. The opportunity and the awful challenge of brave final words is gone. There may be times when we receive news of a terminal diagnosis, and fresh with the sense of it need to break the news to others, but these times tend to come when we are already in the close of our lives, when some preparation for parting will already seem reasonable, even if we had hoped it would not be needed so soon. Illness rarely strikes us down in our prime – the tuberculosis that killed the twenty-five-year-old Keats a few months after he wrote these words is gone from our list of common killers. The frost sets in slowly over years and decades. By the time the end comes our awareness has long been shrouded; the final difficulties are not chiefly for us but for those we leave behind.

'I can scarcely bid you good bye, even in a letter', Keats ended. 'I always made an awkward bow.'[19] For almost all of us the curtain falls so slowly no bow is required: the performer falls asleep even if the audience weep. Of the very many people who I have seen hold the hands and stroke the heads of those who are dying, the comfort brought by the contact, and the distress of the death, has almost always belonged to the person in attendance, not to the one dying.

Diseases

'The same three problems preoccupied the people of twentieth-century China, of medieval India and of ancient Egypt', said a recent book. 'Famine, plague and war were always at the top of the list.'[1] Something to it, not least its picturesque sweep, but the problems that preoccupied people most in the past are those that preoccupy them now: the daily problems of their personal interests, not just those of society and state.* The concerns of individuals tend to be individual concerns, a truism no less robust for the exceptions made by those living in today's war zones of Syria or Yemen. If anything, the focus was even more personal, back when our sense of self was not centralised by mass media. Sumerian poetry is less about famine, plague and war than eating and drinking and love. Disease figured too, but the casual individual deaths made up the daily worries, rarely the plagues that so impress historians. It was in normal daily life, not in its epoch-making

---

* 'I may feel that Europe is finished, that western civilization has had the course, that humankind generally is on the way out, but about my mail I remain hopeful.' Frederic Raphael and Joseph Epstein, *Distant Intimacy*, Yale University Press (2013), p. 230.

exceptions, that the brutal tyranny of microbes over man most held sway.

Mundane life was where the drama lay. 'Confess, Marianne,' says her sister Elinor, in Jane Austen's novel *Sense and Sensibility*, 'is not there something interesting to you in the flushed cheek, hollow eye, and quick pulse of a fever?'[2] Today's television dramas need to rustle up more danger than the world holds to fill their plots and to get their cast into emergency departments. One tongue-in-cheek piece of epidemiology showed that characters in the BBC's most popular television soap opera were eight times more likely to die than viewers watching it.[3] The same gap did not exist between Austen and her readers. Later in *Sense and Sensibility*, Marianne Dashwood gets the reward for her hot-headed love of drama and catches cold. 'Though heavy and feverish, with a pain in her limbs, and a cough, and a sore throat', it was hoped 'a good night's rest was to cure her entirely.'[4] Marianne worsens, the apothecary attends; she rallies briefly then falls into delirium.* The characters gather in concern and Marianne's mother is sent for in case her cold is the end of her.

It takes a lot to make a young person delirious; in a world without effective medicines, their risk of death is high. So when Marianne recovers, her sensible sister feels it:

> Elinor could not be cheerful. Her joy was of a different kind, and led to any thing rather than to gaiety. Marianne restored to life, health, friends, and to her doting mother, was an idea to fill her heart with sensations of exquisite comfort, and expand

---

* To be delirious meant, literally, not to be able to plough straight, to be out of the furrow. Both ploughing and dangerous infections were once the stuff of daily life, the stuff of which words were made.

it in fervent gratitude;—but it led to no outward demonstrations of joy, no words, no smiles. All within Elinor's breast was
satisfaction, silent and strong.[5]

Elinor was Austen's heroine, her model. There was cause for
gratitude and satisfaction in recovery but not for gaiety. To be
reminded of the tyrannical randomness of death, of the easy
accidents waiting to snuff out the young and healthy, was no
cause for a light heart.

This book, and this chapter in particular, is written from the
'First-World' perspective. That's appropriate because it's mine
(and probably yours) and also because the shape of things to
come for the developing world is not so interesting. We know
what it looks like since we are living it. The interest is in figuring out how to help. There are specific challenges, particularly
those of infectious disease and road traffic accidents, solvable
by interventions parachuted in from high-income countries via
vaccines and technology. The fundamental challenges, those of
a poor standard of living, have a solution – raise it – which is no
intellectual challenge to describe, however hard it is to engineer.

Infections of the gut and of the lungs, the sort that have
always killed so many infants and children, will continue to
do so in societies with inadequate sanitation, hygiene, housing,
education, income, emancipation and medicine. In developed
countries they are rare. Diseases of decay now hold their place.
Heart and kidney disease and stroke are primarily the consequences of an ageing vascular supply. Alzheimer's and other
dementias are driven partly by the same, whatever other causes
may also be contributing. Cancer is the decay of control systems
for cell division. Diabetes, the name we give to the behaviour of
our metabolism when its handling of sugar deteriorates, is rarely
the result of a sudden, specific autoimmune disease, the body

attacking essential sugar-handling cells in the pancreas. Diabetes is partly the result of spending our lives happily consuming more food than needed for survival, but while overeating accelerates its development, it may, like atherosclerosis, also be a normal part of ageing.

Into this mix throw other overlapping terms – hypertension, hyperlipidaemia, atherosclerosis, atrial fibrillation and thromboembolism, fatty liver disease, aneurysms; an endless list – all historically seen as things-in-themselves, as specific diseases and maladies, but which more accurately are reflections of the same thing, of wear and tear, and many of them often of a sort of wear and tear that occurs far more often in smokers. The future depends on how we manage and minimise them, how we retard their development.

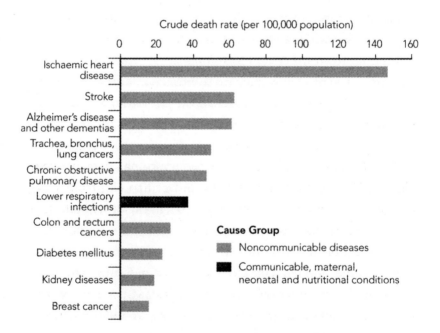

Fig. 4. Top ten causes of death in high-income countries in 2016.[6]

The top ten causes of death in high-income countries (Fig. 4) divide almost entirely into the (overlapping) categories of diseases of ageing and diseases caused by smoking. Deaths from lower respiratory infections (ranked sixth) are the exception. They are not all caused by ageing, with or without smoking, but most of them are.

CANCER

Plot cancer mortality on a graph, adjusted for the size of the population, and one sees a steady rise. This is good news, the result of our success at avoiding death from other causes.[7] If you look at what happens to people when they get cancer, the progress is also apparent – this time it shows as a steady, cumulative improvement in their survival.[8,9] The future will look the same. We will get more cancer and get better at treating it.

Insights from other animals (long-lived tortoises get fewer cancers per year of life than we do, rats far more), from children and adults born with rare mutations, and from advances in understanding our body's ability to fight cancer will continue to be useful. Those from 'big data', from whole-population studies of gene variability, from observational data of what supermarkets record us as having ordered to eat, from what our phones and devices note about our lives, all will add fuel to a fire whose oxygen will remain our ability to test interventions in reliable trials and to see how best to intervene. Progress will continue, and will continue to be slow and undramatic and continue to sum into something very dramatic indeed. It will not be as dramatic as the transformation of childhood cancer but it will tread the same path. At the moment its pace is limited by the practical barriers of the differences between childhood and adult cancers and by the cultural differences in how we test treatments for the two. Our willingness to lift the brake caused by those cultural differences will depend on how acutely we notice that it is slowing us down.

It seems almost embarrassing to offer the reminder that smoking is bad for you. The statement is not novel but it merits repeating. How much the next hundred years are clouded by smoke makes all the difference in the world. Establishing the harms of smoking took a long time. The lag between taking up the habit and suffering from it was so long and the fact almost everyone smoked made the comparison with non-smokers hard to spot. Harms accelerated as production and consumption changed, from pipes and cigars in the nineteenth century to manufactured cigarettes in the twentieth. Even when it became clear there was harm, its magnitude took time to assess. Evidence first arose in those who had smoked little when they were young. Only recently have we acquired the decades of data needed to understand the costs of a lifetime's habit.

Smoking makes life less healthy, crippling it with chronic disease, and it makes life shorter. Smokers are three times more likely to die in middle age.[10] Globally, if people continue to smoke as they do today, with about half of all men taking up smoking and one in ten women doing so, and few of them quitting, then during the twenty-first century tobacco will cause a billion deaths.[11] These figures sound like factoids, a term writer Norman Mailer coined to convey something without truth but one used today to signify meaningless shards of knowledge, statistics that sound impressive but convey little. These figures are not factoids. They are accurate and the result of lifetimes of research work, and they are profound. Smokers lose on average ten years of life from smoking.[12] Smoking cancels out the combined effect of every single improvement in human health achieved over the past sixty years.[13] Given that only some of the gains over the past 60 years are attributable to medicine (perhaps a bit more than half) this lies behind my statement earlier that smoking does more harm than all modern medicine put together does good. In the middle of revising this paragraph I received an email telling me a friend and neighbour, an ex-smoker, has lung cancer. Countless people will have received similar news at the same time. Inbetween submitting the typescript of this book and receiving the copy-edit my mother, also an ex-smoker, was also diagnosed with lung cancer. She will likely die before it is published. The miseries of smoking are not factoids, not even when summed into statistics. They are real because the people that make them up are real.

Smoking briefly in one's youth seems to do little, if anything, to health. Beyond that the costs are real but strongly modifiable – 'Those who have smoked cigarettes since early adulthood but stop at 30, 40, or 50 years of age gain about 10, 9, and 6 years of life expectancy, respectively, as compared with those who continue smoking.'[14] Giving up works.

Certain other aspects of smoking are worth mentioning. Richard Doll, the epidemiologist whose work our knowledge depends upon, commented that 'what you've got to remember is that the directors of the tobacco companies in 1950 were responsible people, insofar as the directors of any firm were, and they were horrified by the idea that what they were selling was killing people'.[15] Worth pointing out: a reminder that those whose work supports tobacco today are not defending a long-standing libertarian tradition but are supporting something murderous and addictive when their forebears did no such thing. 'They are to my mind', said Doll, speaking of those in the industry today, 'thoroughly immoral people.'[16] The question of morality is relevant. Smoking rates are not difficult to alter. Price matters, as a wealth of evidence shows.[17] Politicians, opinion formers and regulators have the power to save more lives than doctors: a fact which is often true, but almost never so clearly accompanied by incontrovertible proof of the action needed.

The government has a role in such matters, in legislating and protecting, mandating and encouraging and nudging. The justification for any intervention must be based upon the magnitude of its impact, tempered by the confidence with which we know it to be true and the amount it intrudes on life. A well-functioning government will be serious about correlating its actions with their impacts and explaining its reasoning to its citizens with a degree of clarity and quantification that is good enough for them to dispute. It is right that tobacco control is taken more seriously than control of meat consumption, another area that has been identified as concerning for human health[18] but where the quality of evidence, and the magnitude of harm it suggests, are both massively less.[19]

Physicians can nag, torment or preach in a professional capacity when they have evidence that doing so is sufficiently helpful to justify its offensiveness. Good trial evidence suggests that doctors nagging people about smoking results in people quitting.[20] Preaching proven to save lives has some excuse. We are prone to viewing illness as punishment.* This is not to

---

* 'The punishment theory [of illness] is deeply erroneous and can sometimes be very cruel. The idea that prolapse of the uterus is a consequence of sexual overindulgence... [is] an example of Aristotle's gullibility and his habitual confusion between what is true and what ought, he felt, to be true.' P. B. and J. S. Medawar, *Aristotle to Zoos*, Harvard University Press (1983), p. 152.

deliver a lecture on healthy living but to highlight how huge a difference smoking makes. It may not match in its interest the sum total of every single medical advance over the past sixty years, but it does in its effect.

Obesity and cancer are linked, too, and obesity is so far from being cured by economic and political developments as to be their herald. Its links with cancer stem from fat being not only an inactive reservoir of energy but a tissue with hormonal and metabolic influences. We'll come to that later.

Hepatitis B and C deserve a mention: a rather apologetic way of introducing two diseases science has made treatable yet which are growing more common. In 1990 viral hepatitis was the world's tenth leading cause of death. By 2013 it had risen to seventh, killing 1.45 million people a year.[21] Hepatitis B is preventable through vaccination, hepatitis C curable through recent advances in antiviral drugs. In the developing world liver cancer is the second most common fatal cancer, principally caused by hepatitis B and C.[22] Cheap vaccines for the former make it a horror that socioeconomic development can be expected to deliver us from. For hepatitis C the undiscounted cost of the drugs required to cure one person in the US comes in at $84,000.[23] In Egypt, where 15 per cent of the population have the disease,[24] the total sum becomes astronomical. These are problems less of socioeconomic development and more of how to encourage the design and manufacture of medicines in such a way as to make them affordable. Two cheers for capitalism. The third cheer is achievable, as it turned out to be when the cost of antiretrovirals for HIV, which seemed similarly unaffordable, was shown not to be. What is not clear is how many of the current generation will die untreated before the problem is solved.

Over the next century more of us will get cancer, despite the improvements we will make in prevention. More of us will die of it, despite treatments also being improved. Those two things will happen because we will live to be older than ever before and because we continue to get so good at avoiding other causes of death. Whatever the achievements in research and development, whatever the steps forward in embedding clinical trials in clinical practice, costs will rise. The latest treatments will always involve new technologies, not yet capable of being mass produced inexpensively, and the costs incurred in researching will be passed on to those few capable of paying. The degree of understanding of specific cancers in specific people – even of specific mutations in specific parts of a single person's cancer – will mean that treatments are ever more individually tailored. The advancing edge of what is possible will become less and less affordable for most. The gap between the care available to rich and poor will widen.

There are grounds for optimism, despite the challenges. The extra money of the rich will fund the developments that a few years later will become affordable to others. That's not because the rich are necessarily philanthropic but because patents expire and efficiencies and improvements spread. The inequality that comes from wealth can never be obliterated – efforts to be that absolute only lead to the obliteration of people – but it can be attacked and reduced and minimised. The endless effort of doing so, in a way that pursues the common good, will be as much a part of our future as our past.

One sees new problems not because they have the dew still on them but because others have passed into the twilight. Cancer, obesity, hypertension and diabetes have always haunted us but never seemed the threat they do now. They always were threats.

They were just harder to spot among the thronging ghouls of infection and trauma.

Between 1917 and 1923 Framingham, 20 miles to the west of Boston, Massachusetts, had been the site of a research project aimed at fighting tuberculosis. In the aftermath of the Second World War the US government saw infectious disease as the great challenge, the chief cause of premature death. For the first time, though, non-infectious threats began to seem worthy of some measure of organised state attention. The first description of the newer Framingham project was recognisably modern in focus and in prose:

> This project is designed to study the expression of coronary artery disease in a normal or unselected population and to determine the factors predisposing to the development of the disease through clinical and laboratory examination and long-term follow-up of such a group.[25]

Not easy to read that aloud and make it sound like one of twentieth-century medicine's most exciting steps, but it was.

The link with tuberculosis was more than geographical. Tuberculosis is a chronic disease and a complicated one. Exposure is a poor predictor of succumbing. Getting ill is a poor predictor of outcome, which varies from complete and cheerful recovery through wan chronicity – pallid ill health aching out over the years – to rapid lungs-filling-with-blood death. The 'factors predisposing to the development of the disease', whatever they were, were known to act slowly when it came to tuberculosis.

It was dawning on people that the sudden events of heart attacks and strokes could also not be understood without understanding their history. Inheritance was thought to matter, as was cholesterol (long noted to be part of the fatty lining that blocked arteries). Lifestyle, employment, wealth and status, dietary and drinking habits, and even 'nervous and mental states' were all considered. Smoking was of so little interest that initially participants were not even asked about it. The US government proceeded slowly. Relations with the medical profession were fractious, not least because President Truman had called for universal health care as part of his 1949 Fair Deal.*

From 'factors predisposing', those in Framingham came to use another term. 'Risk factors' had been spoken of before but not commonly; the Framingham study made the term so popular that it became a part of common vocabulary and common thought. In the 1960s the study was almost closed, threatened by the enthusiasm of those who felt risk factors could be predicted and analysed entirely at the lab bench.[26] The epidemiologists won and the reductionists lost, and the argument was accepted that some properties are best looked for at the level of large groups of people studied over decades, not in dishes of cells over days.

Atherosclerosis, the ageing of blood vessels underlying so many human problems, was seen for much of the twentieth century as a disease of civilisation. Studying biology, anthropology and medicine in the 1990s, I remember it being taught as such. The

---

* In the US, as in the UK, doctors worried that such a system threatened their income. They were right to do so. 'I stuffed their mouths with gold', boasted Nye Bevan, of the deal that won round British doctors. The bribe was temporary and doctors are much more richly paid now in the US than the UK, just as health care is cheaper and more efficient in the UK partly for the same reason. It is notable that British doctors remain supporters of the National Health Service (NHS). Care that is free at the point of delivery and available to all is often better – accept a fee-per-service and you quickly forget the best amount of medicine is the least – and good care is satisfying to deliver. British doctors would profit were the NHS to fall, and hence deserve some credit for wanting it to stand.

teaching often included some sense of a moral recompense. Atherosclerosis was the function of greed and laziness – we ate too much and did too little – and was exacerbated by the stress of modern society, the stress of getting and spending. Our hearts betrayed nature and it was on them that nature revenged herself.

That way of thinking appeals to us now as it did then, and coldly inserts its bony nose where it doesn't belong, twisting assumptions and swaying prejudice, suggesting we must pay for our unnatural modernity. It can be spotted in the preference for vitamins over drugs, or the linguistic sense that pits one against the other as though nature drew a line between them. It's there in the misty fog suggesting that avoiding cholesterol-rich foods is a superior alternative to taking a statin, not a complementary choice. It's there in the notions of organic when applied in its modern way to foodstuffs, and in the hundred descendants of medieval superstitions, from homeopathy to an unwarranted faith in expert opinion. 'Today,' wrote Trotsky a century ago, 'not only in peasant homes but also in the city sky-scrapers, there lives alongside the twentieth century the tenth or thirteenth. A hundred million people use electricity and still believe in the magic power of signs and exorcisms.'[27] I work on a ward where the bays are numbered consecutively but fourteen comes immediately after twelve. Like my colleagues, I have to fight the nonsensical tendency to assume drugs are more powerful when delivered through the invasive power of a drip, a tendency doctors are as vulnerable to as anyone.[28] When a patient is well the tendency is easy to resist. When they are critically ill it is not.

Irrationality lurks in the shadows. The wish to believe natural is best – a wish most honoured by not pausing to think what one means by the slippery idea of natural – faded a little at the dawn of the twenty-first century. We could not escape noticing how effective medicine had become, and while many remained able to construe a manufactured vitamin pill as natural, few managed when it came to aspirin, statins or blood pressure pills.* The notion that atherosclerosis was the evil consequence of straying from the path of natural righteousness faded but remained.

A landmark 1953 paper, showing widespread atherosclerosis in autopsies from US soldiers killed in Korea,[29] made clear the extent of the problem, but its findings were consistent with it being a disease of modern life. So too was a 1999 study taking almost 3,000 American dead, all killed by accident or trauma, all aged between fifteen and thirty-four, and finding atherosclerosis in every one of them.[30]

The idea of modernity being intrinsically bad lingered. In 2004 a respectable paper argued 'our Palaeolithic genome is playing a substantial role in the ongoing epidemics of obesity, hypertension, diabetes, and atherosclerotic cardiovascular disease', and that 'the most practical solution for reducing the incidence of chronic degenerative diseases such as atherosclerosis is to realign our current maladaptive diet and lifestyle to simulate the milieu for which we are genetically designed'.[31]

Realign our lives to the milieu we evolved in and they would be as they were then – nasty, brutish and short. Arguing human problems are best solved by a return to a simpler past usually spells trouble. Whether you picture our past as one of happy primitive communism or natural health foods and blissful physical vitality, the pictures may be pretty but they aren't real. In 2013 a study named HORUS gathered together preserved corpses of 137 people from across history. The dead were

---

* That was regardless of the fact that all three harnessed the natural pathways of our biochemistry, as all drugs do, and that the first derived from a common plant – the shrub spiraea – the second from a fungus and the third from snake venom.

drawn from four continents and four millennia. They included farmers and gatherer-hunters, those who ate mainly vegetables, those who were carnivores and those who lived only on seafood and coastal berries. 'When in the course of human history did atherosclerosis appear?', the study asked:

> Is it a disease of lifestyle? Of ageing? Of another cause? With the doubling of life expectancy across the developed world between 1800 and 2000, atherosclerotic vascular disease has replaced infectious disease as the leading cause of death across the developed world. A common assumption is that atherosclerosis is predominately lifestyle-related and that if modern human beings could emulate preindustrial or even preagricultural lifestyles, that atherosclerosis, or least its clinical manifestations, would be avoided.[32]

Among the Palaeolithic corpses drawn together back across time and space – they had lived to average ages of thirty-two to forty-three – and even with the reduced ability to see the disease that resulted from the bodies being thousands of years old, atherosclerosis was detectably common. 'The presence of atherosclerosis in premodern human beings', the authors concluded, 'suggests that the disease is an inherent component of human ageing and not characteristic of any specific diet or lifestyle.' Premature death from atherosclerosis is as natural as our desire to eliminate it.

VASCULAR AGEING AND ITS COSTS

Vascular ageing is the cause of the bulk of human death and human diminishment.

That atherosclerosis is a universal part of ageing does not mean we develop it universally. We vary, and we study that variation to learn what causes it. Diets and lifestyles matter but individual efforts to diet and change one's lifestyle are largely ineffective, with the pointed exception of quitting smoking. Diet and lifestyle can be effectively influenced at a societal level but while Framingham and other studies have suggested links between diet, lifestyle and vascular ageing, they have not given us the teeth to take many bites out of them.

The half-acknowledged legacy of Framingham is that many of the modern world's diseases are not diseases. In 1970 Framingham showed that high blood pressure gave rise to stroke; in 2001 it showed that pressures just below that, at the higher end of the 'normal' range, did exactly the same, just to a slightly milder degree. It's not that high blood pressure is a disease, nor that high-normal is a-bit-of-a-disease, it's that the higher the blood pressure the quicker blood vessels age. Blood pressure rises as a result of age and as a result of itself, an accelerating tumble towards disability and death. For too long medicine behaved as though one treated blood pressure to a point where it crossed a line and became normal, as though it were a disease like an infection. That was a misunderstanding. Raised blood pressure is ageing in action and one lowers it in order to age more slowly. The same is true with cholesterol, and there medicine embraced the same error. For decades we engaged in a strategy that went by the name of treating-to-target, the notion being that at a certain level normality replaced disease. But there was never disease in the first place, only the normality of ageing. Lowering cholesterol levels is one of the ways we have of modifying it. We have found no level of 'normal' at which lowering them further ceases to have benefit, and it is not for lack of looking.

BLOOD PRESSURE AS A
MODIFIABLE RISK FACTOR

'The normal blood pressure is from 120 to 130 mm. of mercury, but in persons over 50 it is very often from 140 to 160 mm. A permanent pressure above the latter figure may be called high, but there are great regional variations.' So said William Osler in the ninth edition of *Principles and Practice* in 1920.

Osler suggested what the treatment should be: 'live a quiet, well regulated life, avoiding excesses in food and drink', bathe lots, eat less salt, avoid stress. If all that failed, then 'in some instances, with very high tension, striking relief is afforded by the abstraction of 10 to 20 ounces of blood'. Startling to think that in 1920, the advice was for bloodletting, just as it then still was for pneumonia. In sky-high blood pressure, bloodletting would have provided short-term benefit, reducing the amount of blood and hence the pressure. The effects of chronic differences in blood pressure were not apparent to Osler and the medical world of a century ago, hence his suggestion that for many people over fifty figures of 140–160 mmHg were normal. Statistically, he was correct – they were normal in the sense of being routine. Today we would regard them as abnormal, marking the lower boundaries of a disease called hypertension. But it's not clear how much a disease called hypertension actually exists, which was the lesson Framingham was gradually introducing. The higher your blood pressure the faster your blood vessels age; there is no cut-off at which that relationship starts and a disease can be said to begin, only a relationship expressing ever higher levels of risk.

A century ago, the effects of blood pressure on heart attacks were not a part of medical orthodoxy. Heart attacks are mentioned in Osler's book, the greatest standard textbook of his time, but only a few times in the book's 1,168 pages. They do not appear in its thirteen-page table of contents nor even in its index. Heart attacks and blood pressure, to the greatest classifying medical mind in the first decades of the twentieth century, were not major problems.

Osler died the year the 1920 edition was published. By 1948 cardiovascular disease, chiefly heart attacks and strokes, had become such a concern that the Framingham study became the first of many. The higher your blood pressure, they all found, the greater your risk. In 2002 the data the world had accumulated were brought together into a single study, the sum total of sixty-one Framingham-like observational research programmes together enrolling a million people. The huge numbers yielded the power to be precise. For every extra 20 mmHg of blood pressure, people died from vascular disease at double the normal rate. There was no point at which a drop in blood pressure did not further reduce that chance of dying, nor any age at which the relationship ceased.[33]

Why are we not all on multiple blood pressure tablets from youth? Why, if prevention is better than cure, do we wait for the harms of ageing to take hold before starting treatments? These are good questions whose answers aren't good but are clear.

LIPIDS AS A MODIFIABLE RISK FACTOR

Lower your blood-borne cholesterol* with drugs and you profit. The magnitude of the effect is substantial, with a 2–3 mmol/litre (millimoles per litre) decrease yielding a halving of vascular

---

* The fraction known as low-density lipoprotein, or LDL, cholesterol.

risk, the vascular risk in this case not being solely the risk of dying but the combination of the risk of death with that of a heart attack or stroke or something similar.[34] The data here are as reliable as data get. Having studied almost 200,000 people in twenty-six randomised trials means that there is almost nothing we know in medicine with as much confidence as we know about statins, the drugs that lower cholesterol.

In the last quarter of the twentieth century we discovered the power of statins. Now we have drugs called PCSK9 inhibitors that lower cholesterol more powerfully, and one called ezetimibe that does it less powerfully. Nothing to stop us taking the three together; it's certainly not a question of having to pick one. We have other new drugs that also lower cholesterol, and within sight are newer, stranger agents, halfway between traditional drugs and gene therapy, which alter our body's manufacture of the gene products that agents like statins hit. We are likely to soon be able to shut down some of these manufacturing pathways at will, to switch off genes that raise our cholesterol. It can seem like the problem will soon cease to be our technological ability and will swiftly become a question of how far we want to go. 'An ounce of prevention', said Benjamin Franklin, 'is worth a pound of cure.'[35] How far should we go? It isn't simple to know.

Our concept of disease stems from a world in which distinct conditions had distinct causes that could be remedied and removed. Rather than seeing the bulk of modern human diseases as aspects of ageing, we slice them up into names and categories that can be unhelpful even when they are not wholly wrong. Normality can also mislead us, with its statistical implication that variation from an average can serve as sufficient to define disease.

We model our mental ideas of medicines on an almost-fictional notion of antibiotics. A patient has an overwhelming infection from which they will die if left without treatment. Understanding the way the disease works, and having designed a drug to counter it, the patient is saved. A single well-identified problem is matched with its solution and health is restored. If the role of medicine is to cure us in such a fashion, there is something suspicious going on when medicine is also applied when we are in a state of health to begin with.

Antibiotics for overwhelming sepsis, fatal if untreated but exquisitely sensitive to the right drugs, follow the model of fixing a problem and restoring normality. Antibiotics in almost all settings in which they are now actually used do not. Most infections respond to the body's own defences; appropriate antibiotics help hasten recovery and improve its odds, not provide a cure. Most people who take antibiotics would be fine without them and most of those who take them and die would not have been saved by taking more. Antidepressants and antipsychotics, it is worth noticing, possess names reflecting the idea of corresponding to life-saving successful antibiotics. The names have potential as metaphors but they are harmful when taken literally. Most of the time, they are taken literally.

Fixing a traumatic injury that will otherwise be fatal certainly fits the pattern of a disease and a cure but even few surgeries are like that. Most surgical procedures behave like drugs, offering a range of benefits and a range of harms. Most surgery, like most medicine, is about improving the odds of a better outcome. We think of doctors and health care as life-savers, each intervention both dramatic and essential. It would be better to think of them as helpful gamblers, endlessly finessing our chances.

More than ever before, the long term matters. The chance of a middle-aged man benefiting from five years of a statin is small, so small it's generally agreed not to be worth bothering with unless his risk is unusually high. But at the end of five years would he be the same man? With the same blood vessels and the same expectations? We advocate a lifetime of healthy eating, diet and exercise, and we do so without knowing what such choices actually confer beyond knowing they are probably good. For a pill we would never accept such ignorance. Probably good isn't enough – how probably, and how good? And what are the drawbacks? Without quantification we are left with hopes and fears and endless lists of good and bad, the relics of a world where we believed everything either worked or did not, where diseases matched cures, where there was one-to-one correspondence between the danger seen and the action needed. When you are playing the odds, such lists are as useless as a list of horses running a race and a note next to each that they might win or might lose.

Framingham helped. We began to realise we were not looking for causes that were present or absent but for risk factors we all possessed to differing degrees. 'Risk factor' has an appropriate air of measuring the wind and playing the odds, assaulting the hazards of life after a careful appreciation of probabilities. We still improperly speak of risks versus benefits: the phrase is false. It's risk versus risk, the risk of action versus inaction, intervention versus non-intervention, the risk of harm against the risk of benefit. Medicine's job is to determine the odds of the best available paths, to communicate them clearly and to improve them. Whether the risks are worth it is not a medical question but a value judgement for the societies that pay and for the people opting in or out.

The majority of drugs and medical interventions offer a relative risk reduction of the order of 15–30 per cent. That sounds more impressive than it is. It's relative to one's existing risk, which is almost always low, the chance of anything terrible

happening in any one year of our lives being small. Novel mutations, new genetic changes, it has long been noted, are almost
always small: any really big change may have benefits but larger
harms are virtually guaranteed.[36] Complex systems are usually
too finely balanced to offer more, hence the risk reductions of
most drugs being small. Our lives change dramatically only
through the steady addition of small alterations.

Smaller benefits than 15–30 per cent of our relative risk are
perfectly feasible, we just don't normally spot them. To detect
them our trials would need to be massively larger and that has
almost never seemed worthwhile. Ezetimibe, the cholesterol
absorption blocker mentioned above, is unusual in offering a
relative risk reduction of only 6 per cent. It took an unusually
large and long-term trial to detect that benefit without the noise
of normal variation swamping the signal of effect and leading
to a false conclusion that the drug did nothing.[37]

Clot-busting drugs after a heart attack offer a relative risk
reduction of about 30 per cent; rapid angioplasty (threading
balloons and scaffolds down wires placed in blood vessels, so
that narrowings can be expanded and held open) improves
on that by the same amount again. Coronary artery bypass
surgery similarly offers a relative risk reduction of around a
third.* Statins, aspirin, beta-blockers and ACE (angiotensin-
converting enzyme) inhibitors for blood pressure, warfarin and
other blood thinners, diuretics – all of them, in a range of settings, consistently offer relative risk reductions of the order of
20–30 per cent.[38]

---

* If it seems strange that such an obviously life-saving procedure should
offer benefits equivalent in magnitude to taking a statin, it shouldn't. Not
all who have their chest opened up would have done badly if it had been
left alone and some will die from the procedure.

Those relative risk reductions, for people at low levels of absolute risk, are not worth bothering with. If your chance of a heart attack is 1 in 1,000 then, even if a pill had no side effects, the trouble of taking it would scarcely seem worthwhile to drop your relative risk by 20–30 per cent, meaning by a further 2–3 in *10,000* change. Medicine's strategy has been to focus on people who are known to be at high risk. Take people whose absolute risk is high enough and a 20–30 per cent reduction, even spread out over five years, begins to warrant the intrusion of a pill.

This strategy suits the tradition of medicine as the art of treating disease. Lives are saved, heart attacks and strokes avoided: human life made longer and happier, less coloured by fear and tragedy. The strategy works because the interventions add together. Each may offer a 20 or 30 per cent relative risk reduction but they are not mutually exclusive. The benefits from a stent opening up a narrowed coronary artery are of the same magnitude as the benefits from aspirin, a statin, a beta-blocker and an ACE inhibitor for blood pressure. Those benefits add up to at least the sum of their parts. (There is reason to hope that the benefits are more than additive but, because of the way trials are done, no grounds for knowing with certainty.)

For society, the benefits are huge. Keeping people healthy contributes to more than their personal welfare; medicine prolongs productive life more than it extends frail dependence. For society, the 6 per cent relative risk reduction of ezetimibe counts. There are so many heart attacks and strokes that it makes a difference.

The more of these individual interventions we have, the greater the lot of the fortunate and less fortunate will split. Medical care, even in an open-access free-at-the-point-of-delivery system like Britain's NHS, is unevenly spread. Doctors like working and living in nice areas. Richer patients are better at seeking help, understanding it and taking it. The greater the number of individual risk-related interventions we have, the more the medical care received by the wealthy will diverge from that received by the poor. In any system where health care is not free at point of delivery, and available to all, the gap will be wider.

Individualised treatment strategies increase inequalities. Polypills – the contraction into a single tablet of several agents – have long been touted as the answer. The landmark suggestion of them,[39] back in 2003, suggested a combination of a statin, aspirin and three blood pressure lowering agents, presenting evidence that if given to everyone over the age of fifty-five, such a pill would reduce strokes by 80 per cent and heart disease by even more. It would, calculated the authors, add an average of eleven healthy years of life to the span of those who took it. Since 2003 the number of drugs available has risen, as has the estimate of years it would add to average lives.

Polypills mean drugs are more effective as remembering to take them gets easier. They also imply a more scatter-gun approach to shooting at cardiovascular risk. Rather than picking people out, we treat everyone. As an approach, it fits far better with recognising that, in treating cardiovascular deterioration, we are not trying to fix particular diseases, we are trying to prevent age-related deterioration. As a bonus, inequality is reduced.

Polypills open the door for the inclusion of agents whose added benefits are too small to bother with individually. Ezetimibe makes little sense as a pill in a pot, intruding into our daily lives. As an added ingredient in a pill we take anyway, it's a different proposition. As the number of agents rises, polypills will become a necessary practicality even for the richest. As technology improves, individualised polypills will become routine and easy to constantly adjust and deliver. As we get better at treating risk within a five-year period, we will become more interested in preventing risk over the longer term, moving from a five-year view of treatments to a fifty-year and towards a hundred-year view. We will move steadily towards a strategy that really does aim to interfere with the development of athero-sclerosis and vascular ageing from its beginnings. Through ever-improving efforts to avoid heart attacks and strokes – to prevent premature death – we will grow ever more effective at prolonging life and prolonging healthy life. The course of human days will lengthen and it will brighten.

Assuming no global catastrophes, the process will be steadily cumulative. It consists of the medicalisation of life but all of life becomes medicalised the moment one takes prevention seriously, the moment one has the power to embrace health promotion. That does not make every intervention worthwhile, but it does mean the distinction between drugs and lifestyle is dubious. Regarding healthy lifestyles as fine and worthy but health-promoting drugs as the manifestation of evil corporate greed or overmedicalisation is a mistake. Judge interventions on their impact, not on how consonant their origins are with some moral ranking. Two hundred years ago chemists showed that sugar was the same molecule whether it was derived from cane or beetroot: what mattered was what it was, not what it came from. Nothing has an unmixed impact on human life. It's the balance that counts. We regard as insane the minority who reject vaccines as fraudulent conspiracies. When the drugs to alter our ageing process come like vaccines too, as single doses that alter a lifetime's risk, it will be the same minority that objects.

Today there is certainly room among the protestors for the sane. They can point out that our studies have not reliably looked at what interventions do over the very long term. Our research lasts a few years at best. That's a genuine defect in working out what a drug does to promote health over a lifetime, one that stems from unavoidable difficulties in doing the trials. It's not a defect in the argument that drugs which promote health over a lifetime are desirable. We can be very confident what the impacts are of our drugs over the very long term, and make fair guesses about what they would do if we took them before ageing had started to bite. We can be confident they would help, and even more dramatically than their combined impact already does.

GLUCOSE AS A MODIFIABLE RISK FACTOR

The Hindu physician Sushruta, six centuries before Christ, described the honeyed urine that ants crowded to drink. Seven hundred years later, Aretaeus of Cappadocia added a description of those producing it: their flesh and limbs, he wrote, melted into endless urine. 'The patients never stop making water, but the flow is incessant, as if from the opening of aqueducts. Life is short, disgusting and painful; thirst unquenchable.'[40] Diabetes as it was first conceived was an acute, fatal illness presenting with extreme symptoms. The notion that it could be chronic and half-hidden emerged slowly. Deaths from gangrene and pulmonary tuberculosis, wrote the Persian doctor and polymath Avicenna in the eleventh century, were often attributable to underlying diabetes: as with the ears of a hippo, the easily visible part was not so important as the hidden mass beneath.

Before the era of scientific medicine,* interventions for diabetes did not work. Rhubarb and other laxatives, antimony

---

* Not before science, which has always been a part of medicine, but before scientific tests were reliably applied to proposed treatments – before reliable trials.

and ulceration, emetics and diaphoretics were all used – drugs to make you vomit and sweat and defecate. Doctors and patients felt satisfaction in what did not work because it fulfilled the urgency to act. And because life is uncertain and outcomes were not measured in a way that could reliably distinguish the impact of interventions from the play of chance, uselessness went unnoticed. By the end of the nineteenth century, the preclinical sciences of biology and physiology and biochemistry had advanced beyond recognition but clinical medicine had barely changed. There were a wide range of treatments for diabetes and none of them helped. Nor were they all just placebos. Arsenic and uranium nitrate, like bloodletting, were not merely ineffective, they were killers.

Medicines subtract from people's lives whether they work or not. Osler's great textbook *The Principles and Practice of Medicine* specified one of the many diabetic diets inflicted with the best of intentions: '250 grammes oatmeal, the same amount of butter and the whites of six or eight eggs constitute the day's food. The oatmeal is cooked for two hours, and the butter and albumin stirred in. It may be taken in four portions during the day. Coffee, tea, or whisky and water may be taken with it.' He suggested the leftover egg yolks were used to make food for the diabetic's family. Many an oatmeal-hater, gazing up from their porridge and egg whites to their loved ones eating custard, must have felt grateful for the whisky.

With the discovery of insulin, those with type 1 diabetes were saved from the rapid death Aretaeus described but normality was not restored. As the years went by they still suffered. Blood sugar was controlled by insulin injections but control was imperfect. When blood sugar was above 11 mmol/litre the kidney could not retain the sugar, so the urine took on the sweetness ants loved and which doctors had named it for.

(Diabetes mellitus means honey-tasting urine. For centuries the symbol for a physician was a piss pot, and tasting the urine was part of the examination.) If the patient was fasting when the blood was taken – a step taken for the benefit of the test, not the patient – a blood sugar above 7 mmol/litre was shown to be enough to lead to damage to the nerves in the retina and eventually to blindness.

Those two figures, derived from an effort to understand the long-term hazards of imperfectly treated type 1 diabetes, became the foundation for definitions of type 2 diabetes. This was different. Rather than the body destroying the part of itself that produced insulin, in type 2 diabetes the body still produced insulin but became gradually resistant to it. Wealth and obesity were plainly involved. 'Diabetes was so rare among the ancients that many famous physicians did not mention it,' wrote Dr Thomas Willis in the seventeenth century, 'but in our age given over to good fellowship and guzzling down of unalloyed wine, we meet with examples enough, I may say daily, of this disease.'[41] Dr Willis was underestimating the appetite of ages past and overestimating the observational power of his profession: type 2 diabetes had been there all along, physicians had just not recognised it. That they began to do so was partly because of the general increases in health that left them less dazzled by a multiplicity of early disease and death.

Before Framingham, what we meant by type 2 diabetes was the condition in which someone pissed sugar and felt unwell. Framingham showed it was subtler, more insidious. Type 2 diabetes could cause the damage to nerves and eyes seen in those with treated type 1, but the main toll of type 2 diabetes turned out to be earlier death through advanced cardiovascular ageing, a toll that had simply never been apparent to observers before because the heart attacks and strokes were like any others;

they did not look different or as though they were caused by a distinct disease. And they weren't. Diabetes came to be seen now as partly a disease and partly just a risk factor. One might be symptom free and with levels of sugar low enough for one's kidneys to keep the urine bland but that didn't stop the heart attacks and strokes from looming. With the development of new drugs that lowered blood sugar, working alongside the body's own insulin, diabetes became a modifiable risk factor for cardiovascular health.

Increasing medicalisation resulted from growing understanding. In the wake of Framingham and other studies, appreciation of risk factors for early death and disease led to huge proportions of the healthy population being diagnosed as meriting medical interventions. A patient presenting with their sugar levels so deranged as to make them comatose plainly has a disease, but an asymptomatic individual discovered to have a raised blood sugar is harder to describe. There is no suffering – no pathos – unless it be conferred by the diagnosis or the intervention, so such people are not, strictly speaking, patients. Confusion is abetted by language: call everyone with a risk factor for disease a patient and medicine swells until it obliterates all notion of a healthy life, life itself being the essential risk factor for death.

The World Health Organization still sticks to the definitions of diabetes that first emerged: that it begins when fasting blood sugar reaches 7 mmol/litre or a random sample hits 11. That is despite a wealth of evidence showing that blood sugar levels gradually rise as we get older, and that as with cholesterol or blood pressure, the lower the better. With all three, an abnormally low level can certainly harm. We have never reached such a low level for cholesterol in any human being, but it must exist somewhere since cholesterol is essential for life. When blood pressure gets too low you faint. Ditto with blood sugar, if lowered by drugs.

Across the range of normal values found in people as they age, however, there seems no value at which lower values are not better.[42]

Conceived as treatments for a disease when people have no symptoms, interventions make little sense. Pictured as ways of prolonging healthy life, each of mild to moderate impact but all capable of being added together, and they feel different. More than 3 million people across the world die early each year because their blood sugar levels are higher than ideal.[43] The drugs will continue to improve. Implantable glucose monitors and drug delivery systems that function like an artificial pancreas are already in use and the difference they make will only get greater. But even with the technology we have now huge progress is possible.

The reason for declaring someone diabetic, and providing treatment, is not to maintain blood sugar within a normal range but to prolong health and prevent disease. We overdiagnose diabetes as a disease and underdiagnose it as a risk factor, just as we do with high blood pressure and high cholesterol.* But the notion of risk factors was based around the idea of diseases to be avoided on the way to unstoppable old age. When the diseases and the risk factors are the advancing shadows of age, and the interventions an effective way of slowing the going down of the sun, the language doesn't work.

Cardiovascular disease is the biggest burden on human health and as we get better at living longer its importance will only grow. How much we can reduce dementia by reducing vascular disease is uncertain but the answer is certainly 'some' – and the answer to how much we can reduce dementia by other means

---

* Hypertension and hyperlipidaemia, for those who prefer their medical terms in Greek.

is currently, and looks like remaining, 'none'. Where a blocked blood vessel has caused a heart attack or a stroke, a cocktail of cheap drugs cuts the risk of a second event by half over the following few years. The effectiveness of ever larger cocktails, over many more years and started before people have permanently lost a chunk of heart or brain, is unknown. But we know the outlines of it, the lineaments of the future of medicine. The absolute effectiveness per drug and per year will fall as we treat ever more people at ever lower absolute risk. The overall benefits will rise. How much they rise will depend only partly on the new technology of new drugs. It will depend also on the trials we do and how much we adjust our lives and our priorities to pursue the results they offer. Investigating the effects of interventions over decades is not easy but it is important. Our willingness to invest in trials, and in taking medicines when we have no symptoms and will see no benefits for years, will depend on being persuaded by what the trials show such strategies buy us.

A century ago medical textbooks were lists of diseases. Medicine was there to fix problems as they arose. Medical texts of today are similar – certainly more similar than they should be. How much of what medicine does now is about the prolongation of life and the promotion of health? More than ever before, but a better answer is hard to give since we have never had the question in mind sufficiently to collect the information to answer it. Which is evidence of the fact that as a profession we haven't caught up with ourselves.

Infectious diseases

To write about the medical future without including warnings of the horrors of emerging infections and antibiotic resistance would be to ignore tradition so strongly as to yield a letter of reproof not only from the Chief Medical Officer, but also from the Royal Society of Literature.

Could infections re-emerge as a global threat to developed nations, as opposed to a local threat to their development? Might antibiotic resistance make all that has been written about the conquering of infectious illness seem as dated as a papyrus announcing Egypt's triumph over Rome through the defection of Anthony?

New infections always emerge but it is likely their cost can be contained. The Ebola vaccine was no help at all to those in sub-Saharan Africa during 2013–15, but it would be next time, and it requires iron-shod pessimism not to be impressed by the speed with which the vaccine was developed. The same goes for Zika virus. Might seasonal flu merge with pandemic bird flu and cause another plague of the sort that in 1919 outkilled the First World War? Medical students are taught early on that any question beginning 'might', 'can' or 'is it ever possible' should always be answered with a yes. But that doesn't make the yes likely. Flu vaccines take the genetics of the previous outbreak as their model, so the current outbreak is always a step ahead – but that's also to say that the vaccines are never more than a step behind.

New diseases and antibiotic resistance are serious matters but neither is likely to result in the course of future life making a U-turn. At worst, there will be chicanes, at least for those of us in the developed world. New antibiotics are needed but as the old ones fall out of fashion so does resistance to them. A key issue is that the open market which has done so much to promote drug development has a perverse incentive. We want companies to develop new antibiotics and they want to develop them. Should they do so, however, they want to sell as much of their new drug as possible while society would rather it were kept in reserve so no resistance to it emerged. The most useful spur to developing new antibiotics may be a business model that rewards discovery without the need for sales.[44]

Malaria is more worrying. Malaria itself vanishes with wealth, and not because rich people can afford drugs but because a richer society eliminates the ability of the disease to exist. The swamps of southern England and Rome were drained centuries ago but the trend continues; in 2016 both Kyrgyzstan and Sri Lanka were freed of the disease.[45] Where wealth is more limited, drugs are essential. Vaccines work, but only partly, and the best drugs we have are being undermined by the disorganised, ineffective or corrupt ways they are used, particularly along the Thai–Cambodian border, an area whose chaotic social, economic and medical set-up has already given rise to antimalarial drug resistance that has killed millions.[46]

Antibiotic overuse is a problem, in medicine and agriculture. Its harms are real and need to be limited but the urge to say the sky is falling sometimes comes too easily. For all the threats, it is actually lifting and lightening. Leaving aside the hundreds of years of improvement in human health, particular examples of the eradication of infectious disease can be celebrated. They should be celebrated more. Smallpox is gone, save in the deepest recesses of military germ warfare institutes, and the military has quite enough means to kill us all without needing a virus. Polio has vanished from every country whose citizens don't shoot health-care workers (the list of shame reads Pakistan, Afghanistan, Nigeria and Laos, with a recent extra episode in the Congo). Guinea worm is on the way out. Guinea worm may not sound like a lot but its misery afflicted millions. The worms, living in the flesh of people's legs, needed to be twined out gently around a stick from the open sores in which they lived. The medical symbol of the sword and snake is at least in part a sexed-up version of that worm on a stick. How heartening, and what a reminder of the progress medicine never dreamt it would make, that the symbol will soon be redundant.

Exposure to an organism does not create disease; the situation is subtler and more mysterious. It is not clear at all why we sometimes fall ill and sometimes don't. *Neisseria* is a dramatic example: the bug that causes meningococcal septicaemia, a terrifying killer, lurks in many people's noses without causing a jot of harm. Why do some people get ill and not others when all are exposed to the same bug? The spread of a cold, even in a single household, follows no predictable pattern: the finer differences in autoimmune and infective illnesses are beyond our understanding. We are at the stage of being able to give an immune system a big whack with drugs, as though hitting a television to try and get it working, and we can show that doing so in certain circumstances does more good than harm. Drugs designed with increasing ease to hit particular targets, often parts of our immune system that we wish to provoke or subdue, mean our finesse has grown. But it remains orders of magnitude behind tangled reality. Even straightforward infections, understood in great detail at a molecular level, are not straightforward. Exposure to an infection does not lead in any predictable way to illness; doctors on wards fall ill less often than secretaries in offices.[47] This complexity in the setting of simple infections merits being remembered when we reach less straightforward parts of human life, understood poorly or not at all at a molecular level.

Transplantation

Since it was first recognised, AIDS has killed an average of a million people a year. Even if you know someone who made up part of that toll, perhaps especially if you do, you can recognise our imperfect triumph. From a standing start we had effective drugs within fifteen years and delivered them, even to the impoverished, to a degree that seemed initially impossible. Those who die from AIDS today rarely die through a lack of medical ability but as a result of the same socioeconomic problems killing millions more. It is not dismissive of our present flaws and past mistakes to feel that the future, even of emerging infections, is bright. Retroviruses were once barely understood at all; should another emerge, that would no longer be the case. While the number of completely novel diseases will never with certainty reach zero it will tend towards it. Our capacity to respond grows ever more potent.

Had HIV spread in the era before modern medicine, it would have spread more widely. It would also have seemed to become, eventually, a non-infectious disease. A certain mutation protects against it; those with the mutation, of a receptor on the surface of white blood cells, called CCR5, are protected. As HIV spread it would have snuffed out those without the mutation at a greater and greater rate. Soon only those with the mutation would have survived. The mutant variant of the gene would have become the standard. Within generations, the only people susceptible to HIV would be those with new mutations inactivating their inborn protection. At least, such people would develop HIV if it were still around, which it only would have been by then had it incorporated itself into our inherited DNA.

Something, recently, provided the selection pressure giving rise to high frequencies of the protective CCR5 mutation. It wasn't HIV. The mutation exists most in populations where HIV is rare and it got there well before HIV was around. Something over the past years meant that those with the mutation that protects against HIV did better than those without it. We have no idea what that something was. It is entirely possible that other diseases, over the millennia, have shifted from being infectious to being genetic traits.

Along with the less common HTLV – human T-cell lymphotropic virus – HIV is one of two retroviruses known to infect us. A virus, unlike a bacterium, has no capacity to reproduce; it relies on parasitising the cells of its host. A retrovirus gets its name from contravening what Francis Crick described as the central dogma of molecular biology – that information starts in genes and is transformed into proteins. Retroviruses work backwards. Retroviruses insert themselves into their host's genome. When they do that in the cells of egg and sperm, they become heritable.

A remarkable portion of our genetic code is the product of previous infestation. One part in twenty of our genome is viral in origin.[1] This figure, though, is almost certainly an underestimate. It describes the portions of our genome obviously once belonging to retroviruses and which have little or no function.

The figure does not include, because it cannot, portions of us that are retroviral in their origins but which have integrated and altered in such a way as to become a functional part of ourselves and less obviously the intrusion of a virus.

The relevance of mentioning this, in a chapter on transplantation, is that these implanted retroviruses can be found in all plants and animals. Particularly, and for reasons highly relevant to our future, they can be found in pigs.

FROM *CIVIS ROMANUS SUM* TO *CIVIS PORCUS SUM*

The Emperor Diocletian showed an enthusiasm for persecution before acquiring a taste for gardening.* Those martyred under him included the saints Cosmas and Damian, who, in the third century and somewhere near the Aegean, had cut off a man's cancerous leg. Their sainthood resulted from their next step. Unwilling to leave the man a unidexter, and having a recently deceased body to hand, they not only removed the diseased leg but transplanted a new one to replace it. Churches were named in their honour and paintings showed their work. The pictorial appeal was enhanced by the donor being black and the recipient white.† The enthusiasm to depict the miracle hustled away thoughtfulness, to the extent that many portraits show the corpse having its left leg removed to become the grateful patient's right.[2]

---

* In retirement Diocletian was asked to resume the title of Emperor. The allure of the throne was nothing, he said when he refused, compared with being able to grow his own cabbages.

† Any impression of racism should be rejected. The black man had died naturally and it would have been more in keeping with notions of racial purity had the donor also been white.

Transplantation, in other words, has long been half-fanciful. 'Often,' wrote H. L. Mencken in 1925,

> when the newspapers report a child badly burned by accident, with a great loss of skin, they add a tale of heroism about the victim's family and friends, with the names of playmates who have offered to sacrifice skin for the sufferer, estimates of the number of square inches needed, and other harrowing details. On recovery, the whole thing ceases to be news, and we hear no more of it. Unfortunately, such thrilling tales of self-sacrifice are almost invariably untrue.[3]

Mencken was highlighting the fact that journalists in pursuit of a good story were too credulous to be properly sceptical. Doctors were the same. They wanted to help and they wanted to be successful and powerful. That put them in a bad position for scrupulously doubting whether a wound had healed despite their care rather than because of it.

Epistemological advances helped replace confidence with humility, and intuition with testing. Medicine took several thousand years to learn the sceptical technique needed to reliably differentiate hope from reality. Unlike journalism, science has improved since 1925. But then science is based on the notion of progressive improvements, something less certain in other fields of human effort. Not that medicine is incapable of going backwards: when the Italian surgeon Tagliacozzi died in 1599 his technique for rebuilding a person's nose using a flap of their own skin was lost for two centuries. The cost was not only scientific. It meant those disfigured by trauma and disease were left without hope or help. The twentieth century started with years of exciting progress in immunology and transplantation but much of that was subsequently lost and forgotten too, swept away in the wake of the First World War. Ideas died, meaning that people died too.

The development of transplantation was held back by unwarranted deference towards lab bench reductionism and a failure to appreciate the importance of practical experimentation. It was not felt possible to move ahead with transplantation until fundamental problems in immunology – the means by which the body could tell 'self' from 'non-self' and the techniques for altering this – had been determined.

'A problem shown to be soluble is a problem halfway solved', wrote Peter Medawar, adding that 'I am reputed to be – and am often introduced before lectures as – the chap whose work made modern organ transplantation possible.' Medawar was well aware of the impossibility of skin transplants; the body quickly recognised and rejected another person's skin. At a conference Medawar met a researcher whose interest was in studying whether certain traits in cows were most influenced by environment or heredity, an effort undermined by the difficulty in accurately determining whether similar-looking calves were identical or non-identical twins. It was a difficulty easily solved, Medawar told him: perform a small skin transplant. If it takes, the two cows are genetically identical; if it doesn't, they aren't. Medawar was so sure of himself and so expansive ('my mind doubtless unhinged by liquor or by the kind of mateyness that tends to prevail at international conferences') that he offered to do the grafting himself. Unexpectedly, all the grafts took.

The explanation, it turned out, was that non-identical calves share a single placenta. In utero they are exposed to each other's blood. This led to their immune systems learning to recognise their twin as being 'self'. It was for exploration of this mechanism for telling 'self' from 'non-self' that Medawar was awarded a Nobel Prize, sharing it with Macfarlane Burnet, who coined the terminology. 'Immunological recognition of self' was the title of Burnet's prize lecture.[4] The practical impact on the ability to transplant organs from one human to another was, however, nil. 'These early experiments did not lead directly to the successes of modern organ transplantation', Medawar explained. 'Their effect was *moral* only – was only to inspirit the surgeons.' Human transplantation emerged through advances in surgical technique and tissue typing and through the development of drugs damping the immune response that rejected foreign cells. And it emerged through innovative, and often deluded, surgical experiments.

There were understandable qualms about animal experiments, especially when the animals were humans. Many who escaped these qualms did so via the traditional route of surgical arrogance. That had a habit of being attractive to precisely the sort of people who were poor at recognising the real impacts of their interventions. Yet it is not always possible – even in retrospect – to determine which surgical experiments were reasonable to undertake. What good (besides to a surgeon's career) could ever have come of attempts in 1906 to implant people with pig and goat kidneys? We know now the attempts could have led to neither success nor useful knowledge – but could we have known that then? The answer remains a likely 'yes' but needs to be cautiously made. The human-to-human kidney transplants of the 1950s were widely seen as just as pointless, futile and cruel. A contemporary opinion damned them, outraged that a 'pitiable young woman [the recipient] became the needless victim of a needless experiment... which ended in a grave, sacrificed on the altar of the surgeon's ambitions. When will our colleagues give up this game of experimenting on human beings?'[5] They never did, at least in America, and we owe them our success. When early efforts at heart transplantation ran into trouble, Britain embraced a self-imposed moratorium – sensible, given the likely outcomes of early operations, but cowardly and disingenuous since we avoided doing experimental human surgery while waiting for others to do so instead.

Transplantation was studied by many for insights into treating cancer. The two situations shared the essential similarity of needing to understand how the body did or did not keep control of what cells grew within it. Bone marrow transplants, developed in the hope of stopping the rejection of transplanted kidneys and hearts, were incidentally found to treat cancers of the blood. Newly developed anticancer drugs were found to depress the immune system and allow transplantation. Mustard gas developed to kill was found to be a useful therapeutic immunosuppressant, and immunosuppression was observed to lead to the growth of tumours. That latter discovery remains a hazard for those taking immunosuppression and a boon for those studying how tumours arise and escape the body's normal mechanisms of control. The 2018 Nobel Prize for medicine went to two men who showed how stimulating the immune system could help treat cancer.[6]

The twin problems of too little and too much immunosuppression remain key issues when it comes to human transplantation. Alongside them are the difficulties involved in performing a transplant: difficulties more imposing for patients than surgeons. These are big operations with significant risks for even those who are healthy, which many of those needing a transplant are not.

Today we can, and frequently do, transplant kidneys, hearts and livers, portions of gut and pancreas. We transplant bone marrow, bones, skin, the lenses of eyes, lungs: all of these can be moved from one person to another, with a range of successes and a range of benefits and a range of years over which they are likely to last.

More recently, and on a much smaller scale, we have transplanted other parts of the body. Over thirty face transplants have been done, with varying physical and psychiatric results.[7] Hand transplantation has been going on in adults since 1998 and a child recently had both hands successfully replaced.[8] Having someone else's hands or face has long appealed to sensationalist imagination but clinical science has covered ground untrodden by fiction. A uterus transplant enabled a woman born without one to have a child.[9] Another woman received a transplanted trachea: the need for lifelong immunosuppression was avoided by first implanting it in her forearm and wrapping it in her own tissue, which used the foreign material as a scaffold and overgrew it.[10]

Fiction writers did anticipate what happened next. Although there was only a 'slight colour discrepancy', much less than with Cosmos and Damian, surgeons successfully transplanted a penis. The value of the procedure to the young man involved, who lost his own to gangrene after a ritual circumcision, was everything one might have expected. The intoxication of success even found its way into *The Lancet* report of the procedure. 'The recipient reported satisfactory penetrative sexual intercourse at 5 weeks after the operation', the authors noted, 'despite our advice to abstain for at least 3 months.'[11] Think of him as one who loved not wisely but too well.

For a part of oneself to have been transplanted in, to be alien in origin, intrigued the thoughts of fiction writers for good reason. 'The dual psychological impacts on a young man of first losing his penis and then having it replaced, were of concern to us', said *The Lancet* article:

The self-image, which normally has a fairly solid state, becomes fluid again when adding or removing an organ during transplantation. The loss or gain of an organ can have a devastating effect on the ego; it is described as causing a ripple effect on self-image and might induce psychosis, depression, or even renunciation of the transplanted organ. The addition of something as benign as a cardiac pacemaker can induce serious psychological disturbances.

A cardiac pacemaker, thin as a modern phone and a third the size, has never belonged to anyone else before being slipped beneath the skin below the collar bone. It is invisible except in outline but the outline is easily palpable. Some people find the intrusion of a pacemaker too much, and break it from being unable to stop fiddling with it. Not many, but enough to remind us that sense of self is not only a matter of immunology.

Psychological impact, surgical risks and the harms of immunosuppression are limits on the power of transplantation, but the greater limits are the lack of organs. Pleading with everyone to be more reasonable and more generous has been tried; it is worth continuing with, but not worth hoping it will suddenly have an effect it has never before possessed. In the meantime people die not because we lack the ability to transplant organs but because we lack a sufficient supply of them. Two innovations might help. We might build the organs ourselves or we might take them from pigs.

Autologous transplantation

Autologous transplantation is to put something back into the person from whom it arose. A skin graft, taken from a healthy area that will regrow and placed to aid healing in a more damaged site, is autologous transplantation. It dates back centuries. Techniques to reconstruct noses, involving sewing a person's arm to their face so skin can spread while being initially nourished from its blood supply on the arm, are ancient. Noses were damaged in fights, by ritual punishment and by syphilis. Their damage was obvious, hence the desire to fix them. The sixteenth-century astronomer Tycho Brahe lost half his nose in a duel. To cover the deformity he famously spent the rest of his life wearing a brass replacement. Bioprosthetics is a term suggesting brain-enhancing implants of powerful technology, but it also includes false teeth, eyelash extensions, nail polish and brass noses.

Autologous transplantations run from the life-saving to the dishonest and possibly pointless. For the latter, consider the use of autologous transplantation of blood by Tour de France cyclists. A way of increasing blood volume, cyclists donate and store blood, allow their bodies to recover, then add their own blood back: being one's own, the transfusion is harder for authorities to detect. The cheat is based on the notion that the body functions better with more blood than it thinks is optimum, a notion dubious in its logic and flatly contradicted by trial evidence.[12] A boxer withdrawing a pint of their blood to make a weigh-in, before transfusing it back straight after, is being just as dishonest but probably more effective. A patient undergoing extensive surgery, whose blood is collected and reinfused as it is lost, combines effectiveness with honesty. Autologous bone grafting has a decent history, and although it is now being left behind, as new techniques allow the grafting in of foreign material or of stimulants to bone regrowth, it remains useful, particularly in dentistry.

The greatest benefit from autologous transplantation has

come in the treatment of cancers of blood and bone marrow. After removal of some of the stem cells within it, a person's blood-forming marrow is destroyed by drugs and radiation. The aim is to destroy the cancerous cells and the cost is that non-cancerous ones die too. That would be fatal except for the hope of rejuvenating the body's abilities by autologous transplantation of the stored, healthy stem cells. Such bone marrow transplants avoid the risk of immunological warfare between host tissues and those from a genetically different donor.

Autologous transplantation could ideally include transplanting new organs grown whole from starter dishes of one's own cells. Within the nucleus of a cell lie the chromosomes, the tightly wrapped parcels of genetic information. Just as male breasts contain all the material needed to be female, each cell contains all it needs to be any other. Our increasing ability to reprogramme cells means those which were once permanently differentiated can once more regain the power of a fertilised egg. Growing a heart, disappointingly, remains impossible.

Growth of a solid organ requires more than the instructions specifying its design. Cells need the right environment. For a growing heart, that environment is the rest of the developing fetus. The bath of hormones, the impetus of nerves and above all the push and flow of blood are all essential. Growing a new heart is straightforward, but only if you are willing to grow a creature around it at the same time.

Structurally, a liver is simpler than a heart and lacks such a need for developing in response to so many of the strains and stresses provided by a living organism. To grow replacement livers from stem cells is not close at hand but in the next decades it might become so. Most solid organs require more or less the environment of a fully living body in order to grow properly. Guts tend towards the 'more' camp. Watching a baby gently vomit its milk is an immediate reminder that guts have to learn how to work. It may be that a gut grown in a dish could learn later; we don't know. The pancreas is different. The hormonal and immunological glands of the pancreas, thymus and thyroid – in culinary terms, the sweetbreads – may be more amenable to growth in a lab, although the need for them is less. These organs have adult functions that can be replaced to a large extent by technology and drugs.

Other parts of our bodies lend themselves better to the prospect of being grown for us. Cartilage has been made in labs and put back into cartilage-deprived knees since the 1980s,[13] although the fact that it can be done does not mean it always helps. Autologous cartilage from noses, ears and ribs has long been harvested for use elsewhere. Recently, the flexibility of cartilage has expanded as we have learnt to seed it onto artificial scaffolds.[14] Tissue-engineered skin, blood vessels, urethrae and vaginal and bladder walls have all been made and used. The innovations are perhaps more technically impressive than they appear – what is being grown and shaped and transplanted here are not homogenous mats but multicellular organised parts of the body.[15] As we progress, problems with growing hearts may cease to seem so insoluble.

Most arresting among recent examples of autologous transplantation was the construction and use of an artificial trachea. The aim was to make the inoperable operable, to enable surgeons to remove tumours that could not otherwise be touched without leaving people lacking the means to breathe. In 2008 a team took a trachea from a dead donor, stripped it of cells and seeded it inside and out with cells from the patient who subsequently received it.[16] In 2011 they went one better, constructing a 'tailor-made bioartificial scaffold' inseminated with a patient's stem cells. Five months after implantation the patient was tumour-free and the transplant showed 'stem-cell homing and cell-mediated wound repair, extracellular matrix remodelling, and neovascularisation of the graft'. It had successfully integrated.[17] The only hitch was that things may not have been quite as good as they seemed; the excellent results seemed possibly to owe something not only to skill in the doing, but also to fraud in the telling of it. Investigations, resignations and journal retractions have followed.[18] If there was fraud it was persuasive because it took place at the edge of what was becoming possible.

A better way of creating a new supply of organs, more achievable and potentially very much cheaper, is not to build them ourselves but to let others build them for us. It is straightforward to grow a heart as long as you are willing to grow the creature it belongs to. It is therefore simple to manufacture hearts if you are willing to breed and to kill. As billions of bacon lovers know, we are.

XENOTRANSPLANTATION

When my medical world consisted of books, journals, talks and cadavers, in a studentship where college cloisters hid a professor beneath every carved stone gargoyle, a brilliant surgeon gave a memorable lecture. The surgeon had a reputation for unfeeling arrogance. The children he was talking about had been born with major abnormalities of their heart, abnormalities that could sometimes be corrected or partially corrected. The worst thing you could do to such a child at three or four years old, he told us, was to submit them to a major heart operation that did nothing other than extending their distress and ill health before they died miserably at seven or eight. It was an insightful and compassionate comment and I felt a surge of outrage that this surgeon had been maligned. 'By the time they're seven or eight,' he continued, 'you might have grown attached to them. At three or four, it doesn't matter. You just have another.' The reputation, I realised, had something to it. Years later, when I met him in the hospital, he told me that while he was the best heart surgeon in Europe, it was wrong of people to say that he was the best in the world. Of course that might well be true, he explained, but it was important to be humble.

Cause and effect are often difficult to tease apart. There are certain characteristics associated with certain professions. Within them, too. Just as classical musicians joke about the characters of viola players, and all musicians joke about timpanists, so medical specialties offer character traits that harden into archetype. The surgeon told us how many small children died each year as he operated on them, as his hands were inside them. It wasn't clear to me then, and still isn't now, whether he became a good surgeon because he was unable to see these kids as human beings, or if he stopped seeing them as fully human in order to become a better surgeon.*

Efforts to move parts of one animal into another have been made for centuries, usually so poorly that even those who did them were unable to accurately judge what happened. In the 1700s Jean-Baptiste Denys transfused people with blood from sheep and calves until it led to him being tried for murder, after which he beat a retreat from medical practice. Under the

---

* Another surgeon, a friend, told how his junior had suggested he didn't give a damn about any of his patients, he merely wanted to perform the best and most appropriate surgery on them that he could. 'She's only been working with me for a few weeks,' he exclaimed proudly, 'and she's realised already.' A man whose self-esteem relies on them doing a good job can be reliably excellent.

guidance and supervision of surgeons whose insight was as bad as their observation of external reality, and in whom those related failures were explained by their arrogance, the nineteenth century saw patients receiving skin grafts from rats, pigeons, chickens, rabbits, dogs, cats and even frogs. Early nose reconstructions might have involved sewing a patient's arm to their nose but these obtuse experimentalists went further: some early recipients of skin grafts tolerated being laid in bed with a live sheep stitched to them. None of the grafts worked but few noticed. In the sea of normal human variation, where many things got better despite bad treatment and many failed despite good, no one grew wiser. Early in the twentieth century patients received implants from the testicles of chimps and baboons and felt the benefits. Had they received the ovaries of sea urchins or small bits of Lego it would have been all the better for the chimps and baboons and no worse for the people. Several hundred procedures were performed with many men reporting astonishing degrees of rejuvenation. The moral is not that they were fools but that true effects are hard to determine and traits of personality easily misunderstood when taken to be simple properties of biology. The notion that a man's 'zest for life', his mix of libido and general gusto, can be reduced to the level of a hormone and adjusted like a volume dial has a treacherous appeal.

The cornea can cloud over, blocking vision. Corneal xenotransplantation has been performed since 1838. Over the course of the nineteenth and twentieth centuries people received implants from pigs, sheep, rabbits, fish, a 'barn fowl', cows and a gibbon. One of the rabbit xenotransplants, in 1888, is reputed to have been partially successful.[19] The reported failure of the other attempts suggests a seriousness of observational power from the surgeons involved. The nineteenth-century success with the rabbit may not entirely have been due to optimistic mis-interpretation. The cornea is unusually isolated from immune rejection. For that reason, we are more confident than ever that corneal transplants from other animals really will soon work.[20]

Interest in xenotransplantation was dampened almost entirely by the emerging understanding, in the middle of the twen-tieth century, of tissue rejection. During the 1960s chimpanzee kidneys were repeatedly transplanted into humans with dismal results. Attempts made with baboon kidneys fared even worse. Chimps seemed attractive sources for organs, but limited availa-bility and doubts about the ethics of using them stopped serious investigation.

The ethical justification for continued attempts was that temporary successes were sometimes enough. 'One of the indications for the use of the heterotopic cardiac transplant is temporarily to support a failing heart in the anticipation of its recovery when all other measures of support have been unsuccessful',[21] wrote Christian Barnard and colleagues in the 1970s, reporting on their experience of xenotransplantation as a bridge to recovery. Heterotopic was the term of the day for 'xeno' and the baboon and chimp hearts they placed lasted four days. Further attempts should only be made, they reasonably concluded, when a very short-term success could lead to long-term benefits – when there was imminent hope of a failed organ spontaneously recovering or a human donor soon becoming available.[22]

Alexis Carrel, winner of the Nobel Prize for innovations in reattaching blood vessels when moving organs around, expressed the view in 1907 that 'the ideal method would be to transplant in man organs of animals easy to secure and operate on, such as hogs, for instance'.[23] Pigs are cheap and plentiful. Physically, they are the right size. Unlike chimps they grow quickly. The ethical questions about harvesting organs from another species are minimal when it is one we already raise and kill for chops, especially given that pigs kept for organ donation will be looked after more carefully than their edible brethren. The notion that unstressed animals produce better meat has always seemed strange – what if it turns out not to be true? – but is plainly true for surgeons looking to harvest organs. Anaesthetics and the absence of fear and pain have physiological benefits.

Two practical barriers prevent the use of pigs for xenotransplants. Pigs, like humans, contain retroviruses. They have lots. What might pig retroviruses do in a human body? What is harmless for a pig might not be so in a person. The risks seem small – pig organs might not transmit infection and even if they did the infections might do no harm – but we don't know. For pig organs to be given to a handful of people, who would die without receiving them, such risk might be acceptable. If pig organs are going to become an industry, allowing us to transplant earlier and more often than we have previously dreamt of, we will need to be more confident.

Second, pig tissue is rapidly rejected. Our bodies register it promptly not merely as foreign but as very foreign, as not kosher. It may never be possible to develop immunosuppressive treatments capable of preventing such rejection without leaving us fatally vulnerable to our fecundly unsterile world. The goal instead has become to genetically change the pigs. That might allow us both to delete the pig's retroviruses, something we're making excellent progress towards,[24] and to make the pig's cells more human. The immunosuppression required could be steadily diminished as we got better at doing that. To make pigs as human as a normal donor would only be the starting point – we might hope to make them so closely match their recipient as to make all immunosuppression unnecessary.

Portions of pig pancreas – the portions producing insulin and thus treating type 1 diabetes – have been transplanted into non-human primates and survived for almost a year. Kidneys have lasted for seven months, hearts for two and a liver for one. Lungs have lasted a week.[25] The problems of rejection, of infection, even of the way organs might grow differently once within a host from a different species, are all hurdles we cannot currently jump: but they look jumpable.

If organs are made to match so well that immunosuppression is barely needed, or not needed at all, the number of people who might benefit from transplants would increase massively. Massively, and enough to transform human life expectancy, but with limitations all the same. Transplants are big operations and elderly bodies do not cope with big operations well. For those in whom one organ has failed early, transplants can be wonderful. Less so for those in whom the frailty of age means everything is in decline.

CRISPR, our current technology for gene editing, was developed in 2012. Although precise compared with what came before,[26] it is imprecise compared with what is needed. It has off-target effects. Genes can get inserted or altered in the wrong place, with unpredictable results. We are held back by the technical difficulty of gene editing but the difficulties seem surmountable. Xenotransplantation appears to lie in the realm of the imminently achievable.

Transportation

The best part of a hundred years ago, car-makers proposed digging up the roads and laying tracks. Put cars on tracks, the theory went – and the theory was sound – and you could automate them. Jams would be gone, crashes a distant memory; the world would be swift and safe. The idea would have worked, too, had it not involved that detail of digging up all the world's roads and replacing them, accompanied by the other small detail of junking all the world's cars and replacing those too.

We age, we weaken and we fail to cough: saliva and food go down the wrong way and we get pneumonia. Weak to begin with, pneumonia carries us off. But it needn't be that way. There is no reason why the nose and the mouth need join up as they do, no reason why the tubes and orifices we use for breathing should be, for a few short but error-provoking inches, the ones we eat and drink with. Our salivary glands produce a litre or more a day and the saliva drips down a tube that leads not only to our stomach, but also to our lungs. The best evidence for evolution is found not in its perfections but in its cobbling-togethers, its compromises and failures. Creationism fails to explain bodges. The reason our lungs and our stomachs share their treacherous union is that way back in time, when we filtered water for food and filtered it for oxygen too, the design made sense. It made sense when it started and, ever since, it's been stuck. Nature makes no giant leaps. The luck of new mutations can no more discard hundreds of millions of years of fundamental design than the world could have contemplated tearing up its roads and starting again.

Road traffic accidents kill as many people each year as HIV or tuberculosis. Globally, when you die, there's a one in fifty chance it'll be a car that kills you. Between the ages of fifteen and twenty-nine, it's the most likely reason. The pandemic of diabetes has a toll similar to road injuries.[1] Of the sum total of human wealth, 3 per cent is obliterated by the costs of road traffic accidents.[2] Increasingly autonomous cars rarely feature in medical journals, even when they devote page after page to calculations of how to reduce premature death. Something about it doesn't grip.

Really, they should. Before the end of our lives, road safety will be unrecognisable. Estimates range from a massive reduction in deaths and accidents by 2040 to it becoming impossible, by then, to kill someone with a car even if you deliberately try. Seatbelts, impact protection, the design of bonnets and bumpers, daytime running lights and high-level central brake lights all help. Evolution, which cannot anticipate, will never reach a better design unless every intermediate step is better too. Re-engineering our infrastructure can be done with forethought, but inertia can be too great a cost to overcome. Mutations cannot ease away the union of our breathing and feeding tubes because it is too embedded in our design, just as roads are too embedded in the infrastructure of our daily lives to rip them up wholesale in one go.

Autonomy in cars helps because it requires no giant leap. Parking sensors, cruise control and electronics monitoring tyre pressures and engine performance are all useful in themselves. So are collision-sensing and avoidance systems. Vehicles that can help in some situations begin to be able to handle themselves temporarily in others. Autonomy, like salvation, comes by increments.

Deaths on the road get little medical attention. Each one is an accident – it happens because someone screws up. Accidents are easy to tolerate, oddly, when they are so common as to feel normal. Some cars take diesel and some petrol, and some people who drive cars forget which. The accidents could be avoided if people were not occasionally dumb, which is to say that the accidents can't be avoided at all – except that they all could, if pumps and tanks were redesigned so that petrol tanks and diesel nozzles couldn't connect. If that was a change that could be made through gradual steps it would already have happened.

By 2030 the World Health Organization estimates that annual road traffic deaths will reach 2.5 million, exceeding those of malaria and tuberculosis combined.[3] The actual figure is likely to be hugely lower but then the World Health Organization overlooks autonomous vehicles entirely. That's a remarkable omission, but it's one shared by the medical community in general. Doctors feel removed from automotive engineering in a way they do not from vaccine development. That matters. Complacency about the direction of travel should not equate to indifference about the time of arrival. Our love of breakthroughs leaves us vulnerable to 'disenchantment around marginal gains'[4] and it is those that make history. When it comes to accepting and welcoming and encouraging the risks of harm from autonomous cars, risks no less real for being so much smaller than those of human drivers, regulations and public interest are essential.

Marginal gains add up to more than marginal change. Autonomy in cars will increase over the coming years until it reaches a tipping point where cars do not merely help us drive but drive for us. That's a problem if being a driver is your living. Fully autonomous cars will change the way we live and commute and plan our landscapes and our homes. And if a car will be there on demand, it's not clear that you'll need to own one.

All of this is not merely a First-World solution, any more than road traffic deaths are only a First-World problem. Developed countries have a near-monopoly on the design and manufacture of cars and even when they do not their regulations sway how it gets done. Increasingly, autonomous cars will be everywhere. They won't get everywhere equally quickly but they'll get there all the same, and they'll be designed so that even if some of their systems fail, the others will still work. Socioeconomic development will remain the best cure for socioeconomic ills but the price of preventing a road death can be small, from $7 when installing a speed bump in Africa to $135 for a fence in Bangladesh[5] while the total cost of accidents can reach 10 per cent of a developing nation's gross domestic product.[6] But should Africa install no speed bumps and Bangladesh no fences, some of the road safety being acquired by richer nations will still trickle down.

Other aspects of vehicle development affect public health. The shift to electric reduces pollution. To say that in the near future the air we breathe will be more than ever the stuff of life is to speak literally. Adolescent boys will be less likely to kill themselves while learning how to become men. Mobility and social isolation will alter. A great proportion of the ageing population, for whom driving is difficult or unsafe, will regain their freedom. Social isolation has more than social costs, and isolation – in those too young or old to drive, in those for whom car ownership is prohibitive but rental per ride affordable – will be reduced. This brave new world shall be, as Humphrey Bogart said, the stuff that dreams are made of.

Sex

Most chapters in this book deal with subjects that are the domain of professionals. Sex is best left to amateurs, a statement not so easy to make about the treatment of cardiovascular risk.

It's a relief to find how little medicine has to say about human sexuality. This chapter *should* describe patterns in human sexual behaviour and consider variations and patterns of it geographically and historically. That information, happily, is not available. For all that Kinsey and others have taken snapshots, there exists no epidemiology of sexuality, no reliable chart of prevalence and incidence. From pregnancy and disease and other sources we can make inferences but there is not much to them. Sexual activity, for example, plainly starts for many at below the age when the law says it should. Rates of coital frequency can be estimated,[1] which should provide fun material for journalism but can only be a distraction when it comes to matters we really wish to think about. 'My marriage was like the marriage of other people', wrote Trollope in his autobiography, 'and of no special interest to any one except my wife and me.'[2]

The interest we find in our own sexual lives is not easily augmented by peering into those of others. Prying has a habit of seeing everything through the distorting lenses of prurience; adolescents telling each other about their early sexual experiences are unlikely to be telling the truth, and even when they try their efforts will most likely be distorted by having an audience. Being grown up does not involve discovering what everyone else is up to so much as accepting that it's none of your business. Voyeurism is not an aid to happiness or good sense.

There is precious little to report of genuine value about the sex lives of our fellows – at least not directly. There is a reason why art works by hints, and pornography is not art. When Justice Potter Stewart of the US Supreme Court famously defined pornography – 'I know it when I see it' – he left open the suggestion that here, too, the eye of the beholder mattered. The converse of prying being bad is that intimacy depends on privacy. The lack of information about human sexual activity, in contrast to the wealth of data we have about other aspects of people's lives, is heartening.

APHRODISIACS

The name links them to Aphrodite, Greek goddess of love, but aphrodisiacs pre-date her and pre-date the Sumerian goddess Inanna on whom she was modelled. Gauging the future of aphrodisiacs in human lives involves taking the measure of our past relations with them.

In the oldest existing medical text, erectile dysfunction is fought with henbane, animal brains, beans, dirt, sawdust of pine and willow and juniper and sycamore, acacia juice, flaxseed, onion, oil, goose fat, pig's dung, myrrh, salt and ox fat. Bandaged together to the wilting penis they brought it new life.

If an ancient physician declared a problem treatable, yet

failed to treat it, there were consequences. The Sumerian legal code of Hammurabi stated such doctors might not get paid. In some circumstances injury was added to insult and the injury took the form of them having their hands cut off.[3] This had the power of concentrating the medical mind wonderfully. Where there was little or no chance of success, the correct action was to declare that a problem was not treatable and to refuse to try. The ancient wisdom and natural ingredients the Ebers papyrus lists must have worked. If they hadn't, the prescription – and perhaps the physician – would not have survived.

For those unable to afford the mix of ingredients listed in the papyrus, and the physician to bandage them onto the disappointing penis, another treatment was available. It was simpler but, as the Greeks warned, it could cause so powerful an aphrodisiacal frenzy that it needed to be used with care.[4] The aphrodisiac in question was lettuce.[5] Romaine, in fact, which for those unfamiliar with their salad varieties is not a round lettuce but a proud upright one. To Egyptian eyes it looked phallic. That, and the fact it oozed an opaque milky-white sap when cut, formed the mental link.

Those who could afford it went for the mixed ingredients of the penis poultice. If the contents of that should by any chance not seem varied enough, the history of aphrodisiacs contains more, many more. Many are exotic while others, like lettuce, have lost the exoticism they once possessed. Soon after its introduction to Europe, it was widely understood that an ageing libido could be restored by a rare and special tuber from unimaginably distant shores. Hence the greedy invocation of Falstaff, the old goat, to 'let the sky rain potatoes'.[6]

Only one explanation accounts for so many different agents working, and then, as cultures change, ceasing to work and being replaced. Of all the vast array of aphrodisiacs with which people have draped, dosed and sprayed themselves, none has the slightest actual effect.[7] None work, that is, in the manner in which people have believed them to, through some pharmacological effect. There's an opportunity missed every time one shucks an oyster in the belief it contains some special chemical, not least when a seduction might fail if the target of one's lust prefers parmesan to molluscs. The message is more than that we fool ourselves when it comes to sex, or that the flux of human variation makes it impossible to spot a placebo from an effective drug without structured experiments. The message is that we are strongly attracted to false biological explanations for traits of character and culture.

The insertion of slices of chimp testicle into older men, to restore their libido, 'can be looked upon as the Viagra of the 1920s'[8] said one historical review – a useful comparison to bear in mind when we jump forward and consider the Viagra of the modern era... Viagra. The little blue pill is not a lot to look at but its cultural impact has been huge. When we consider its actual pharmacological effects, could there be less than meets the eye? Developed in the hope of dilating blood vessels, and thus being an effective treatment for high blood pressure and the angina caused by narrowed coronary arteries, Viagra went through the normal process of investigation for a promising drug. Early on it was given to a small number of healthy volunteers, an experiment designed not to test its effectiveness but to ensure its safety and check for unexpected side effects.

A number of these healthy young men, the experiment revealed, did indeed experience some side effects. The drug gave a minority of them an erection.[9] That led to a different kind of excitement for drug company Pfizer, in the form of sales of billions, and prompted the manufacture of similar agents that work via the same molecular route but stay in the blood for longer, meaning sexual spontaneity could be unplanned. It also helped reinforce our powerful belief in the idea of performance-enhancing drugs. Recreational use of Viagra and similar drugs is common. It is hard to know how common, since it is illicit, but a Brazilian study found that 9 per cent of healthy young Brazilian men had used them[10] and in Argentina the figure was 22 per cent.[11]

When given to healthy young men, Viagra makes erections easier to obtain, firmer and longer lasting. It confers more intense orgasms and reduces the refractory time following them, accelerating recovery. Super stuff and not necessarily a trivial boon to human life. But placebos, in the same trial, did all those things too.*[12] Viagra can have an effect on physical problems but its effect on psychology is greater, both when there is no problem to begin with and also when there is. 'It achieves success rates of up to 80 per cent in patients with organically caused dysfunction, and more in patients with predominantly psychologically caused disturbances.'[13] Striking that the drug should be even more effective when used in those with no physical problems. Why should this be? And why should it be that Viagra's erection-causing effects in healthy men were picked up accidentally in a study that wasn't looking for them, but are absent in other studies set up precisely to investigate them? Could it be that Viagra's effectiveness is a mirage, and that its biochemical power is no more than is to be expected of someone swallowing a salad – dressed with sufficient expectation of effect – of lettuce and potato?

---

* The trial did show one difference, namely that the period of physiologically enforced flaccidity after an erection was reduced more by the drug than the placebo. It is not clear if this effect, which was marginal, was real or just the upshot of looking for lots of different things in a sea of normal variation. Roll the dice enough times and you get double sixes.

The widespread use of Viagra by healthy young men is certainly testament to the preoccupations of young men and the power of placebos. Pharmacological aphrodisiacs, including Viagra for those in good sexual health, do not generally work.[14] That is, drugs to enhance and improve upon normal human sexual function are figments of our imagination. Drugs can certainly alter human sexual function, and improve it in some ways at the expense of others, but none acts to simply improve it and none ever will, since our sexuality is not itself the simple product of any single biochemical pathway, and that's all a drug can change. Those drugs whose aphrodisiac impact is real work in the same way as all the other effective aphrodisiacs, from longing to love: they work on the mind. Alcohol is the most common. 'Studies examining the effect of alcohol on female sexual function are very limited with inconclusive results'[15] is a statement that finishes well but starts badly. To suggest few such studies have been done is to ignore a vast body of informal work on the subject. Mind-altering drugs like gin modulate our experiences in the same way as love, empathy, imagination and food, drink, clothes and music. The idea that drugs are out there, in our pharmacies or in our futures, to turn us into sexual superheroes, is not a new one nor one that will ever get old. In the future we will continue to believe in such things and continue to be fooled by them. We shall not find them because they cannot exist, not in the way we imagine them. The idea of them rests on a simplified conception in which psychological traits possess a one-to-one correspondence with a biological switch or state.

Does Viagra actually work at all? The accumulated evidence says it does. Such reviews can be flawed. Viagra and similar drugs cause side effects; in a placebo-controlled trial if someone taking the pill notices the side effects, even unconsciously, they will have some realisation they are not on the placebo.

If they can tell the difference, the trial isn't testing the difference between the drug and a placebo, it's testing the difference between people who know they're not being treated and people who know they are. The result can be a false positive, the appearance of an effect simply because the power of the placebo has been stripped away – in order for it to be a good comparator, in order for a placebo to be a placebo, people need to be unaware of whether they are taking it.

The reviews of the evidence of Viagra are limited in the extent to which they describe whether patients could tell whether they had been given placebos. They are limited both because they do not describe this in detail and because they are reviewing evidence which has not been published in its entirety. Many trials done by drug companies are not made public. Might such distortions of the evidence have resulted in the appearance of chemical effectiveness where none exists?

It's possible, but there's reason to think not. The side effects of Viagra are common but not that common. In one review, 12 per cent of people noticed flushing, 11 per cent headaches and 5 per cent some indigestion.[16] That compares with an overall success rate for the drug of improved erections for one man in every two that took it.[17] For a drug to have a useful effect in half the people who take it is incredibly good. Even if a quarter of people are able to tell by side effects whether they have been given Viagra or placebo, that shouldn't account for one person in two having a better time of it on the drug.

For the first time in human history, we have an aphrodisiac that works partly as we imagine it to, at least in those with a problem to begin with. But that hasn't stopped us imagining it works in ways it does not, especially in those who had no circulatory problem holding them back. Viagra works not because it enhances human sexuality but because it eases a certain circulatory problem by which age constricts it. Small and limited improvements, fretted with side effects and drawbacks, are all we can expect from any single medical advance. Even then, intense care is needed if we are to reliably distinguish real effects from observational error, hopeful fantasies, the play of chance and the corrupting hands of vested interests.

With so many Viagra-like drugs approved for men, and such a big financial market for them, there was an obvious next step. Female sexual frigidity was established as a formal psychiatric diagnosis back in 1952. To be dis-eased by lack of libido, to have it subtract from one's life, is worth attending to whether you are female or male. Declaring it a psychiatric illness is a different thing, and not necessarily a help to taking it seriously and thoughtfully. As the winds of fashion reshaped the sand dunes of psychiatric terminology, the term changed. The most recent alteration was from 'hypoactive sexual desire disorder' (HSDD) into 'female sexual interest/arousal disorder'. The shifting terminology meant a label in search of a market and the market was big.

Enter flibanserin, a drug developed to treat depression.[18] Flibanserin had been judged and found ineffective. Spotting an opportunity, Sprout Pharmaceuticals bought the rights. They tried getting the drug licensed for the treatment of HSDD. They failed, since the drug didn't work.

Undeterred, they tried again. This time Sprout helped fund and organise an advocacy campaign, arguing the previous rejection of flibanserin was a sexist dismissal of women.[19] 'For the millions of women with HSDD,' wrote a leading female academic, 'the FDA (Food and Drug Administration) must overcome the problem of institutionalised sexism.'[20] The International Society for the Study of Women's Sexual Health noted the twenty-four drugs already approved for male sexual dysfunction and reported that 'two-thirds of women polled believe it's inappropriate that the score is 24–0 when it comes to federal approval of treatments for desire, arousal or orgasm dysfunction in men vs. women'.[21] Neither statement, curiously, noted that its author was funded by Sprout.

In the wake of such advocacy, flibanserin was approved for use in the USA. The drug showed minor improvements in sexual happiness, consisting of one additional 'satisfying sexual event' per two months. This was criticised as trivial, outweighed by the drug's known side effects and potential harms.[22] There were other reasons for concern. This is a drug that was fixing no known biochemical or physiological error. A review of all the evidence noted the quality of data on which its weakly positive conclusion rested was 'very low'.[23] The review listed its many concerns about how the poor standard of the studies made their conclusion suspect. Researchers had shuffled the outcomes they were looking for, literally moving the goalposts. (Starting out by measuring increases in sexual desire and interest, the study found none whatsoever – so promptly switched to measuring something else, 'satisfying sexual events'.) Another issue was that it was not clear if the patients taking flibanserin were capable of working out if they had been prescribed the real drug or a matching placebo. Side effects were common and participants were carefully warned what side effects to expect from the actual drug. Without the patients being blind to their allocation, there could be only the false appearance of a control group. Placebo effects on sexual function, as one would expect for experiences that are subjective and modulated by expectation, are huge. Without decent blinding, a weak positive result for flibanserin might even mean the drug *worsened* people's sexual lives in a way just barely compensated for by the placebo effect of knowing they were taking it and that it was meant to work.

Forty-eight hours after receiving licensing approval, for a drug whose minimal benefits were widely viewed as not justifying its side effects, and whose benefits may be the illusory result of poor trial design, Sprout sold the rights to flibanserin for a billion dollars.[24]

Intelligence, libido, happiness, industriousness, humour, kindness, mercifulness – for none of these, or anything like them, will there be drugs, machines, rituals, devices or neurotransmitters that allow us mastery. Traits that are properties of human personalities and cultures need to be approached as such. Normal libido can be undermined by lack of hormones, and in those cases it can be fixed by adding them. That cannot be extrapolated to believing normal libido can be enhanced by adding extra. Intelligence can be undermined by lack of hormones – insufficient thyroid hormones in youth lead to the mental disability once called cretinism* – but adding more does nothing helpful. We are persistently over-credulous, and our credulity is another property that will not, despite advances in technology, ever become one that can be tackled with a drug or by gene therapy or some implantable bioprosthetics.

Various statistics, unreliable but suggestive, describe patterns of homo- and heterosexuality in different settings. There are even data, a minimal amount, on changes over time.[25] None of this adds much to the impression one gets anyway, that we live in a world that has grown more tolerant of sexual variation,

---

* The name comes from the Swiss French word for Christian: it was meant to be a reminder that those affected were human like the rest of us.

and where sexual variation has perhaps increased as a result.

For 150 years at least we have been reaching puberty earlier than ever, the result of better health favouring more rapid growth,[26] but at the same time we have become more protective of children, more concerned about early sexual activity. Nothing to regret about either trend, but the stress between them seems worth remarking. Adolescence has been described as a period in which one can practise, relatively safely, for adult sexual life. For evolutionary biologists the notion is based partly on the fact that fertility starts low. This description is accurate but the evolutionary account explaining it is probably false. The eye is capable of perceiving minute amounts of light – an experiment in 2016 reported people detecting single photons.[27] Strict evolutionary explanations would describe the selective advantage of being able to do this. Such explanations reduce an observation ('humans can sense a single photon') into a discrete characteristic. But attributes are often not just things-in-themselves but epiphenomena. An eye designed to perceive light best in a particular range will show an ability to perceive different amounts of light across a distribution. The extremes – the greatest and least amounts of light it is capable of differentiating – are side effects of the centre of the distribution over which the eye has evolved to function. We are not capable of perceiving single photons because that trait has been selected for, we are capable of doing it because such an ability is the contingent effect of an eye designed to see best at greater intensities of light. Human fertility follows the same normal distribution. Relatively low early fertility is probably not a thing-in-itself, but the rising start of a curve.

Evolutionary explanations of sexuality are not normally useful and they are often not correct. Despite efforts to identify a gay gene, none has been found, nor do patterns of sexuality suggest it is more genetically determined than one's tastes in politics or footwear. Science can say very little about what sort of behaviour is best, and next to nothing about what's right. It can peer at these things inasmuch as they cause or reduce happiness and unhappiness, or measurable degrees of sanity and mental illness.

The ages at which we are able to have children will continue to stretch. Parents will continue to have full responsibility for their children without full control; earlier puberty will not, therefore, be without earlier pregnancy. Greater ability to control the hormones that modulate fertility will give us more power to make fertility last or to resurrect it when it has fallen away. Nothing in this technical ability, or in the scientific knowledge that underpins it, will tell us what we should or should not be doing.

Sexual activity does not stop when fertility does. There is a divergence in our species between recreation and procreation. Unlike most other mammals, where females are sexually receptive only when fertile, libido in humans is uncoupled from ovulation. This assertion is not disproven by the fact that careful experiments can show cyclical links between ovulation and female sexual interest. The uncoupling of libido from fertility is amply demonstrated by the need for careful experiments in order to demonstrate any link at all. Sexual life continues as we age, unless impaired by decay or frailty.

Monogamous creatures have lifestyles that are similar for the two sexes. Therefore they look more alike, being built to do more similar things. Those creatures we use as cultural symbols for sexual fidelity, swans and turtle doves, are good examples. Chimpanzees and gorillas are not. Neither are monogamous and both have larger males with large testicles relative to their body size. As with lions and deer, the male's overall size and power is not there because of extra responsibility for hunting and gathering: it's there to fight other males in order to gain females. They fight and die in order that their offspring may live. Humans follow the usual mammalian pattern of being sexually dimorphic, with males averaging out as larger, stronger, faster and shorter lived.

There is some relevance of this to our lives today and in the future. The risk-taking and rivalry of adolescent boys seems absolutely part of a half-playful, half-serious jostling for position in a competitive social hierarchy. The greater cardiovascular risk of men is related to their physical power: they can do more at the cost of wearing out more quickly. Such considerations may be helpful when exploring the two, in thinking how to modulate them, and in shaping our expectations for how much we can realistically change without ceasing to be ourselves.

It does nothing to take away from the interest of these observations to note how limited their implications are. If we could establish that we are fundamentally polygamous (or polyandrous), we could make a case for being suspicious of social mores that hold monogamy as the most likely route to a well-lived life. But biological fundamentals and human history are different things. The physical traces of having been recently polygamous tell us little about far more evolutionarily recent human lives and nothing certain about our own. Despite our sexual dimorphism, rates of cheating, based on DNA fingerprinting of offspring, are remarkably low, of the order of 1–2 per cent.[28] That compares with figures an order of magnitude higher in birds whose lifestyles are supposedly monogamous.[29] Our recent past fails even to predict the current reality of our lives; we should not look to it to discover what lives we wish to lead. To look for moral lessons in our genes is to muddle up categories best kept separate.

★

The appearance – the constituents and constitution – of each sex is not only a reflection of the life it needs to live, it's a reflection of the sensibilities of the other. We select for what we like and what we love, and by selecting make it.

Darwin wrote of the evolution of aesthetic appearances and the capacity to appreciate them. Sexual selection gave rise to 'the law of battle' but it was 'taste for the beautiful' by which that battle was fought:

> If female birds had been incapable of appreciating the beautiful colours, the ornaments, and voices of their male partners, all the labour and anxiety by the latter in displaying their charms before the females would have been thrown away; and this is impossible to admit... The case of the male Argus Pheasant is eminently interesting, because it affords good evidence that the most refined beauty may serve as a sexual charm, and for no other purpose... the male Argus Pheasant acquired his beauty gradually through the preference of the females during many generations for the more highly ornamented males; the aesthetic capacity of females advanced through exercise or habit just as our own taste is gradually improved.[30]

The biologist St George Mivart protested that 'such is the instability of vicious feminine caprice, that no constancy of colouration could be produced by its selective actions'.[31] Mivart's bruised appreciation of female character did not give rise to the only disagreement. Naturalist and explorer Alfred Wallace differed from Darwin in believing firmly in human exceptionalism. What was true for us was not necessarily true for other species. Their intelligence had evolved through natural selection, ours had not. We were driven by a taste for beauty, they weren't. 'The only way in which we can account for the observed facts', he wrote, 'is by supposing that colour and ornament are strictly correlated with health, vigour, and general fitness to survive.' He did not mean to include in 'fitness to survive' the broader notion of 'fitness to survive, charm and enthral'.[32]

Our tastes lead us to select for potential, whose boundaries and contents are not defined by genetics, even though their capacities are underwritten by them. To say that a human has balls can be a great compliment, assuming one is speaking metaphorically. And to speak metaphorically is a reminder that being able to do so is part of the imaginative capacity we have inherited as a result of our forebears bringing it into being through finding it, generation after generation, attractive. To say that our children are our loves incarnate is not to speak metaphorically at all. We are the cumulated manifestations of our ancestors' tastes. 'I must study Politicks and War that my sons may have liberty to study Painting and Poetry Mathematicks and Philosophy', wrote the second American president, John Adams, to his wife. 'My sons ought to study Mathematicks and Philosophy, Geography, natural History, Naval Architecture, navigation, Commerce and Agriculture, in order to give their Children a right to study Painting, Poetry, Musick, Architecture, Statuary, Tapestry and Porcelaine.'[33] Adams would not have written that way had he not believed his wife had a high opinion of the worth of such thoughts, or if he had lacked a desire to display to her the colours of his mind and character.

If women had been designed from scratch there would be no monthly menstruation. It sits in our lives as a relic of our descent from creatures with periodic oestrus, sexually receptive only in their moments of fertility. As sex became less strictly directed at conception, more a part of maintaining the pair bond needed to spend years raising children, the split between fertility and libido widened. A woman's breasts and buttocks persist in our species in precisely the way a male peacock's tail does in theirs. They are advertisements of sexual maturity; gloriously (in the eyes of their beholders) wasteful uses of metabolic resources, not efficient parts of physiological design. Breasts in other apes appear only when breastfeeding; in humans, permanent fat appears at adolescence to mimic that appearance. Will changing human tastes lead to changing human bodies? Perhaps, but there are no obvious trends to extrapolate from; there is nothing new under the sun here.

Medicine cannot create beauty or character or fulfilled sexuality but it can help prevent their blemishment. Dysfunction becomes more treatable. The failure to find sexual satisfaction is no longer purely a private or domestic tragedy, rather a problem that can sometimes be tackled with the help of professional aid (or aids, come to that). The heartbreak of childlessness for those who fervently long for children, and the tragedy of losing pregnancies and children that have been so devoutly wished for and loved, has been diminished. It will continue to be.

Some 15 per cent of women do not have children.[34] Nor do all conceptions lead to live births. In the first few weeks after conception, fetal loss generally goes unnoticed – a painless and slightly late period is interpreted as being just that, if it is noted at all. For that reason, we have no firm idea how many spontaneous abortions occur so early. It is not even clear the extent to which we would view them as being spontaneous abortions. These very early failures of pregnancy are often due to wildly abnormal mutations: the more abnormal they are, the more they will end before they have properly begun.

To lose a half-developed early placenta, containing little or no organised fetal tissue, is not obviously to lose a baby, not when one is unaware and has not invested one's imagination in hope. Estimates of how many conceptions are lost before they are known vary hugely; in some, the number lost form the majority. From about five weeks of gestation the odds of success, of being born alive, become massively in the baby's favour. Around 80–90 per cent survive.[35] In the early deaths and failures to thrive, evolution retains wide room to operate, as it does in the various fates of our genes as we age and reproduce. Modern life will not eliminate this, nor will technology.

A child growing into itself, full of the self-renewing energy of youth, hides with its own vigour the enormous odds, 'the play of chance, the capricious fate that energised the inevitability, the number of strokes of luck'[36] it took to make it. 'I wonder sometimes, how did Dad meet Mum, and how did they conceive of me?'[37] Nothing is more unlikely in retrospect than the sexual choices that resulted in those most contingent manifestations of all, ourselves. Which is a useful reminder that sexual life is about much more than an act of intercourse, as anyone who has brought up children will fervently vouch. The time it takes to make a baby, sang Billy Bragg, could be the time it takes to make a cup of tea: but the cup of tea is not asking to borrow your car twenty years later. 'Everything in the world is about sex, except sex,' goes a famous quote, 'and sex is about power.'* The first part is partly wrong: blue-green algae, happily asexual, would see things differently. The second part, happily, is just wrong. It's about what you make of it. The tastes of our ancestors, over generations, have made us.

---

* The derivation is unclear.

Height

At different elevations a man can vary in character:

> Perhaps some that fume away in meditations upon time and space in the tower, might compose tables of interest at a certain depth; and he that upon level ground stagnates in silence, or creeps in narrative, might at the height of half a mile, ferment into merriment, sparkle with repartee, and froth with declamation.[1]

That was the view of Samuel Johnson, or at least it was his view in the moment when he wrote it. My spirits rise – the vertical ascension is impossible to avoid – at the thought of the good doctor's prescription. I know I would not profit from the cavern or the ground floor: a view from a high window lifts me more. This feeling may be, though I doubt it, partly a reaction against my normal state of life when walking on a crowded pavement. It is certainly something, that sense of being above the fray, which I rarely experience in a crowd. I am, no getting over it, short.

No man can avoid his bias and few can be sure they have the measure of it. It was only towards middle age I realised

I had been walking about with a mental half inch added to my actual height. I don't recall adding it and don't believe I did so deliberately but deliberation is not the issue. When I used to row and we lifted the boat from the water and above our heads, it was occasionally so far above my own particular head that my fingertips could not touch it. I consoled myself knowing that had I been born in times past, I should have been a comparative giant. I was not so much short as a visitor from the eighteenth century, that most thrilling of times. Keats was only five feet tall. His words, heard from his lips, would have lifted me into a ferment of sparkling thought but I would have had to stoop to hear them. Height has risen over the ages. Sadly, it turns out, my own estimates of its rise, as we will see in a moment, fall short.

More interesting than caricatures about the effect of height on personality are when we find people unswayed by their stature: the tall man who does not domineer, the short one whose confidence is self-contained and measured against no one else. We don't doubt that height issues us with a challenge, even if we don't swallow the idea it has an obvious determining effect on who we become. At least, we don't swallow that idea when it comes to ourselves – we have a different standard for others. 'I never think myself qualified to judge decisively of any man's faculties', wrote Johnson, 'whom I have only known in one degree of elevation.' But with the mild daily exception of the effects of shoes, no more is available.

Of the intersection of height and social traits, the most straightforward relationship is that wealth and health lead to each other and both contribute to stature. Records of height open windows onto the state of societies. Parts of the people who were born long ago are still around, and much that history forgets these bones remember. Taking a thousand male skeletons from AD 200 to 1850, one study compared shifts in height to those of wealth.[*2] How much the two move together yields insights into equality. When a country does well and average people do not grow, the wealth is at the top.

What have the Romans ever done for us? It turns out that among other things they made Britons richer, healthier, taller and more equal. From the start of the third century through to the end of Roman rule in Britain, heights grew 3 cm from their Neolithic average of 167 cm. That Neolithic measurement was itself a remarkable 2 cm above that of the ancient Egyptians.[3] The development of agriculture, commerce and civilisation in Egypt was not accompanied by enough equality to match that offered by a life gathering and hunting in temperate Britain.

That's not a judgement on the kindness of primitive communism versus the unfairness of societal development. It is an observation about contingencies, not necessities, as the Romans proved. Being colonised was good for Britain. When the invaders left, height fell until, by the end of the Saxon era, it was close to its pre-Roman low. Another wave of violent immigration, coupled with enthusiastic repression of the Saxons, had a marvellous effect, and the Normans lifted height once more. A warm few hundred years played a part – as subsequently did the reversing effects of colder weather in the 1300s, combined with an exhaustion of agricultural fertility. From 1400 height rose again, reaching 174 cm midway through the seventeenth century, with wages rising and the economy flourishing.

Then, in the era just before industrialisation, something

---

* The paper is not comprehensible on why women were excluded. 'The morphology of male and female bodies is different and girls are more resistant to adverse conditions than boys.' The former point will have struck interested observers already while the latter suggests that female data would provide a useful comparison.

about the inequality of society and the labour it required (the working year had doubled from 165 to 330 days) worked out badly. It is not clear quite why height fell from 1650 to 1850. Itching to blame it on factories and urbanisation doesn't fit. London was exploding only by the late 1700s, the other new industrial cities even later. And from 1850, when Britain was properly industrialising and urbanising, heights began climbing. They reached levels never before seen and they are rising still.

At about 173 cm, I would have to visit Roman Britain, or be transported back into one of the more miserable setbacks Britain has experienced since, to be taller than average. Were I to change country rather than time, the options would be more open. Heights have been rising across the world in modern times almost everywhere; Bangladesh and Myanmar are the exceptions. Born in the 1970s, I exceed the average height for men of my generation in those two countries, as well as in Haiti, Zimbabwe, Yemen, Egypt and the Democratic People's Republic of North Korea. It is not only because patriotism trumps vanity that I stay English and stay short.

It is not true that the taller candidate in an American presidential election is more likely to win,[4] but it is true that candidates are taller than their electors.[5] It plainly does not follow that as the height of Americans continues to rise, more will run for office. Does it follow that those seeking the highest office are genetically superior?

Heritability describes the extent to which variation in a trait is genetic. Height is highly heritable. Getting a feel for heritability when it comes to a trait like height helps when it comes to thinking how it applies to intelligence, health and other characteristics. That's important when considering our potential to adjust them. The extent to which variation in height is genetic – its heritability – has been seriously investigated, in a quantitative way, for over a century.[6] Most estimates for the heritability of height, in the developed world, give a figure of about 0.8. That figure also happens to be the one most commonly given for intelligence.

Estimates are made by comparing the impact of shared genes and shared environments. The ideal example is of identical twins separated at birth compared with identical twins who are not. Such twins are in short supply. Their scarcity, and their desirability when it comes to making such estimates, are not the only reasons they have been fraudulently invented over the years. They have been invented out of our obstinate wish to view through the narrow lens of heredity what is best understood in a broader manner.

A measurement of height is its own self whereas a measurement of intelligence, an IQ test, is not intelligence but a representation, an aspect, a potentially useful abstraction of a complex trait into a single quantitative measurement. IQ measurements have enough consistency that we can be confident they are measuring something, and we are confident that part of what they measure is a part of intelligence. No one suggests human intelligence is summed and captured in a number. Height is different.

When a study suggests that height has a heritability of about 0.8, it is saying that 80 per cent of the variation seen in height has been determined by genes. The statement is more limited than it seems. It is not telling us that genes contribute 80 per cent to the determination of height, and environment 20 per cent. It is not even telling us that genes contribute 80 per cent to human variation in height. It is telling us that in the population studied, at the moment of the study being done, genes contributed 80 per cent to the variation in height and environment 20 per cent.

Human height has risen over the past few thousand years without changes in genetics being responsible. The historical variation in height – or the current geographical variation – exists despite historical and geographical variation being almost entirely environmental. A heritability estimate can be sky high, in other words, and genes can still not matter as much as environment. Imagine a field of wheat spread out across either side of a hill and down along a valley, with the soil type changing halfway along. The variation in growth will be almost entirely due to the environment. The heritability estimate of height for that wheat will be low. Take the same wheat and plant it under cover in a controlled setting, with identical soil and sunshine throughout, and the heritability of height rises to 100 per cent.

Human height is less straightforward than that of wheat. Nutrients and parasites influence the growth of people and wheat alike but cereals do not also have shifting patterns of behaviour, culture and thought. In poorer environments human height is less heritable. In the developing world estimates tend to be 50 or 60 per cent rather than 80 per cent: a different environment means genes are less important. The changes need not be dramatic. A few decades ago we had the same genes and we were not then hungry or cold or suffering from a lack of clean water or proper toilets. Yet over those decades we have grown taller. The explanation is hidden in the unknown interactions of endless combinations of genetic and environmental influences. We get a sense of their overall effect but we do not understand the detail and it may be that the detail is so literally endless – there are so many potential combinations of effects – that it is unknowable.

We do not know what would happen were our environment to change. In a different setting, the genetic heritability of height might be altered. Even if a change of context left the heritability estimate of 80 per cent unaffected, that change might alter which parts of our genome and which parts of our environment were the ones that mattered. With no change in heritability, different environments might mean that some people who would have been short became tall and some who would have reached the heights remained squat. Mendel's famous experiments with peas, where single genes gave rise to predictable colours or shapes, are not good representations of how most genes work. His experiments are used as examples not because they represent the way most genes work but because they are easy to teach and understand.

Seven hundred genes at around 400 places in our genomes have been found to contribute to genetic variability in height.[7] The number of permutations and combinations of these variants is astronomical. Even so, they are a small part of the story, even the strictly genetic story. Taken together, they account for only a fifth of the witnessed heritability seen at a single point of time, and even less of that seen over generations.[8]

A small number of these variants exert strong effects – eighty-three have been discovered with an influence of up to 2 cm each.[9] That sounds impressive but it does not predict that the variants will hold true in different environments. Plus it should draw our attention back to how little the 700 variants put together explain – only a fifth of heritability, so it is not the case that a few of them contribute 2 cm each and together they explain everything. There is no 'gene for height', nor a hundred of them nor even a thousand. A recent study argued that the reason our analyses missed so many of the genes that contribute to height was because the contribution of each gene was so small. The authors presented a third of a million mutations that together, they estimated, explained a bit under half the variance in human height.[10] Another recent paper showed that a third of the variation in human height was explicable on the basis of 10,000 variations. 'The results are consistent with a genetic architecture for human height that is characterised by a very large but finite number (thousands) of causal variants, located throughout the genome but clustered in both a biological and genomic manner.'[11] True, but not useful. That the genome is organised 'in both a biological and genomic manner' is a tautology, and it is not much more than to point out that thousands of variants are involved in determining human height. With only 20,000 genes in our genome, that was always going to be true. And all these variants are fluid in what they do and how they interact. Those genes making a big difference in one setting may make no difference at all, or a difference in the other direction, for a child raised in the house next door or born the day after or with different habits. The interactions, even when they can be understood, are not stable.

In any social class people who are taller than their peers are more likely to ascend. 'People moving to a higher socioeconomic class are on average taller than the class they leave and shorter than the class they join.'[12] The taller you are, the happier and more educated you are[13] and the more you earn.[14] Height, rising by 0.5–1.0 cm per decade since 1900,[15] represents realised potential. But what is true on average – that height and success go together – is unreliable in making predictions on a smaller scale, on the scale of individual lives. The notion of the short-man complex, originally used to explain away Napoleon's behaviour on the basis of his height,[16] is alluring for its simplicity and not for its power. The interaction between height and fate is full of interest, but the interest is obliterated by assuming altitude is destiny. But we know height matters and we wonder how that reflects and shapes and twists our societies.

Bringing together separate studies in order to combine them

into analyses of greater power and reliability began in the final decades of the twentieth century. Its origins lay in the effort to determine the effects on human health of interventions to prevent heart attacks, interventions whose impact was too finely balanced to be clear from individual studies. The technique was given the name of meta-analysis. Richard Doll, who had pioneered these studies, felt the term needlessly Greek and obscure, a piece of jargon both off-putting and unhelpful. He lost his argument that the studies should just be called over-views and the name of meta-analyses has stuck. Countless small studies look at the effects of height on health and, as expected from countless small studies, their conclusions vary. The best overview of all the data, the meta-analysis combining 121 studies with over a million people, provides our most reliable verdict.[17] Those who are taller live longer.

How much of this is association and how much causation?* Height is the result of good health and therefore a marker of it. Taller people have a lower burden of cardiovascular disease and that means they live longer. But taller people die more often from cancer and more often from blood clots on their lungs. Since they go against the flow, these harmful relationships look causal. It may even be the case that being taller, overall, is bad for you. It might be that height is bad for you in itself, but a marker of other things that are good. We can't know and it doesn't matter, except for the value of bearing it in mind when indulging in fantasies of genetically engineering children to make them taller.

Evolutionary explanations for the advantages of height note

---

* Those teaching the subject use the joke that is told of a woman who attends a lecture on the difference between association and causation. She tells a friend that before hearing the talk she did not understand the difference and now she does. 'It must have been a useful lecture', says the friend. 'Well,' the woman replies, 'not necessarily.'

that healthy people are taller. They conclude it makes sense for us to value the tall more than the short and hence evolution left us regarding people we look up to as people to admire. Hence the oft-proven observation that taller people earn more money. The story sounds good but a good study suggests it isn't true. The extra earning power of tall people is real but it is not their adult height that matters. If you control for the height they were as teenagers, their final height ceases to have any link with earnings.[18] Employers don't value people differently because of their final height, then, and they can't do it on the basis of height in adolescence because that's not known to them. What they value, what earnings seem to depend upon, must therefore be either the cause or the effect of being tall at sixteen.

What is the source of the premium of being tall as an adolescent? The study's authors found family resources, financial or otherwise, were not responsible, and they noted that height differences in identical twins at sixteen also predicted different adult earning power.* Other analyses also pointed to height at sixteen being the cause of future differences, not the effect of some other factor that caused both. If social or financial capital resulted in tall height, they would exert their effect relative not only to one's height at any age, but also to the height of one's parents, who on average will have shared in this capital. Neither was true. Nor was height at sixteen a proxy for health before or after. Surprisingly, the authors also found no link between teen height and self-esteem. What they did find was that taller teens were more socially active – from sports to academic clubs to dating. That, they believed, was the cause. Those who are taller at sixteen acquire a social capital they never lose.

---

* Identical twins vary in height even when raised in the same house, but not usually by much.

The advantages of height do not come from being tall but from being taller. At a formative age that yields a gain to the spirit that is never lost.

Outside of health considerations one can still be – I am a little pleased to report – too tall, and not just to squeeze without discomfort into a seat on a plane.* The taller a tennis player, the better they are at serving but the worse their returns.[19] There is an element of doubt about why. Serves come first. You win them if you can. If you can't, you return. Are the shorter players better on the counter because their lower stature gives them an advantage or because it's forced them to acquire one? The answer influences our opinion of them, and of their taller competitors.

The repetition of heritability estimates in thoughtless ways has given rise to the false sense of them telling us something interesting and important and useful. Except in limited settings, they don't. The effect of noting heritability is often to simplify and exaggerate, cloud and confuse. Heritability estimates – that 80 per cent of height and intelligence are genetic – give a false sense of reality to mistaken ideas. They satisfy the urge to respond to a puzzle with an explanation and a number.

The increase in height across history represents a human good. Not all lives and lifestyles are equal. There is no superiority from altitude, any more than from being closer to the earth. But height marks wealth, of the sort that means one suffers less disease and deprivation and enjoys more life and longevity.

---

* 'Rejoice not when thine enemy fallest', says the biblical book of Proverbs. Good advice. But taller people live longer, make more money and have a tendency to peer down at us shorter citizens. One is allowed a flush of pleasure seeing them bump their heads on low beams.

The notion that some societies are better than others is true when one looks at their heights just as it is true when looking at their levels of infant mortality. I am taller than men of my generation from – to repeat the list – Bangladesh, Myanmar, Haiti, Zimbabwe, Yemen, Egypt and the Democratic People's Republic of North Korea. Those countries have more in common than the average height of their citizens.

Height will continue to climb and we have no clear idea how high. Shorter people will remain but they too will get taller. Drugs to increase height already work but surprisingly little. Giving growth hormone can be powerful when correcting a deficiency but deficiencies are not to blame for normal variation in adult height. Adding the drug to someone whose levels are fine does little or nothing. We can be thankful for that; if it wasn't the case, the fear of being below average might trigger a drug-induced race for the heights. As it is, neither drugs nor gene therapy can do that.

'Which of you by taking thought can add one cubit unto his stature?'[20] Ilizarov frames work, if you really want to be taller – these are pieces of engineering that form thought into artifice. They are the steel circles one can position round a leg, their spokes embedded through the flesh and into the bone at their centre. Snap the bone between the two anchored circles and then keep gradually stretching them apart as it regrows: one ends up with longer bones. It's a technique for restoring height after an accident, when a chunk of bone has been destroyed and would leave someone with legs of different lengths. Some have used the frames cosmetically in order to stretch their legs. We are too sensible for that to become as common as the use of dental braces. If it turns out to be true that height is a marker of health but a cause of ill health, will we produce drugs to restrict our growth? We could do that. The end of physical adolescence brings growth to a close; the parts of the bones where growth takes place seal and cease. One can induce that early. But we are a long way from having any warrant for thinking we should.

So long as the environment changes, so will we, and since we are creatures that change our own environments our heights will never be fixed so long as we remain ourselves. Every aspect of our lives affects every other; our genes whirl round in the storm of circumstance. In his 1962 book *Mankind Evolving*, the geneticist Theodosius Dobzhansky wrote of height as an exemplar of attempting to understand a human trait from a genetic perspective. 'It is sometimes said that the genes determine the limits up to which, but not beyond which, a person's development may advance', he wrote:

This only confuses the issue. There is no way to predict all the phenotypes that a given genotype might yield in every one of the infinity of possible environments... we do not know how to obtain the evidence needed to determine how tall [an infant] may grow in some environments that may be contrived to stimulate growth. It is an illusion that there is something fundamental or intrinsic about limits, particularly upper limits... limits are elusive and hard to determine, most of all when the environmental conditions are not specified... Even at the risk of belabouring the obvious, let it be repeated that heredity cannot be called 'the dice of destiny'... The evidence of genetic conditioning of human traits, especially mental traits, must be examined with the greatest care.[21]

The last point is critical. Something as simple as height cannot be effectively understood, predicted or manipulated from a genetic point of view. How much more true, then, for other, subtler expressions of human life.

Breadth

'Gritty realism' emerged as a phrase in the 1920s. It sim-mered until the late 1970s when the popularity of the term came to the boil.[1] Setting itself out as superior to class-ridden complacency, it is a misleading idea, as mean-spirited ones often are. Its implication is that optimism is false and the world is not a fundamentally cheerful place in which happiness is spreading and progress being made, that such views are the pretences of those enjoying their own privilege and wilfully blind to the downtrodden whose misfortune is the source of privilege for the lucky few. Reality is only reality when the grit dries your mouth and wets your eyes.

In such a spirit, the global rise of obesity is proof. What is all the triumph of medicine and the supposed benefit of liberal, wealthy industrialised life when we are all swelling into tumescence? The world is sick and anyone who says otherwise ignores the rise of diabetes, of weight-related disability and early death, of millions of lives blighted by the free market and mass production.

The rise in global breadth, the rise in the average human circumference, is bad news, but it's a piece of bad news dwarfed by an immense amount of good. Those who are overweight would live longer, healthier lives if they were slim but they are overweight because they live in a world granting them more health and longer lives than the one that gave their ancestors no choice but to be skinny. Obesity is a global problem. The fact that it now so often affects the Second and the Third Worlds is not a grim mark of how our pollution spreads but a happy reminder of how far and fast we have come and how widely the benefits spread. The happiness goes only so far: countries with enough wealth to suffer from obesity but without the riches to properly treat diabetes pay a vast price in shortened and blighted lives.[2]

Fatness and good humour go together sufficiently often for us to notice their constellation. Both flourish in an absence of want and the presence of an appetite for life. The British cleric Sydney Smith (1771–1845), an enormously fat man himself, combined the two in full Falstaffian manner. 'Going to marry her?', he exclaimed, on hearing of a proposed wedding to a woman of similar dimensions to himself:

> Impossible! You mean a part of her; he could not marry her all himself. It would be a case, not of bigamy but trigamy; there is enough of her to furnish wives for the whole parish. One man marry her! – it is monstrous! You might people a colony with her; or give an assembly with her; or perhaps take your morning's walk round her, always provided there were frequent resting places, and you were in rude health. I once was rash enough to try walking round her before breakfast, but only got half way and gave it up exhausted. Or you might read the Riot Act and disperse her; in short, you might do anything but marry her![3]

To an extent – a lesser one – he also made fun of himself for his own immensity. A doctor advised him to take long walks on an empty stomach. He agreed but replied, 'Whose?' After dieting he wrote to a friend saying, 'If you hear of sixteen or eighteen pounds of human flesh, it's mine. I feel as if a curate has been taken out of me.'

Being overweight has not always been regarded as something solely miserable. Cheerfulness keeps breaking through. Being fat can seem a mark of great appetites and being thin the physical result of antipathy to life. Shakespeare's Julius Caesar warned of the dangers of lean and hungry men; French gastronome Brillat-Savarin offered advice for the improvement of thin female gourmets, who he knew (correctly, given the fashion of his day) wished to be plump. If we say today that our weight is the product of blissful domestic contentment, few would imagine us skinny.

Modern abhorrence of fat comes partly from the puritanism that abhors indulgence as a moral shortcoming. This is Protestantism with a waspish American twist, the sort that believes in egg white omelettes and cannot describe a pleasurable meal without mentioning what it does to arteries. The grain of truth is that there are shortcomings associated with excess weight and some really are moral. Deplorable as it is to immolate oneself with hunger out of masochism or a sense of superiority, it is also a flaw to be always snacking. To never allow oneself to get hungry, to always expect all food and drink to be sweet: the man who does so may be grown up and admirable in every other way, but here he is childish.

Sentiments about sentiments, speculations about the way we view weight, are necessary for understanding our concerns over the rise in human weight and the ways we might modulate both the concern and the rise. Consider the use of surgery not as a tool to cut out disease or heal wounds but as a technique to directly reshape our bodies and lives. Breath-taking transplants, tissue engineering and bioprosthetics come effervescently to mind. So they should, they're real, but they're niche and will remain so. Surgery for obesity, on the other hand, is real and we can do it and we mostly do not. It is a gap that is difficult to explain except by virtue of sentiment.

The world is fat. Over a third of us qualify as overweight (a BMI – body mass index – above 25 kg/m^2) and a quarter as obese (a BMI above 30).[4] While weight may be beginning to level off in the world's richest countries[5,6] it is still estimated that by 2050 the majority of humans will be obese.[7] Huge amounts of effort have gone into researching ways of helping people lose weight. The result has been minimal. We have got better at labelling and swaying the manufacture of processed foods and our efforts here have been useful. When it comes to designing interventions to help individual people lose weight, they have not. An industry of medical research exists that achieves very little, other than to support a large number of careers producing strings of publications suggesting that diet and exercise are good for us but which do nothing to help us achieve them. Even the best diets make little difference. An overview of all our knowledge showed that diets, regardless of which were chosen, helped people lose 7 kg (15 and a half lbs) of weight after a year.[8] Diets achieve these minimal results in trial settings but in real life they do less and the effect of advising people to follow them is even less again. 'This seemingly obvious distinction is often missed', noted one paper.[9] Accumulated medical knowledge shows that adding in exercise to a medical trial of dieting helps people shift only another kilo[10] while drugs, with all their side effects, get rid of a further 2–5 kg (4 and a half to 11 lbs).[11] These figures are not good. Obesity for an American man of average height begins at 93 kg (205 lbs). Combined successfully and continued lifelong – which is beyond anything seen in the trials – these interventions together amount to losing little more than 10 per cent of body weight. Even for someone who had only just crossed into the realm of being obese, that's not enough to bring their weight down to a desirable level. The combined effects of dieting, drugs and exercise, even when exaggerated into an unrealistic experimental ideal, still aren't enough.

Surgery to reduce weight – to reduce the absorption of food or the capacity of the gut – performs better, much better. It reduces weight by an additional 26 kg (57 lbs).[12] That's enough to drop our average American from the borderlands of obesity to the healthiest range possible, and to do so in such a way that they have a realistic chance of staying there. Diet, exercise and drugs combined scarcely add up to what could accurately be called a treatment, but surgery has such a powerful effect it seems like a cure.

First used in 1956[13] bariatric surgery was carried out 146,301 times worldwide in 2003,[14] a 266 per cent increase on five years before.[15] That means 'of the patients qualifying [by being overweight] for surgery, only about 1 per cent are receiving this therapy – the only effective treatment currently available'.[16] In 2008 the number of global bariatric surgery procedures rose to 344,221[17] but by 2011 the figure actually fell, to 340,768.[18] Our best treatment for obesity is being used less while the number of people who are obese is rising.

Being overweight is not in itself a disease, not unless it's extreme. Instead it is a condition in which your chance of bad things happening – heart attacks, strokes, diabetes, cancer, even depression and a reduced ability to exercise – is more likely. Treatments for obesity must be judged not on what they do to weight but what they do to health. Intensive lifestyle interventions, for example, have been shown in a high-quality trial lasting a decade to help overweight and obese people lose weight but also to make no difference to their survival or health.[19] It seems inconceivable that the lack of difference seen is due to a lack of benefit from losing weight – instead it must surely be a consequence of even the best trials being still too small and too short. But that conviction is based on faith and reason rather than hard evidence. We do not know what effect weight-loss drugs have on whether people live or die or get ill or stay well over the long term,[20] an absence all the more remarkable given our previous experience of harms from such drugs, many of those harms having appeared late and caused the drugs to be hastily withdrawn.[21] Drug trials for statins, antihypertensives and other agents aimed at lowering cardiovascular risk tend to recruit thousands or tens of thousands of people, to last for years and only to be judged useful when they demonstrate their impact on death and disability. Trials of interventions for weight loss, whether of diet or exercise or drugs, rarely do any one of those things and scarcely, if ever, do all. The quality of the knowledge they produce is poor because so are the studies themselves. We know how to do better studies and elsewhere we demand them. Why do we not do so here?

The magnitude of weight loss resulting from surgery, and the small amount from other approaches, almost justifies the notion of surgery being 'the only effective treatment currently available'. Data exists showing that bariatric surgery can have impressive effects on blood pressure, blood lipids and remission of type 2 diabetes.[22] Bariatric surgery is surprisingly safe, given that obese individuals are not ideal surgical subjects, with a perioperative mortality rate of 0.3 per cent.[23] But that rate, and the fact 4.3 per cent suffer major harm around the time of their surgery (from blood clots and extended hospital stays through to needing to go back to theatre to reoperate and fix problems),[24] is not innocuous. How does it compare to the number of lives surgery saves through avoiding weight-related problems like heart attacks, strokes and diabetes?

Remarkably, we have no idea. Trial evidence is too sparse and too short term.[25] Observational evidence is encouraging. It extends beyond two decades[26] and suggests a large drop in lifetime health-care costs,[27] but really reliable long-term knowledge of the impact of weight-loss surgery is poor.[28] It is better than the even scantier and shorter term evidence we have about diet, exercise and drugs, but it is terrifically poor nonetheless. There is no other area of medicine where a huge global health problem has a range of treatment options that we have completely failed to investigate in order to determine their impact on people's lives.

What explains the gulf between our enormous concern over obesity and our poverty of effort when exploring how actually to tackle it? It is astonishing that drugs are used without us knowing if they have serious long-term harms – or any long-term benefits. The short-term impact of weight-loss surgery is so much greater than all other options that it should have been seized upon with all the seriousness science could bring. Instead its evidence base comes from data that are short term and for which the number of patients enrolled into all the trials ever done comes out to less than the number included in one recent new trial of a blood thinner.[29,30] The lack of evidence is not because weight-loss surgery, although promising, is new. A review of over 200 studies of it noted that 'these publications [only] summarise short-term evaluations, results, and complications'[31] and that better evidence was needed. That review came out in 1976.

We seize with enthusiasm on interventions that have been shown not to work, like high-protein diets.[32,33] We take seriously efforts to reduce sugar intake, confident (correctly) that they matter for public health even though successful interventions here cut body weight not by the tens of kilos needed but by hundreds of grams.[34] A recent academic review of global obesity, a prestigious one in a leading medical journal, noted in passing the apparent importance of weight-loss surgery and then, while issuing multiple demands for interventions relating to diet and exercise, never mentioned it again.[35] It is worth repeating that regulations to reduce sugar intake through limiting sweetened drinks, capable of reducing people's weight by a few hundred grams, quite properly receive huge attention. Weight-loss surgery, where the loss is twenty-six *thousand* grams, does not.

Whether or not to blame people for being fat is not the province of medicine. But taking their health seriously is, and it is striking how consistently we have chosen to focus on offering advice that is of no help in place of doing so. What would a world look like where we did not properly explore the medical tools available for weight loss because we believed obesity was not a medical problem but a moral failing? It would look very similar, surely, to the one in which we live.

Surgery for obesity might work superbly. The comfortable arguments that people should eat less and do more somehow take the place of action. Unhealthy lifestyles are more palatable to us as moral failings than as technical problems with technical solutions. Sydney Smith's mockery of a fat woman would not be tolerated today, no matter how convinced we were of his willingness to make fun of himself for the same reasons. Being non-judgemental has become too important. Medical writing was once full of discussions of the duty of doctors to combat moral evils and weaknesses. The same changes that have stripped Smith's type of humour from public dialogue mean such discussions no longer appear in medical journals or medical textbooks. Contemporary discussions of obesity studiously avoid being judgemental. The result is possibly that we are being influenced all the more by views we still possess but do not acknowledge. We have avoided the problems of obesity treatments by never considering them seriously. Being thoughtfully judgemental might be preferable to a thoughtlessness that allows prejudices to emerge unseen in our choices and omissions.

In the past, people have found plumpness desirable and slimness off-putting. That fashion seems unlikely to come again, not in a world that so values svelte youth. Even if our pills could obliterate the health costs of being fat, there seems no immediate prospect of painters once more viewing pudgy bellies as more beautiful than flat ones.

Is there the possibility of developing medical interventions to increase metabolism, not only solving fatness but positively allowing and encouraging gluttony? Such an intervention already exists in the shape of exercise. Surgery may keep us in check and give us the health benefits of a lower body mass, but what of pills to take the place of the gym? The changes that occur when we exercise; could they not be mimicked pharmacologically, leaving us not only slim but lean and hungry too?

For the foreseeable future the answer is no. Our habit is to equate exercise to a single chemical – endorphins are often invoked – but exercise affects our body in a multitude of ways that relate not to one pathway or chemical messenger but to a numberless host of them. They will not be mimicked in our lifetimes, not effectively.

Sceptics of progress might pause to consider that a modern obese diabetic on a full range of appropriate pills is still healthier by far than their slim ancestors. Nor do the pills help cause the obesity they ameliorate: people do not opt to lead unhealthier lives because they feel drugs save them from having to do better.

Breadth will continue to swell, not only because the world is getting richer and happier and better fed but because being overweight spreads in the manner of an infection. It's the power of a norm. Being overweight spreads through communities via webs of friendships; we put on weight when those we admire are already plump.[36] 'Smoking- and alcohol-cessation programs and weight-loss interventions that provide peer support – that is, that modify the person's social network – are more successful than those that do not', noted the paper that discovered this. 'This highlights the necessity of approaching obesity not only as a clinical problem but also as a public health problem.' Make fun of people for being fat, as Smith did, and might you make them more likely to be slim? What if being judgemental were shown in a reliable trial to help people lose weight? To make people feel bad might be justified if it actually made them better. We would certainly not wish merely to make people more miserable about a condition they could do little about. Except that this is what we already do, not through politically incorrect jokes but through endless advice about diet and exercise. The advice is easy to give and hard to follow and its net result is not to help people lose weight but only to make them more miserable about not doing so. Smith's humour may be less cruel and more useful.

Gristle

A sarcophagus is named for what it does. Leave a body in one for long enough and there's nothing left but bones: it's called a sarcophagus because it eats the flesh. Life, too, is a sarcophagus. In old age people waste away and in extreme old age they do it extremely. Their temples sink and their cheek-bones protrude as the muscles of their face dissolve. Arms and legs lose their bulk and between the bones on the backs of their hands the years plough deep furrows.

From the foot of the bed (doctors like talking of what can be recognised from the foot of the bed), such signs are unmistakeable. In younger people there may be a cause that can be addressed, some lurking disease to be cured, but in old people there often is not. The emaciation is not malnourishment. These people have a poor diet without fail but the reason for it is usually that they have lost their appetite. They are cachexic, sarcopenic, emaciated, suffering from muscle-wasting and the withers: the terms multiply and the flesh fades.

Synonyms signal more than a condition being common. Scrofula, the King's evil, phthisis, consumption, the white plague – the host of terms for tuberculosis testified both to its importance and also to how little we understood what caused it.

In poorer countries tuberculosis is still common but it is now rarely called anything other than 'TB'. We understand it and hence the need for synonyms has gone; it has coalesced into a single comprehensible condition. The flesh-eating aspect of age has not.

Reshaping human life through modifying cardiovascular ageing has a clear trajectory. It will go on accumulating effectiveness, accumulating small increments and altering our expectations of healthy life. Our hearts and brains will stay healthy to an extent our forebears could not have imagined. When it comes to gristle, to cartilage and bone and muscle, our understanding and our power is more limited. Each of us gets only so far in life before wincing, clutching some part of ourselves that always worked smoothly before, and wondering what a joint like that could be doing in a kid like us. Against the development of arthritis we have got nowhere. Glucosamine is a popular over-the-counter treatment. The least reliable evidence says it doesn't work much and the best says it doesn't work at all.[1] The same goes for other similar over-the-counter pills marketed as being helpful.[2,3]

Replacing joints has been around so long that it feels ordinary. The difference it makes to people is not. It has become more important as it has grown routine. Peer into the future, though, and no artificial muscles wait for us, nor drugs to rejuvenate the ones we have as they weaken. The small joints of the hands and feet remain painfully disabling for many, and cannot easily be replaced; our power lies in cloaking the symptoms. Not something which has changed much: morphine is the oldest of effective medical interventions. Newer painkillers are more effective at making money for those holding the patents than in supplementing the ones we already have. The back pain that troubles so many is recalcitrant. A host of effective treatments exists but from surgery through to injecting worn vertebrae with body-friendly cement, they tend to be no more effective in trials than the sham procedures they are compared against.*

Modern life, which we are so accustomed to blame for our ills rather than thank for our blessings, is not often held responsible for higher rates of osteoarthritis, which we are more inclined to link with the wear and tear of our forebears' hard lives of manual labour. We know arthritis existed throughout human history since we have found it in fossils.[4] Higher rates today have been attributed to modernity's benefits – living long enough to get arthritis and eating and weighing more, straining our joints. The attribution might be wrong. With arthritis, modern life might actually be the baleful presence we elsewhere so often and so falsely see it as. Even if you account for us getting older and fatter, osteoarthritis has still been getting more frequent – it has doubled in the past sixty years.[5] It is unclear why.

As we age our skin thins and breaks, our joints decay, our muscles wither and our flesh wastes. The effectiveness of medicine in other areas, particularly in ensuring we do not die before old age, means more and more of us live to encounter these problems and live to dwell with them for longer. There may be nothing intrinsically unsolvable about the ageing of gristle, but we do not know. Here there is no light. For the foreseeable future, these problems do not lie in the realm of the soluble.

---

* A curious result is that private back surgery in the UK pays particularly well. Were the operations more effective, the NHS would provide them. Since it doesn't, the trade in doing them for an added fee is brisk.

Power

'These three words represent a programme of moral beauty', explained Pierre de Coubertin. The words were Citius, Altius, Fortius and the motto was that for the Olympics he founded in 1894. As conceptions of moral beauty go, Faster, Higher, Stronger was blunt. To strive, to seek and not to yield might have been better, but sport has always slipped easily from desiring excellence and victory for oneself into wanting to inflict defeat and failure on others. The difference is vaster than empires and its effects may not always be visible, usually they are. If the spirit of the competitors is not clear in their striving they are probably not engaged in sport. Watching Usain Bolt sprint is to share in the glory of what humans can do. Watching him glance sideways and slow down as the race closes is to taste what it feels like to be satisfied with leaving people behind.

Until 2008, the notion that exercise made you happy via endorphins was based on noticing that people said exercise made them happy, that their endorphin levels increased and that both could be prevented by opiate-receptor blockers. (Endorphins = endogenous morphines, meaning opiates.) This all sounds very persuasive and science-y. But the same could be said for levels of adrenaline as for endorphins, or for potassium (released by exercising muscles) or carbon dioxide, and again the effects of these things can be reversed in such a way that you will feel bad as a result. In 2008 new evidence arrived. Brain scans of ten people showed that after two hours of running there really were changes in their brains consistent with endorphin activation. 'Impressive', said one neuroscience professor in a report on the research. 'This is the first time someone took this head on', said another. 'It wasn't that the idea was not the right idea. It was that [previously] the evidence was not there.'[1]

The findings were interpreted as showing that endorphins were responsible for an experience that the scan actually only indicated they were involved in. Scanners might one day get good enough to show evidence from people's brains that they reach too easily for bad reductionist explanations of human experiences. But that would be substituting scanners for thought, since we do not need scans to tell us that. Talk of endorphins tends strongly towards devaluing what they are – part of the convoluted process by which physiology becomes psychology – while fetishising what they do, namely playing some part in happiness.[2] The notion that endogenous neurotransmitters affecting opiate receptors are involved in our experience of exercise is not a silly one; clearly they are. What is foolish is the notion they explain it. Scientific jargon sometimes offers only the masquerade of helping clarity of our thoughts.

Endorphins do seem involved in subduing the pain that builds up as a race progresses, but endurance athletes neither show on their faces nor report in their words that extreme exertion leads to pleasure and bliss. 'Shut up, legs!', the Tour de France cyclist Jens Voigt is reported to have said while racing.

It was not their cries of joy he meant to silence.* Supplementing endogenous morphines with exogenous ones – giving them the drug – demonstrates the same point. The happiness created is not the one we have in mind but one that comes at the expense of the minds we have. As a step to making the human race happier, the intoxicating effects of morphine and Heroin are not widely seen as a success. It is entirely reasonable to suggest we will find new ways of drugging people into happiness. They will look like the old ones. There is no genetic or pharmacological or surgical switch to make us exactly as we are only a bit more cheerful. There isn't even an easy cultural way of doing that, but at least there are an infinity of difficult ones.

Snatching after technical language and pantomime bio-chemistry matters even in the field of sport. We rest decisions and behaviour on scientific explanations that aren't scientific and don't explain much. We structure training programmes and make choices, swallow supplements and take drugs, all with only a tenuous idea of what we are doing.

In 2017, for the first time, a reliable study was carried out on the effects of erythropoietin, the hormone that prompts the body to produce more red blood cells, on competitive cyclists. The fact it took so long was not because the drug is banned in competition. It took so long because we were content believing that a drug that increased the viscosity of blood must be good for athletic performance – we were content with an untested simplification of an intricate physiological system. Looking back at the drugs abused by Tour de France cyclists would have warned us, if we had been willing to be warned. Over the years it has been clear that the enthusiasm to cheat outstripped

---

* If it hurts me, he is said to have consoled himself, it must be hurting the others twice as much. The latter comment makes one like him less.

knowledge of what worked. Ether and alcohol no longer have much pseudoscientific allure as performance-enhancers. But the notion that more blood was better has lingered. Is there a case to suspect that evolution has let us down by filling our veins with less than the optimum amount? It's a possibility, since natural selection may have opted to reduce our performance in order to make gains elsewhere, in efficiency or cost or in resistance to disease and ageing. But it's not reasonable to assume our guesses will be correct. Doing that is taking our body to be more predictable than experience tells us it is. There are many experts who know that erythropoietin and other drugs help, and many winners, like Lance Armstrong, who we can see have won because of them. But history is full of experts that were wrong, and of those who swallowed ineffective and harmful potions and yet did well. Leeches were used for precisely those reasons. The response of a cancer to a chemical is a simpler process yet as we have seen half of all new trial drugs, even after performing well in animal and human experiments, turn out to do more harm than good. Experience and expert opinion are no guide. Simple explanations are often no explanations at all. 'World is crazier and more of it than we think,' wrote Louis MacNeice, accurately.

Only after decades of use, in which erythropoietin was vested with all the aura of scientific power and all the confidence of expert opinion, was the experiment conducted to see if it worked.[3] The authors of the 2017 study noted that the previously existing experimental support for the drug's power was so poor as to be absent:

> The evidence for the performance-enhancing effects of [erythropoietin] in high-level competitive sports is rather scarce. The evidence constitutes of small, often uncontrolled

studies, in arguably unrepresentative populations and is often inappropriately expressed only in exercise parameters that mainly evaluate maximal exercise performance.[4]

Evaluating maximal exercise performance, some brief test of power produced on a bike in a lab, isn't enough. It's a soft outcome, an unreliable surrogate for the hard outcome of sporting success. Maximal performance doesn't win the Tour de France, only sustained performance does that. Drop an elephant onto someone's knee as they are pressing down on their pedal and the force with which that pedal gets pushed down will increase massively. Their maximal performance will briefly rise. It does not follow that one cycles more quickly with elephants on one's knees. Erythropoietin increases haemoglobin levels and various performance measures dependent on them but it does not follow that this helps with performance overall.

The trial took forty-eight elite cyclists and randomly allocated them, in a blinded fashion, to two months of injections of erythropoietin or to matching placebo injections. At the end those given the erythropoietin had thicker blood with more haemoglobin and scored better on two short-term measurements of performance. On another laboratory measurement of performance over the slightly longer term (forty-five minutes) there was no difference. To measure results overall, on the outcome that matched the goal of the cyclists, a proper Tour stage, the participants raced up Mont Ventoux. It was there the cyclist Tom Simpson died in 1967, having taken both amphetamines and alcohol in order to improve his performance. Both amphetamines and alcohol have good short-term effects on athletic performance but their effect on something as prolonged as a cycling race up a mountain is less sure. They certainly have drawbacks.

The study found that whether the cyclists had been given the placebo or the erythropoietin made no difference whatsoever to their ascent of Mont Ventoux. Just as with a thousand medical interventions before, the fact that the drug was known to do something effectively, the fact people had seen it work and the fact people understood the mechanism by which it did work, did not stand in the way of the greater fact that it didn't work at all. Theory, expertise and observation have no power to figure out the truth of interventions on a system as intricate as the human body. Only structured, randomised, blinded trials will do. The lessons of science don't suit our wishes. If they did, they would not be lessons and science would need no method.[5]

Historically, we would have had, as a species, less blood in our bodies than we have today. Frequent infections, a poor diet, lack of iron – a host of factors meant normal haemoglobin concentrations were much lower, just as they are still lower in poorer countries. It might be the case that athletes do better in today's richer societies, with more blood and more erythropoietin, but it doesn't follow that it's true. There was nothing stupid about the idea that erythropoietin might make cyclists faster. The stupidity came from believing that because it might, that it did: from the overconfidence that meant we believed an idea without appreciating how important it was to test it, or how rigorous such tests needed to be. Might there be situations in which less erythropoietin and less blood gave one an advantage? There might. Maybe even in the Tour de France. Each litre would carry less oxygen and carbon dioxide but each litre would be easier to pump and more likely to match the composition of the blood our circulatory systems evolved to expect.

★

Science handled properly – rather than as window dressing – will continue to help us go faster, stronger and higher. Olympic records keep falling. Part of the improvement comes from the fact we are healthier and more numerous, part from the fact that professional sport is not something we have taken seriously for very long. Efforts to screen and encourage children with athletic potential are recent. Permutations and combinations of training regimens are being refined. It is not surprising records are broken so regularly. It implies no evolutionary process, no change in the gene pool.

Are there limits to what evolution could accomplish, given time? Even in the absence of any genetic engineering technology, given enough generations and resources and the sufficient subjugation of freedom, could we select for humans to become ever faster, stronger, higher? Overlooking the manpower shortages – the global deficit in mad scientists and the modern decline in the number of dictators[6] – selective breeding could help. Humans are not masters of anything save for intelligence and a capacity to sweat* and there seems no hard roof even to those. But enforced selection over generations, though, has limits. We see that in pedigree animals, from dogs to cattle. The largest dog breeds are notorious for joint problems, while all start developing a host of issues once inbred enough, from behavioural problems through to smelly anal glands. The law of unintended consequences runs riot after only a few generations.

The body with its tangled interactions is not so easy to

---

* The latter is due to being functionally hairless. If you have fur, sweating is like getting wet while wearing cotton – not a good way of controlling your temperature. Being able to sweat so superbly helped facilitate our rise in intelligence, temperature control being critical for the brain. But our lack of fur did not give rise to intelligence, only meant it was possible when pressures selected for it.

re-engineer. Improve one bit and you create consequences, some of which you will not be able to anticipate. Horses have been intensively selected, over multiple generations, for speed. We have the records of their times, over set distances in known races, going back two centuries. While trends suggest some room for improvement over short sprints (distances we have not historically focused on), improvements over medium to long distances appear almost finished. Horses seem as fast as selective breeding will ever make them. For the past few decades, speeds, in the three races that make up the US Triple Crown, have been broadly flat.[7]

Horses need to live as well as race, and to race they need to have lived first, and to have trained. Mutations that would increase their flat-out running speed, at the expense of the life needed to get them to the start line, will not prosper, even if selected for. Another sort of limitation comes in the form of balanced polymorphisms, where a desirable quality is derived from a blend of two genetic factors. If they give an optimum result when evenly mixed, selecting for either would disrupt and balance and slow the horse. Physiology is full of trade-offs. As creatures get bigger, their theoretical speed increases yet their actual speed does not. The theories are based on calculations of the power produced by ever more muscle. They fail because it is hard to predict the constraints that pull tighter as size grows, constraints of power delivery and of blood, flesh, bone, heat regulation and countless other factors, some known and some not. Just as elephants are slower than cheetahs, so the tyrannosaurus probably lagged behind the velociraptor.[8] As human height continues to grow, it might not follow that sports that now favour the tallest will continue to do so.

Women are 21 per cent faster over 1,500 metres since the Second World War and over 60 per cent faster than they were in the marathon; men are improving too but they have been competing fiercely for longer so the improvements are smaller – their 1,500 metre time is 14 per cent quicker over the past century and their marathon time 23 per cent so.[9] Stats from other disciplines tell the same story of improvement, even if not yet of a plateau. In the 1966 World Cup final, the German players passed the ball some 300 to 400 times and got it to reach its target 78 per cent of the time. In 2014 the number of passes almost doubled and accuracy rose to 86 per cent.[10]

Humans will continue to get faster and stronger, even if not forever.[11] With a rising population there is more variation to draw from and the extremes will stretch. Training regimens, with or without effective drugs, will get better – the lack of experimental rigour in sports science suggests room for improvement. More importantly, the sheer increase in human health means more records to come. A hundred years ago many of the great athletes came from the upper classes because others did not have the opportunities. A hundred years hence countries now too poor to make the most of their citizens may be rich enough for those citizens to make the most of themselves. That height is still rising in even the richest countries suggests that, there too, our physical capacities continue to expand in ever more nurturing conditions. Faster, higher, stronger seems a poor programme for moral beauty in itself but a rich reward for general improvements in human lives.

Will genetic engineering make a difference? Efforts to edit our genes are not beyond us – they are in front of us, already fumblingly usable. The same interplay of influences that stops horses getting faster with each generation will limit our power. No single gene equates to success in sport, nor any handful of them. We might make a few changes here and there but their effects will be small and unpredictable – it would take a generation each time to see if they match the ineffectiveness of erythropoietin. The subtleties of creating physical genius will happily remain out of our reach for the foreseeable future. Speculating on what might be achieved by a world beyond that becomes removed too far from fact. It has its own interest, but that's what science fiction is for.

A concern for physique dates back to the emergence of vanity, roughly a second before the development of sexual repro-duction. Lord Byron's battle to stay muscular was neither the first nor last. Sedentary people with sedentary jobs do not have the bodies of those who hand-ploughed their fields any more than such ploughmen had the shape of those who spend half a week on a bench-press.

Trends in muscularity are framed by biology but not decided by it. As our bodies have changed our biology hasn't. Could we develop pills to give us muscular bodies without the need for exercise? We already have: a bodybuilding, rugby-playing acquaintance referred to them as vitamin S. Anabolic steroids give us muscles we have not done the work to deserve. Such drugs are not sold over the counter. That's not because we judge that people should have the shapes they earn. It's because the drugs enhance only some of the effects of exercise. They give an appearance of vigorously powerful health that is only muscle deep.

New drugs with similar effects will have similar side effects. They go together. The suite of stresses imposed on the body by exercise are not easily reproduced. What about a drug to help speed your metabolism and burn fat? We have that too and amphetamines are also not widely advised for the pursuit of health. Muscular power is no more reducible to anabolic steroids than happiness is to endorphins: something of both can be produced using drugs, and very effectively so in the short term, but nothing close enough to properly suit.

Might it be we will soon develop a new drug that will do much better than anything we have had before, a drug to make us more lastingly muscled and trim and healthy, less plump and indistinct? Vanishingly unlikely. Drugs like antibiotics have effects that seemed miraculous. They really were 'magic bullets', hitting their targets with precision and power. Antibiotics aim at parts of bacterial cells that are essential for them and non-existent in us: the potential for accurate targeting was there as a result. When it comes to the countless interdigitating processes that direct our bodies, no magic targets exist. We have evolved to become strong and slim in certain conditions and to lose muscle and put on fat in others. Those capacities are based on no single biochemical thermostat. They are the results of the thousand different processes by which the varied parts of our bodies constantly adjust themselves. Even exercise gives no standardised results. Rugby produces a different physique from mountaineering and within the physical shapes they produce lie deeper physiological differences.

With all the genetic variability of billions of people, no single mutations have been found that make the difference between a forty-four-pound weakling and a hulking Charles Atlas. What we share instead are a host of genes that mean the choice is up to us and depends partly on the exercise we do: hence the success of Atlas's training programmes. Nor, with all the money that has been poured into investigating drugs to slim us down or bulk us up, has much been achieved. We are not even at the stage of having a range of small but sound interventions to build upon. Those interventions may well happen in our life-time – the firmer identification of genetic variations that add a percentage or two to svelteness or drugs that reduce a little the softening effect of a life spent sitting. Nothing more can reasonably be expected.

There are trends in human muscularity as there are in human fatness. They should not be muddled up in misty fantasies of future human evolution. Our evolution continues at the same pace it always has. No predators or catastrophes are needed, only for some of us to have more children than others. Tracing the trends is not a matter of asserting that only now have women fancied good-looking men and men returned the favour. The issue is noticing that the trends that matter here are not biological.

What sort of bodies we have in the coming century, the shapes and forms we desire and seek, will be determined by taste and circumstance, not drugs or gene editing. As with so much else, what matters is not strictly our genes, only the roomy capacities they grant us. Our intelligence gives us a potential that is not unique save in its extent. It confers an ability to operate on the basis of an inheritance not to be found in our genes.

Culture

Genes give you pleasure in exertion and delight in athleticism. They also give you abiding joy in sitting, resting and eating. To say they give you these things is stretching it since what they give you is potential, and potential is unpredictable. The many gene variants that alter your potential do not alter that. There are so many of them that they do the opposite. Genes that have some effects in certain environments have different ones in others. Life is a lesson in genetics and the lesson is the absence of predetermination. We are not built to lead one particular lifestyle but to be capable of many. Genes, environment and choices are the trinity that shapes us and we shape them in turn.

Not all of the environment that matters is biological. The physique of heroes in Hollywood has been influenced by the popularity of American football. Big pectoral muscles matter. In most sports the increase in power they offer comes at the cost of bulk. In American football the increase in bulk is part of the reward, so long as you can possess the tonnage of a hippo but still accelerate like a startled water vole. The pecs and biceps of Captain America are too large to suit soccer, cricket and most athletics. But America has Hollywood and American football benefits from bulk, so the common worldwide image of the masculine man is someone whose upper body is unsuited not only to normal life, but even to the needs of most sports. 'How is society possible?', asked Georg Simmel in 1910.[1] It is possible through the possession of norms, traditions, knowledge. The shape of American bodies has been altered by ideas of the ideal just as life expectancy in Mogadishu has risen because of changing norms of hygiene and nutrition. Survival after a heart attack in Belgium has gone up not only because of drugs and surgery and angioplasty, but also because Belgians live healthier lives in ways that include drugs and surgery and angioplasty but are not limited to them. What gets passed down along with our genes is our culture. It has been our environment for so long that our genes and our decisions are shaped in expectation of it. We cannot escape it and would not be human if we did. No man is an island, preached John Donne, and his young contemporary Thomas Browne agreed. 'There is no man alone', he wrote; 'every man is a Microcosme, and carries the whole world about him'.[2]

The particularities of our cultures are side effects, epiphenomena of our cultural capacity. Evolution has not selected for religious belief: it has selected for minds capable of it. Culture is constrained by our genetic inheritance but the constraint is not tight. Very occasional counter-examples – like our strong distaste for incest – do not change this. That humans have a capacity for aggression is plain, sufficiently so that there is some interest to evolutionary stories about how deeply it might be a part of us. The interest is extremely limited. It does nothing to help us understand why some cultures are obnoxious in their aggressiveness or horrific in their violence. Culture needs to be understood from its own perspective, not from that of biology, which must remain as having little of interest to say of it. The culture in Russia changed when the Soviets lost power but the changes did not stop the country being Russia. Habits learnt through years of repression, dishonesty, autocracy and ignorance have lives of their own. In 2005 a Russian man was more than five times more likely to die before fifty-five than a British one and alcohol was chiefly to blame.[3] That was culture, not genes, cutting lives short. Since then the situation has improved and the toll from alcohol has been cut – the culture has been deliberately and helpfully changed.

When maths, laws, song, poetry, accounting and consumer protection appeared in Sumerian society they changed it and changed the people in it and those yet to come. From the concept of the number zero to the tradition in British schools of devoting Wednesday afternoons to sport, culture shapes lives. Culture was what Karl Popper referred to as world 3.[4] World 1 was the physical world, world 2 our internal mental one; it was world 3 where the action was, where human minds and ideas and experiences met across countries and generations. Were it not for world 3 a human born today would be no different from one born 50,000 years ago. Because of world 3, we are: we think differently, see differently, live differently. There is no unique value in Popper's terminology; many other terms have been coined to describe culture. To talk of inheritance as exosomatic or exogenetic provides the reassurance of dressing up in Greek what can sound plain in English.

'I feel most deeply that the whole subject', said Darwin of religion, 'is too profound for the human intellect. A dog might as well speculate on the mind of Newton.'[5] He did not mention that if Newton had ever had a dog, that's exactly what the creature would have done. The difference between us and other animals is one of degree, even though the degree is extreme. To be struck by what is beyond full comprehension is the property of any thinking mind. Nations are made up of the people who belong to them but there is something in the idea of Britain or the USA, France or Germany or any other country that contains some notion of national character, something belonging to itself. We believe such things exist despite being uncertain what they consist of. Our notions are half mythical, but then nations and cultures are made up of myths as they are of people and history and traditions. Culture is the phenomenon produced by a functioning society, impossible to pin down precisely because it is the shifting product of lives, memories, habits, ideas, geography, climate, literature and tradition.

Anthony Trollope wrote of 'the Upper Ten Thousand of this our English world',[6] the nineteenth-century aristocracy who set the tone. For Shelley, it was instead poets who were the unacknowledged legislators of the age. Today we might be inclined to nominate reality TV stars, wincing that our times have declined so much. 'Men do always, but not always with reason, commend the past and condemn the present', wrote Machiavelli, and 'extol the days in which they remember their youth to have been spent.'[7] No age goes by without leaving complaints that things are not what they were. The great foaming wave of pop culture crashes over us but most withdraws. It seems unlikely that someone looking back from a hundred or two hundred years hence will feel intruded upon by celebrities in the way we do today: at least, they will not feel intruded upon by ours. It is fitting that we are more aware of our problems than our successes, for our successes require less of our attention. But the temptation of noticing all the things that are going wrong is to overlook how much goes right. That leads not only to a needless loss of cheerfulness but to mistaking the character of the world.

★

As some societies are better than others when measured by the health of their citizens, so some are better in the lives their people live. When the mass sexual assaults took place in Cologne and other cities in Germany on New Year's Eve 2015/16, attacks perpetrated almost entirely by immigrants, the concern was not solely in relation to the individuals harmed. It rested on fears that the country's norms were being threatened, that mass immigration might degrade them. Attitudes to sexual assault vary, as do those to female empowerment, and while people vary as to what they believe few vary in believing that the differences matter. Relativism has limits. A culture that holds a woman has less right than a man to walk down the street without abuse or assault is inferior to one that does not. So is a culture where people are attacked for being immigrants, as many were in Germany after the sexual assaults with which they personally had had no involvement.[8] Up until the First World War, women had the vote only in Norway, Finland, Australia and New Zealand. They did not get it in Switzerland until 1971. Democracy has spread, and where it grows it is rarely uprooted. Progress is real. Its foundation is the conviction that some forms of life are better than others, some norms more admirable, some traditions and cultures superior, some scientific theories more truthful. Language, too, is not all equally valid. It requires discrimination. It is a question of style whether language should be clear or clichéd, but the choice is not between two equal styles but good and bad. Cliché makes it easier to offer an opinion and harder to think. Language is better when it does the opposite.

Neither the taste of a pineapple nor the global trade in them can be predicted or explained by knowing the atomic constituents of pineapples or the people trading them. Biology is based on physics just as humans are based on genes, but physics is no more capable of explaining biology than genes are people.

Nor can you 'add up the attributes of individuals and derive a culture from them'.[9] Different levels of organisation need to be approached in their own terms. Cultures need to be judged on their own basis, not on that of the atoms composing them. The geneticist Sydney Brenner gave an example from biology:

> Advances in X-ray crystallography, electron microscopy and nuclear magnetic resonance methods allowed us to determine the structures of large numbers of protein molecules and even complex protein assemblies, but the problem of going from the one-dimensional polypeptide to the folded, active structure remains unsolved and may even be insoluble.[10]

He said that because he knew it to be true, and both his ability to say it and his ability to see it were the result of the culture he was born into and the history of the world that had created that culture.

Humans are not alone in having inherited norms and ideas. Pods of whales hunt in certain ways and chimps and monkeys learn from their parents to hunt and gather and use tools. The frequency with which a driver on a rural English road hits a pheasant is a cultural phenomenon, and the culture responsible is partly that belonging to the pheasant. Reared en masse to be shot, they grow up without adults to learn from. Their response to cars, from trying to run ahead of them to bolting onto the road when one approaches, is part inborn stupidity but part cultural ignorance. Other birds have more opportunity to learn by example. Many animals, like us, are cultured, they are just not cultured like us.

Great attention is paid to the timing of when fossil human bones became anatomically modern. When did our skeletons become so similar to their current form to suggest humanity?

There's nothing wrong with asking, so long as we keep in mind the proper question, the one we would ask if we could. Our chief interest is not in skeletons but people and the chief characteristic of people is their capacity for culture. When did humans acquire it? The notion of a single answer – a year, a date – is plainly wrong. Our evolution, the evolution of our bones and skeletons and lives, did not stop when our capacity for culture emerged, nor are the two things separate. Natural selection continues to operate, as do the forces of random genetic accident that aid and abet it. Our capacity for culture helped create itself and continues to do so. The notion that our ancestors were less capable in such matters glitters with the attraction of possible truth. Step back far enough in time and the possibility becomes a certainty. But the glitter, the false glitter, comes from any notion that there might be a gene for culture, one that made it spring into being. There isn't, any more than there is a book one can read to acquire it. Culture begins when you cannot remember where it was that you learnt something from. That's not my idea but I genuinely can't remember where I read it. Genes interact in rich and unpredictable ways and so do traditions and norms and the rest of our cultural world. Attempting to trace the sources of the culture in our genes is like attempting to study atomic physics in order to work out the principles of painting: there's a lot to learn and little of it helps.

What happened to human evolution between the appearance of anatomically modern skeletons 150,000 years ago and the beginnings of preserved, written, abstract thought, the poetry and law and maths and economics of Sumeria? The hardest things to explain are often those that did not happen. In medical history, it has been noted, there was an inexplicable gap of 200 years between the development of the microscope and the recognition of germs.[11] Why did writing and poetry and maths and economics not emerge sooner? It may not have been a genetic change. They just may not have occurred to us. Looking forward, the innovations it is hardest to predict are not those which rest on breakthroughs yet to happen. Many of those breakthroughs we can contemplate even though we cannot yet achieve. What is hardest to predict are those breakthroughs we are capable of already but have not thought to make since we have not conceived of them.

Culture and tradition are the temporal expression of experience and shared self-consciousness. The sociologist Edward Shils wrote of how 'the present and the past of the society are experienced as parts of the same thing'.[12] Our sense of self comes from our sense of others, past and present, real and imagined. Read Keats and Shakespeare – just grow up in a world familiar with them – and life is altered by their achievement. 'Man is a noble animal, splendid in ashes, and pompous in the grave'[13]: we affect others even after our death. We don't have to be Keats or Shakespeare to do so and they realised that. It was sensitivity to others that made them. In Willa Cather's *Death Comes for the Archbishop*, the hero is served onion soup. 'I am not deprecating your individual talent, Joseph,' he tells the friend who has cooked it, 'but, when one thinks of it, a soup like this is not the work of one man. It is the result of a constantly refined tradition. There are nearly a thousand years of history in this soup.'[14] Culture is itself 'a soup thousands of years in the making'.[15] It is unpredictable. Partly one judges it by its fruits. To point out that Hitler, Göring and Goebbels were cultured is not a nicety of speech but a truth not nice in the slightest. Culture plants seeds and sows ideas and in its fecund blend something new emerges. Trends are never guarantees. Concerts of the best of human music, representing some of the finest expression of high culture, were organised by the Nazis at Auschwitz.[16]

Our genome and our bodies are 'not an array of optimal adaptations to their immediate surroundings, but complex products of history, not always free to change in any direction that might "improve" them'.[17] The same is true of our exogenetic baggage, our culture. Sociobiology, by which people have attempted to understand sociology at the level of biology, has a good record of going down the wrong track. Practitioners first picture human behaviours as single traits – homosexuality, racism, aggression – then produce stories in which the trait offers a selective evolutionary advantage. Behind each trait lurks the idea of a gene. The idea is misleading. Culture is vital for the future of medicine but it has to be approached on its own terms, and technology will not change that.

'The notion of hierarchical levels that cannot be reduced, one to the next below, is no appeal to mysticism', wrote Stephen Jay Gould.[18] 'A claim for the independence of human culture is not an argument for fundamental ineffability.' His analogy was with the *Mona Lisa*. The painting might be dependent on the particles of paint from which it is made, and the pigments might be of interest, but 'only a fool would invoke such chemistry to explain the essence of the lady's appeal'. It is not always helpful to look too closely at the constituents if one wants to understand the picture: Rembrandt pulled people away when they put their faces too closely to his paintings.[19]

Saying that cultures cannot be judged or approached biologically is a reminder they need to be tackled culturally. Not everything or everyone is equal and some ways of looking at the world are better than others. Without discrimination, we are all eyes and no sight.[20] Some differences matter. 'We have no higher duty, and no more pressing duty, than to remind ourselves and our students, of political greatness, human greatness, of the peaks of human excellence', said the philosopher Leo Strauss:

For we are supposed to train ourselves and others in seeing things as they are, and this means above all in seeing their greatness and their misery, their excellence and their vileness, their nobility and their triumphs, and therefore never to mistake mediocrity, however brilliant, for true greatness.[21]

He was speaking to his students about Winston Churchill, who had died the day before.

Culture shapes the lives we live not only on the grand stage of world history but at every level. At the midway point of my professional medical life, I have explained to several thousand people the implications of their heart attack. The coronary angioplasty or bypass surgery, the drugs for lipids and blood pressure, the improvements in diet and exercise: I have gone over these things so many times that a conscious effort is required to make sure that I am speaking to people rather than reciting a cliché to them.* All the armamentarium of modern medicine, I explain to the smokers, even the glittering drama of surgery, adds up to less than quitting. For an individual the key choice is social and psychological, not medical. For society it is cultural:

---

* There is no difference in the words spoken, only in the music of the voice. The difficulty is that a doctor is only good in a technical sense when they are treating a problem they have seen a hundred times before. Which is to say that the mark of a fully trained doctor is to be slightly bored. Keeping going as a doctor can lead to one either switching off one's intolerance for boredom – pomposity and self-satisfaction are great tools for doing this, and those driven to them by professional demands merit a little sympathy for their sacrifice – or tolerating boredom and covering it up, which comes at a cost. The best solution, achieved by all of us some of the time, is to use the mental freedom that comes from scarcely having to think about the technical problem to think instead about the patient. Meeting people is more permanently interesting than treating diseases. But one no more wants a doctor excited to see one's disease than a pilot eager to fly a plane still unfamiliar to them.

what steps are we willing to take to discourage smoking and limit the freedoms of smokers? Even problems that can be completely understood on the molecular level of pathophysiology are not necessarily best approached in that way.

Cultural judgements have to be based on cultural value. Matthew Arnold, 150 years ago, urged his readers to hone their discrimination. He pointed out the example of those whose cultural level was poor despite worldly wealth:

> Consider these people, then, their way of life, their habits, their manners, the very tones of their voice; look at them attentively; observe the literature they read, the things which give them pleasure, the words which come forth out of their mouths, the thoughts which make the furniture of their minds.

Arnold wanted people to recognise the worth of what they lacked and to itch for self-improvement. 'Thus culture begets a dissatisfaction', he concluded, 'which is of the highest possible value.'[22]

For William Hazlitt, writing when the French Revolution (which he believed in) licensed the radical rejection of hierarchies, some seemed to him to remain indispensable. 'Where there is no established scale nor rooted faith in excellence, all superiority – our own as well as that of others – soon comes to the ground.'[23] To have any opportunity for serving and pursuing the superior parts of ourselves we must learn to recognise them, to make judgements. The alternative is that 'by applying the wrong end of the magnifying glass to all objects indiscriminately, the most respectable dwindle into insignificance, and the best are confounded with the worst'. That abuses and errors of judgement will occur has to be accepted unless all attempts at judgement are abandoned. 'I would rather endure the most blind and bigoted respect for great and illustrious names', concluded Hazlitt,

> than that pitiful, grovelling humour which has no pride in intellectual excellence and no pleasure but in decrying those who have given proofs of it, and reducing them to its own level. If, with the diffusion of knowledge, we do not gain an enlargement and elevation of views, where is the benefit?

To live in a world where we are not constantly aware of the ways in which others are better than ourselves is to live in stifling poverty. Culture gives us the opportunity for perceiving the superiority of the best parts of ourselves and the best of those we meet and the best of those who have ever lived. These qualities matter even if our sole aim is to prize culture for extending health. They matter even more when wishing to make the most of it.

Underpinning our lives, culture merits respect for what it offers and what it is. The eighteenth-century naturalist Georges-Louis Leclerc, Comte de Buffon, believed that wherever a text mentioned the Creator the capitalised name could be replaced by 'Nature'. Yet he wrote to a friend declaring that 'when I become dangerously ill and feel my end approaching, I will not hesitate to send for the sacraments. One owes it to the public cult.'[24] And when the end came he did so. That may have been the fear of an atheist in a foxhole but more likely it was something more common and finer. The rituals and traditions of society, be they as ridiculous as a shirt and tie, matter. They do so because they are our inheritance. We know we are engaged seriously in an activity when we notice our interest in those who have engaged in it before; the doctor with no interest in medical history is no more to be trusted than the footballer who cannot talk with awe of those who came before them. When we are serious about an activity we enter into community:

> In this way a man who is interested in the art of war not only acquaints himself with the performance of great generals, but he has an admiration and enthusiasm for them. So, too, one who wants to be a painter or a poet cannot help loving and admiring the great painters or poets who have gone before him and shown him the way.[25]

The evolution of our cultural existence is not hard to explain; the trend that produced it is clear. 'The characteristic which is so vital for the human peculiarity of the true man – that of always remaining in a state of development,' wrote Konrad Lorenz, 'is quite certainly a gift which we owe to the neotenous nature of mankind.'[26] Neoteny is holding onto youth. Not by aping the clothes and manners of the young but with our hairlessness, small teeth and large heads, with our delight in learning and our capacity to take delight. Humans are biologically neotenous and it is a nice question to ask whether the natural selection of neoteny was driven by physical or mental advantages. The question cannot be answered on the basis of what makes the difference now. Intelligence and culture count more than thin skull bones and a loss of a bony eyebrow ridge but that does not mean they provided the initial benefits. Evolution makes do, it takes advantage of whatever material comes up. If a body retaining some physical aspects of juvenility has a survival advantage, natural selection will likely find herself dealing with a mind that has the same. Playfulness and a willingness to learn may have been accidentally selected for as side effects of a developmental pattern favouring limbs that were short relative to torso size, a pattern that has advantages against the cold. Once selected for, though, these properties become subject to direct selection themselves. Recognising our neotenous nature can be a helpful reminder to make the most of it. Muhammad Ali was on to something when he said the man who views the world at fifty as he did at twenty has wasted thirty years of life. But that is to move from evolution to psychology. Neoteny describes a trend that resulted in us becoming who we are, not a moral force that tells us who to be. A dislike of wasting our power has to be its own justification for fighting to retain our pleasure in thought and learning. To conceive of neoteny as moral justification for behaving at fifty as we did at twenty would be not only a failure of judgement and a lost opportunity, but also a category error.

No gene for neoteny exists, any more than for honesty, although with the former we can find some genes whose effects contribute directly enough to interest us. (Understanding when they emerged might provide some evidence as to what parts of neoteny were selected for at different times in our past.) In contrast a genetic approach is unlikely to yield anything of value in understanding honesty, for all that honesty has a genetic substrate by being based, like all traits, on our biology. We can even note the recent evolution of a trait encouraging honesty, that of the whites of our eyes, which makes our gaze and our attention more obvious to those around us.* They come at the cost of displaying our interests and attention whether we wish them to or not, but the benefit they provide, the trust

---

* A characteristic that can be hidden to some extent by some serious emotional dissembling. Or more effectively with technology – a case of science influencing culture – in the form of shaded glasses.

and shared understanding they buy, is worth the price. Such an explanation is another of the sort Stephen Jay Gould called a 'Just So story'. It is not without value, but its value depends on whether we find it persuasive. It cannot be subjected directly to testing and so it is not science.

Of all the influences that will shape human lives in the future, culture is the most important. And culture itself is constantly reshaped, not always in a manner beyond our control. Good and bad acts reinforce themselves. The Polish Jew Janina Bauman escaped the Warsaw Ghetto with her mother and sister and hid among her gentile countrymen:

> Some time and several shelters passed before I realised that for the people who sheltered us our presence also meant more than great danger, nuisance, or extra income. Somehow it affected them, too. It boosted what was noble in them, or what was base. Sometimes it divided the family, at other times it brought the family together in a shared endeavour to help and survive.[27]

The ability to shape culture was apparent to the Germans too, hence Himmler's 1943 efforts to seize for the fatherland a prized copy of Tacitus's *Germania*, a much-fetishised early account of the German people. Ideas, he knew, made history. Hence also the Nazi encouragement of Polish anti-semitism, and the care taken to make sure that while food was scarce, vodka and pornography were not.[28] The notion of the virtuous Pole contains some power to form such a person, just as the notion of English fair play and personal freedom does something to bring them about. In the cultural world qualities really do come into being by virtue of our belief in them. Buffon was right to embrace the comfort of a loving God. Hollywood's large-chested male heroes, like its female ones, portray an image that is not quite real but do so in such a way as to make it more so. They do the same when those heroes and heroines are braver and better than us. We may benefit from the movies we watch just as we may be owed some credit for the tastes they reflect. Heroism and virtue may seem silly guides to real life but they are not silly ideals. A sense of history and of virtue comes from an appreciation of how it is the world has been improved, and pointing out the ways it has happened over the centuries helps bring future gains closer.

That we have culture is genetically determined – what sort of culture we have is not. Genes explain nothing about the differences between cultures, our chief interest and our most practical one. Genes do not explain culture any more than biology explains psychology. Insights are limited to the grandiose and meaningless or the precise and trivial. Everything is what it is and not some other thing, and pretending sociology is neuro-physiology is a shortcut to thoughtlessness. When sociology looks too injudiciously towards biology for ways of explaining things, just as when biology reaches too eagerly towards physics, the results are nonsense at best. When the reaching out is judicious it is most often not enlightening (perhaps, 'our culture is dependent on our biology'). The power to understand sociology and anthropology at a biological level is as limited as explaining plant biology through quantum physics. Plants are made of subatomic particles but it does not follow that this is the way to understand them.

The Sumerian inventions of writing and money are abstractions that advance our capacity to think. Our cultural wealth is a form of artificial intelligence. When we watch or read or hear thoughts and ways of thinking they leave us able to participate. Great athletes can offer something of the same: when we watch them we feel part of their physical power or grace and are lifted. They form part of our collective self-consciousness, they expand our communal sense of human capacities. The best of culture adds to our lives just as the worst subtracts. Knowing the difference matters. Collecting information about the world is inferior to searching out the best in it, the parts most worth knowing.

Understanding how consensus and collective self-consciousness work is not essential. They continue whether we understand them or not. But the problems of groups and how they relate to each other will continue to dominate society, whether we approach them through instinct, politics and culture or through sociology or psychology. We can be confident that biology and medicine and the hard sciences will be of little help and, more likely, will contribute harm by offering the false appearance of insight.

The liberalism that took fire in the 1960s increased our ability to see cultural value we were previously obtuse. But it has come at the cost of our confidence when differentiating between the lastingly worthwhile and the ephemeral. We have usefully downgraded the power that prejudice and custom exert, but our profit has been mixed with loss. 'Without the aid of prejudice and custom,' Hazlitt noted, 'I should not be able to find my way across the room.'[29] The canon of great literature, for example, is less agreed upon now than it was a hundred years ago, and even when there is agreement, the fact that it is in name only, and represents no deeper conviction, is demonstrated by that literature going unread. A hundred years ago the great poems in English were not only broadly agreed upon, they were also known: privates as well as officers fought in the First World War with copies in their backpacks and in their memories, and as a result their experience of the war was shaped by their common possession of high culture.[30] Technological changes and mass media play a part, diluting much of what was once agreed upon as being most of value, but the part they play is on the stage of culture, not of technology. The future of culture is, as always, uncertain, and equally as always it is worth fighting over. Being clear about what it is that we value and wish to fight for is a good first step. Noting how some cultural traits mean people live longer, healthier or happier lives can support us in making our judgements.

Class and inequality

Class differences power health differences. That has been plain for as long as class differences have existed, which is certainly longer than we have. Power, class and competition are strong influences on society. The collision of individuals is the fundamental force: that power, class and competition are best understood as the secondary phenomena produced by living societies is as plain as noting they are not unique to humans. Social status affects health in other species too, and in fact seems to do so in all of them that have societies.[1] It was wrong for some to conclude from nature being red in tooth and claw that human communities needed to be the same: an analogy is not a requirement. But differences will always result in struggle, even if only through competing tastes and ideals. Complete equality is impossible without complete lifelessness.

Concerns about social classes leading to genetic divergence – concerns about social inequalities being magnified by the processes of natural selection – are more recent. They do not date back to the early evolution of microorganisms, only to the development of human communities. What 'they' will do to our society is a question that would have begun to form as pack animals began to think. Modern concerns about classes or groups polluting or outbreeding us are not new; they were shared by the ancients (albeit with more focus on cultural attributes and less on skin colour).[2] In the nineteenth and again in the twentieth century they only felt new. That was because they had been dressed with the trappings of genetics by Galton and other nineteenth- and then twentieth-century scientists keen on justifying their prejudices with eugenics.

Distinctions and inequalities are found wherever animals form societies or plants communities. The question is how to manage them. In Britain life expectancy for newborn boys born to the highest social class is six years longer than for boys in the lowest; for girls the gap is just under three years.[3] London has long been an example of a city where rich and poor live close together, meaning the expectations of a baby born in one street differ wildly from those of its neighbours. Maps from the eighteenth century show it. So do ones today of life expectancy as it relates to different stops on London's Underground, from ninety years for those near Knightsbridge, to seventy-five around Whitechapel.[4]

Inequality is harder to measure historically, our pre-Roman and Medieval ancestors having not had our modern aptitude for form-filling. The children of British monarchs, dukes and duchesses between the fourteenth and seventeenth century lived largely as long as commoners.[5] The figures, with life expectancy at birth rising from twenty-four for men and thirty-three for women in 1330, to forty-five and forty-eight by 1779, are massively skewed by infant mortality. Those surviving the first five years of life, the most dangerous, would have had a decent chance of three score and ten. Equally, the virulent nature of infections meant wealth was less protection from the infectious hazards of other people's situation. The example of Prince Albert's death from typhoid in 1861 is often used, the queen's consort succumbing to that disease of poverty as fatally as any slum dweller.

Large class differences in longevity began appearing from the eighteenth century. By the middle of the nineteenth the top aristocrats had life expectancies of fifty years for men and sixty-two for women compared with the British average of forty. Since then inequality has decreased not only relative to overall life expectancy but in absolute terms too. We are less bounded by the position we are born into. Progress can stall and recede and even when underway it can be intolerably slow, but progress has nevertheless been made. Shils referred to 'the movement towards equality and particularly the diminished deference granted to properties like descent, ethnicity, occupation, wealth and authority in modern liberal democratic societies'.[6] Compared with 1750, 1850 and 1950, the leap forward has been great.

Society is no longer so strongly identified with its brightest and best – or at least the meritocracy of celebrity pays less attention to science and high art than to the glitterati – and its worship of its richest and most advantageously born has softened. Much has been gained by the change in both cases, but even in the latter there have been some losses. The general hankering after aristocracy suggests a lingering fondness for the idea of an upper class, a fondness with more to it than a fantasy of being a resident of Brideshead or Downton Abbey. The great stately homes are often beautiful. They would never have existed but for an inequality capable of spanning generations. Inheritance taxes have made the world fairer at the cost of reducing the number of landscaped mansions. It is a more than reasonable price to pay but it remains a price.

Inheritance taxes have recently declined, a promising sign for stately homes but reason for concern that inherited inequality will rise. Inheritance taxes 'pit two vital liberal principles against each other. One is that governments should leave people to dispose of their wealth as they see fit. The other is that a permanent, hereditary elite makes a society unhealthy and unfair.'[7] Such problems need compromises, continually adjusted in the light of ongoing arguments based partly on the evidence of practical results. Health inequities are useful measures.

In 1872 Francis Galton set out to investigate prayer.[8] He noted that people of all faiths believed in it but few faiths believed in the prayers of others. He also spotted that doctors rarely prescribed prayer as a means of cure nor made it a key part of their own intervention: 'To fully appreciate the "eloquence of the silence" of medical men, we must bear in mind the care with which they endeavour to assign a sanatory value to every influence.'[9] He noted that stillbirths, when published in the newspaper, showed no correlation with whether the parents were religious, despite religious parents, during the anxieties of pregnancy, being likely to pray. His chief conclusion, however, was drawn from his observation that people across the Empire prayed for the health of their monarch. He compared the longevity of royalty with that of clergy, lawyers, doctors, tradesmen, naval officers, army officers, men of letters and science, artists and gentry and lower members of the aristocracy. Members of the royal family, he showed, died younger than all. Galton did not conclude that prayer was useless.* Might 'the conditions of royal life... be yet more fatal... [such] that

---

* This is partly because he noted its utility was not solely in fulfilling the wishes it articulated. 'The mind may be relieved by the utterance of prayer. The impulse to pour out the feelings in sound is not peculiar to Man... There is a yearning of the heart, a craving for help, it knows not where, certainly from no source that it sees. Of a similar kind is the bitter cry of the hare, when the greyhound is almost upon her; she abandons hope through her own efforts, and screams – but to whom?'

their influence is partly, though incompletely, neutralized by the effects of public prayers'? Possibly.[10]

Showing a relationship does not prove a causal link, nor prove in what direction it might run in. Health influences wealth but not as much as wealth does health. Those in poorer health are more vulnerable to dropping out of their class. Downward social mobility has to be something that fair societies encourage, since without it there can be no mobility at all and status has to be fixed and hereditary. But fair societies will also seek to make mobility meritocratic. The nature of that meritocracy, and how to pursue it, can never be definitively settled but we certainly do not like it to include the random effects of illness and disease.

There is a social gradient to health in olive baboons as there is in British civil servants. Spend more on health care, and health is often unchanged as a result. Spend on reducing social inequality and health gets better. Some societal traits are as influential on health as blood pressure, diabetes and hospitals. Education, wealth and personal freedom – through not only the freedom from repressive laws, but also the possession of personal autonomy – are aspects of health care. When Reverend Malthus noted the tendency of populations to enlarge he found his factual observations leading to political arguments. Given human appetites, the population would always come up against a check and left alone those checks would be war, famine and disease. Political solutions were needed to direct human lives down better paths. They still are and always will be. Continually adjusted compromises are needed for insoluble but unavoidable problems. Equality of opportunity conflicts with autonomy. There are no perfect solutions. Autonomy and equality of opportunity are meaningless if they consist only of the opportunity to be the same as everyone else.

Relative inequality matters. It does not melt away when people possess a certain level of food, income, housing or anything else, which is to say we cannot solve its problems by all getting richer. 'Stress, self-esteem and social relations may now be one of the most important influences on health', said the *British Medical Journal* back in 1992.[11] It sounds like the sort of sociological conclusion one is wafted towards by wishful thinking, not driven to accept by evidence. But the evidence repeatedly suggests it is true.

Wanting to see if inequality mattered even when incomes were astronomical, researchers hit upon a group in which economic poverty was non-existent. Perhaps other studies had failed to pick up on subtle differences in wealth, with some people able to afford healthier lifestyles. Here that question would be off the table. Only differences in social status would be left. They compared actors and actresses nominated for Oscars with their colleagues who had been in the same films and were of the same age and sex.*[12] Those who won Oscars not only lived longer than those who had never been nominated, they also lived longer than those who had been nominated but had not won. The 'results suggest that success confers a survival advantage', noted the authors. The difference came out at an added four years of extra life. The health benefits of winning an Oscar were roughly equivalent to the impact of completely abolishing cancer.

Something about social success is good for people, and not in a way ever likely to be replaceable by a pill, injection or gene. We are unable to eliminate social hierarchies and unable

---

* The exception was for 1951, when Katharine Hepburn was nominated for her role in *The African Queen*. She was the only woman in it.

to hope we can abolish their effects through pharmacology or genetics. How much they shape our lives is modifiable, but it depends on policy and sociology and culture.

Mobility can be geographical as well as social. Some of this accounts for the greater inequality between London Tube stops than between the top and bottom social classes. Migrants from poorer countries have lower life expectancies than those of the nation they move into. They also have greater expectations than the nation they leave, a difference not all down to the benefits they gain by moving. By being the ones who make the move they mark themselves as different. Host countries receive those with the advantages that let them move. Some of those advantages are inherited monetary wealth and the social privileges that bring opportunity; others are ingenuity and initiative.

Social class and income matter, as do differences of religion and ethnicity, diet and exercise and smoking and lifestyle. Education counts too, particularly a woman's: something about female empowerment is good in an immediate and direct way for human health. This is not something we have traced to an enzyme or DNA sequence, nor will it ever be.

Another form of inequality does have a simply biological cause. It makes a difference, from country to country, of five to eight years. Inequality in this regard is not getting better as the years go by: not only are women living longer than men, as they always have, their advantage in absolute terms has grown. Since 1841 life expectancy in Britain has doubled and a woman's advantage over a man's has doubled too (Fig. 5).[13] Male advantages in other spheres reduce our interest in attacking this inequality. It is certainly modifiable. It may be genetic and may manifest through risk-taking behaviour (particularly in

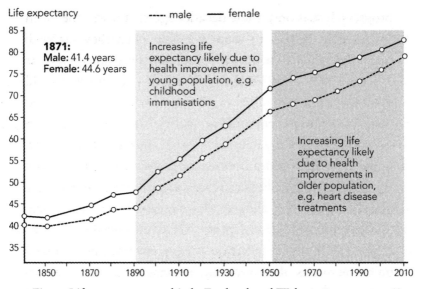

Fig. 5. Life expectancy at birth, England and Wales, 1841 to 2011.[14]

adolescence) and in higher cardiovascular risk from middle age, but those can be reduced without the need to change our genes. Male advantages in power and earnings should not prevent us paying attention to male disadvantages in dying young. That would imply a willingness to trade what should not be tradeable. No part of progress on any of these issues should be dependent on progress elsewhere.

For all the discrimination and inequality and unfairness that remain in modern life – along with the uncertainty over how much is acceptable* – it is easy to overlook the enormous pace

---

*   The vast majority of drugs were discovered and developed by dead, white, First-World men, just as most books taught as part of an English literature course were written by them. That represents the results of centuries in which the talent and genius of many were suppressed or suffocated to our mutual cost. The future brightens if we do better. For now, though, if we altered pharmacies and libraries to offer strictly equal representation, the world would be more equal but not better.

of progress. It was only a few decades ago that it was the norm for women in Britain to stop working when they married. We have had only two female prime ministers but fifty years ago, before Mrs Thatcher became the first, even one would have been unthinkable. The notion that society is weakened by female empowerment still lingers in obstinate pockets and in reactionary nostalgia, but it has evaporated beyond the bounds of what would have seemed realistic to imagine even fifty years ago. It is unclear to what extent the benefits of more sexual equality include the fact that our world is in many ways a kinder, gentler place now than even a few decades ago. On a small scale, bullying at schools has gone from being relied upon as the means of turning boys into men into being deplorable and carefully watched out for. On a large scale, war and violence have declined.[15] Certainly we are kinder and gentler, more cautious and more risk averse. No coincidence that over the past centuries, murder rates have plummeted.*[16] Ever greater value is put on human life. Seatbelts in cars, doors on the back of buses: safety first, safety everywhere. We fight wars without wishing to have our soldiers die and we agonise over, rather than celebrate, the lives they take and lives lost as indirect consequences.[17] We also put soft-cushioned floors down in playgrounds, and the two are connected. My own hospital hosts tours of schoolkids to teach them how to avoid minor injuries, and in the basement mortuary the British war dead from Afghanistan and Iraq have undergone careful post-mortems in the hope of improving battle armour and survival.

Diminution of infectious disease made this possible. Random

---

* That this is less so over the past fifty years does not undermine the notion that society is going to get increasingly kind but it may suggest we cannot rely on that trend to lower murder rates further.

misery is less normal. We get more risk averse as we get better at managing risk. Heartbreak is reduced and risk-reducing intrusions become an ever greater part of our lives. We will become ever keener to use medications that lower risk by amounts that today seem hardly worth bothering with, ever keener to reduce hazards at work and at home, in peace and at war. One of the prices will be an increased sense of needing to stick with instructions and follow protocols.* Adventurousness is one of the factors that gives adolescent boys a greater chance than girls of getting themselves killed. We will curtail it. Much will be gained, much lost. We will make our world tamer and safer. Adventure will not be lost completely. Too much always remains in the daily strife of domestic and professional life. But we will be less like Odysseus, smiting the sounding furrows with our oars in search of battle, and more Telemachus, his son, working 'by slow prudence to make mild / A rugged people, and through soft degrees / Subdue them to the useful and the good'.[18]

Socioeconomic success reduces fertility. The need to have more children as insurance for those that die dissolves with falling infant mortality. Barriers to contraception fall and opportunities for women expand. So does the importance of children's education, the need for them to be thoughtful and capable rather than another pair of hands for the endless demands of manual labour. Relationships change. Over the past fifty years, across the developed world, university-educated parents have

---

* In the 2003 film *Pirates of the Caribbean* the modern young heroine accuses one of the pirates of breaking their own protocols for behaviour, the Pirate Code. 'The Code is more what you'd call "guidelines"', he replies, not being so modern in spirit, 'than actual rules.'

begun spending more time each day with their children than parents who did not go to university.[19] The seeds of inequality and unrealised potential are not all sown by tax policy and schooling.

Falls in fertility, and lower fertility among the better off and most educated, have given rise to concern, from anxieties about the checks to progress by the unwashed masses of the recalcitrant poor, through to their impact on ongoing evolutionary trends, through to worries about racial purity and racial degeneration. These concerns crop up repeatedly. It was the Spanish aristocracy's concern over dilution of their *sangre azul* by Moors and Jews two centuries ago that gave us our term 'blue blood'. The British politician Enoch Powell, despite having superbly condemned those seeking to overlook the British murder of Kenyans on the grounds that the latter were lesser people, articulated an exaggerated view of the long history of racial anxiety when he expressed his fears about black immigration to Britain with a Roman quotation, suggesting that 'rivers of blood' would result. Nor have the twentieth-century's mass slaughters burnt such fears from our minds; the American desire for a wall with Mexico is driven partly by concerns over American culture being swamped by illegal immigration, and David Cameron, as prime minister, spoke similarly of the 'swarm' of migrants seeking to enter the UK.[20] Less developed nations have higher birth rates but that merely suggests global overpopulation is best dealt with by ensuring development for all. The recurring notion that lower classes, or less desirable racial or religious groups, will outbreed their betters and subtract from the quality of societies, is different.

To the extent that a lack of education, culture and civility is a threat to society the solution is to worry not about differential birth rates – no liberal society can do much to change these

– but about differential opportunity. From a society in which the lower classes could not read we have one in which they can excel – against the disadvantages of their birth, and against disadvantages we worry have increased in recent years, but nevertheless against disadvantages that have been vastly reduced.

Does society's success depend on the reproductive triumph of its most successful members, or will its ideals work out their own salvation in the next generation regardless of whether the rich have fewer children than the poor? Putting the same concern another way, will entrenched inequality lead to increasing genetic differences between those of different social classes and ethnic groups? Do different cultures and experiences of opportunity sum up, over time, into a genetic parting of the ways, one that might create new races and even a new species? As an immediate prospect the notion belongs to the lunatic fringe, but as a distant possibility it is more persuasive. The fear that the differences between us have been or will become biological is there in the genetically divided castes of Aldous Huxley's *Brave New World* and David Mitchell's *Cloud Atlas*, and a thousand other books besides. It is there in every notion of races containing peculiar genetic attributes, positive or negative, from criminality to industriousness, running speed to musicality or violence. Some traits are expressed more in some races than others: the statement is a tautology since we define a race by virtue of being a group in particular possession of a trait. Skin colour is what we often have in mind. If variation in the shape of a nose can be genetically inherited, is it not wishful thinking, or ideological blindness, to argue that there is no possibility that something like intelligence or character might be too? And if such an inheritance is possible, does it not become correct to suppress or avoid what is worst and to encourage or support the best?

'At the time the book was written,' Galton wrote of his first edition of *Hereditary Genius* in 1869, 'the human mind was popularly thought to act independently of natural laws'.[21] The book considered the implications of the ideas that Galton's cousin, Darwin, had put forward about the human mind as the product of natural selection. Given the heredity of traits, and the many successes of selective breeding to enhance them in agricultural animals, how should societies respond? The idea of blood running true, of traits passing down a human lineage, had new vitality.

The belief that classes or races are genetically more or less desirable rests on the belief that our fate lies not in ourselves but in our genes: that the spread of genetic variation in a population accounts for identifiable traits in society. Such beliefs are inconsistent with the unpredictable intricacies bridging the genetic code with the characters of people and communities. Class, inequality, civility and culture cannot be understood through genetics.

That one level of organisation cannot be reduced to another is not because we lack knowledge, nor because of some spiritual quality incomprehensible to science. It is because certain patterns only exist, only make sense, at certain levels of organisation. They come into being as we ascend a hierarchy from quark to atom, molecule, gene, cell, organ, organism, society and culture and history. No level represents truth any more than any other, only an arena in which certain properties exist and are subject to certain approaches and description and understanding. Traits we prize or detest in certain groups or cultures may be apparitions of prejudice and misunderstanding or they may be real, but they are not real at the level of genetics.

'If you ask a physicist what is his idea of yellow light, he will tell you that it is transversal electro-magnetic waves of wave-length in the neighbourhood of 590 millimicrons', wrote Schrödinger:[22]

> If you ask him: But where does yellow come in? he will say: In my picture not at all, but these kinds of vibrations, when they hit the retina of a healthy eye, give the person whose eye it is the sensation of yellow... The sensation of colour cannot be accounted for by the physicist's objective picture of light-waves. Could the physiologist account for it, if he had fuller knowledge than he has of the processes in the retina and the nervous processes set up by them in the optical nerve bundles and in the brain? I do not think so. We could at best attain to an objective knowledge of what nerve fibres are excited and in what proportion... But even such intimate knowledge would not tell us anything about the sensation of colour, more particularly of yellow.

Who we approach for a description of yellow depends on what part of it interests us. A physicist is not less correct than an artist. Their responses refer to different levels of organisation. Ralph Waldo Emerson was wrong when he said there was no history, only biography, just as wrong as he would have been had he said there was no society and only individuals. Skin colour is a trait which can be analysed at the level of races, if one defines races by skin colour. Usually, one has in mind other traits as well. The trouble is those traits are often only half in mind, and even when fully conscious any association they may have with levels of epidermal melanin is often either fictional or cultural or both, and its cultural part cannot be understood via biology.

Morality, intelligence, educational achievement, aptitude, talent, genius, character and ability: for none of these things is there a gene or even a cluster of them. Genetic variability from person to person makes a pool of genetic variation within a population, a pool which neither racial nor class differences demarcate. People tend to marry those like themselves but the tendency is mild. The internal genetic divisions in even the most rigid caste-driven and polarised societies are lines cut by a knife through water.

In 1873 Galton, struck by the difference between races, wrote to *The Times* with a constructive suggestion. China had shown through its history 'a remarkable aptitude for a high material civilisation'. The contemporary state of China was unimpressive but only since 'a temporary dark age still prevails, which has not sapped the genius of the race'. Galton suggested the Chinese be invited and encouraged to settle in Africa. 'The gain would be immense to the whole civilized world if we were to outbreed and finally displace the negro'.[23] In *Guns, Germs and Steel*, Jared Diamond described how accidents of geography and ecology were responsible for civilisation developing where it did. Galton's point is swept away in the wake of Diamond's knowledge. But might similar arguments be true today? Might some of the socioeconomic plight of African nations – a failure far from complete but completely real – be down to inferior genes? In an era of gene therapy, if genetic differences were responsible, they could be fixed. What historically has appealed most to those with a racist faith in biological determinism could, if shown to have some basis in genetic reality, become a tool for black empowerment. If the barriers that hold Africa back are genetic, the solutions might be too.

The logic holds but not the premise. Genetic variation in a group – any group – is greater than that between groups. None of this variation comes close to explaining the traits we want it to illuminate, those of culture and psychology, ability and personality. Fleeting correlations of no practical significance do not even hold true from one setting to another. 'The problem is not that knowledge of such group intelligence differences [between black and white or between men and women] is too dangerous,' wrote Steven Rose in a *Nature* letter titled 'Research into group differences isn't wrong, just pointless', 'but rather that there is no valid knowledge to be found in this area at all.'[24] When it comes to the length of our femur, the size of our nose or the shape of our eyes, genetic differences provide a window of understanding we have cracked open a fraction. It does not follow that genetics stands ready to open such windows onto less physical and more complex traits.

Human characteristics like intelligence and culture, morality and imagination, compassion and thoughtfulness reveal no genetic variation at a racial level. That is not because people have not looked. They have. It is because that is not a level at which these properties appear.

Genetic variation between even the two most separate and isolated groups of humans on the globe – the Inuit and the Khoisan bushmen, for example – provides no route into understanding the differences in their histories and cultures. That has major implications for those who worry about the future effects of differential breeding rates. The genetic difference between one class and another in the same country is minuscule. The argument would be easier if one could replace 'minuscule' with 'absent' but one can't; it isn't true. Any two groups, whether selected by skin colour, class, earlobe size or just the roll of a dice, will contain genetic differences – that's the nature of random variation with so many genes to play with, and it is enhanced to a tiny but real degree by the fact that people tend to marry those like themselves, even down to matching for earlobe size.[25]

But genetic variation between widely separated racial groups offers only confusion for those wishing to understand the traits of history or culture or of almost all of those belonging to individuals. Those looking for genetic technology to alter societies are going to be disappointed. With no gene for educational achievement, marital harmony or creative power, no pursuit of those qualities can be based on injecting anything into anything else, at least not when we are thinking of pipettes, eggs and genomes. Injecting enthusiasm into a growing child, or supportive norms into a society, is a different matter. Those worried that the future of their societies will be determined by the different breeding rates of classes or groups or races need to recognise that their concerns are not genetic. They may or may not exist, they may or may not be real on a cultural or societal level, but at a genetic level they are a fantasy. Cultural differences are important enough to be taken seriously, which means not mistaking them for biology. When you misuse genetics to try and explore culture you shine a beam of darkness intense enough to obscure what light there was in the first place.

Autopsies of Ötzi showed what was in his stomach and what his body was made of; they give few clues about what was in his mind. What were his values, and the thoughts he harboured? How much were they determined by the qualities of the society he lived in? How much was his access to the best of that society limited by his social position? 'When Tocqueville, visiting America in the early nineteenth century, said that the new democracy was imaginary, he didn't mean that it was illusory: he meant that the haves and the have-nots could share the same condition, even if only in their minds.'[26] Wondering about Ötzi means wondering about his culture. All culture is imaginary. It might be written down but it isn't real until someone reads it and the letters on the page become ideas in their mind. What makes it culture is that before it was in their mind it was in someone else's.

Genetics is genetics and culture is culture – every thing is what it is, said Bishop Butler, and not some other thing. One of the advantages of taking care not to confuse genetics and culture is the freedom to think more clearly about what is valuable about the latter. Culture's value is in the society it makes. One where people live longer, happier lives is better than one where lives are brief and miserable. Freedom, thoughtfulness, kindness and creativity are better than their opposites. These differences are not in our genes and cannot be adjusted with genetic technology.

The numbers of those excluded from civil society has shrunk. As society has developed it has required more from its citizens. Literacy spreads when people need to be able to read to do their work, and when they learn to read for that reason they read for other reasons too. Translating the Bible into languages that common people could read was a brave move by the imaginative, and an unavoidable consequence of society improving. The question was when, not if.

Amartya Sen pointed out that famines do not happen in open societies. Absolute poverty, a part of daily life throughout human history, has become a solvable problem for developed societies. Relative poverty is different. When we see health inequities we worry. We worry not only because they are bad in themselves, but because they suggest society is unequal in other ways too. Health inequities represent lives cut short and limited by illness, and they suggest that those same lives are blighted by limitations of opportunity that restrict not only life, but also liberty and the pursuit of happiness.

Automation poses a problem for a society maintaining a

large class of unskilled people. If these people were genetically different from others, incapable of acquiring more sophisticated skills, the problem of inequality thus produced would be unsolvable. Automation will remove the need for many types of work – it places no limit on the amount of work that needs doing. The work that needs doing is not limited to that needed to satisfy our physical needs but is bounded by our desire and imagination. Automation entails the need to train people to function at a level above that of shelf-stackers and taxi-drivers, just as our predecessors altered their societies to take seriously the need to train people above the levels of illiteracy allowed by agricultural economies. Shelf-stacking and taxi-driving are no more dishonourable than ploughing by hand, only as vulnerable to becoming equally as redundant. Automation and robotics will lead to the elimination of large numbers of menial jobs. That has the potential to reduce drudgery and free people for more interesting lives, but if steps are not taken to make sure that such lives are opened up to them, they will be freed from honourable drudgery only to be condemned into unemployment. The point is that we no more need to be constrained by existing class differences and inequalities than we need to leave the outcome to the unregulated winds of a free market. We have deliberately improved before. Preparing for the close of the Second World War, President Roosevelt signed into law the GI Bill, meaning the troops came back with an opportunity to start their lives again with a better education. It worked. The Australians had achieved the same after the First World War. Even the most ardent supporters of free markets understood that some things worked best if organised by the state: they understood that because no one close to the military, which in those years was everyone, could reach any other conclusion. SNAFU was a Second World War acronym but no one suggested the war could be fought better by private individuals making their own decisions.*

Social realism and gritty reality are terms which suggest that those who really understand what's going on in the world should feel bitter about it. To a degree they should, since the suffering and the unfulfilled promise are real. But it is also true that society and its opportunities have improved beyond the expectations of our ancestors. Future improvement is not guaranteed but it seems likely – the trend is there – and it becomes more likely if we are confident in its potential and perhaps still more so if we are aware of how bad the alternative could be. Reality is gritty but it is also cheerful. Genius can appear from anywhere but we knew that anyway. If it weren't inexplicable, it wouldn't be genius. The real grounds for optimism lie in the ordinary. The more fortunate classes do not perform better in the world because they have better genes, they perform better because they are more fortunate: they are the recipients, generally speaking, not of unique and unexpected combinations of genes but of the more predictable benefits of inherited wealth, position and opportunity.

Some benefits, including some of health, will always depend on relative advantages. It's not enough to succeed, quipped Somerset Maugham; one's best friend must also have failed. But mental and cultural success are not necessarily like that. Fewer and fewer opportunities for the less skilled would be a calamity were it not for the fact that the less skilled have all the potential of the most. Automation has the chance to

---

* The Australians had achieved the same after the First World War. The Australian Imperial Force Education Service, set up in 1918, aimed to 'help each individual soldier in mind, character, and occupation, and by doing so to help the future of Australia after the war'. 'A.I.F. Education Service – A Splendid Scheme', *The Mail* (Adelaide), 346, 10, 1918.

be disaster or success and will undoubtedly be some mix of both. It will mean ever fewer seats in second class but the efficiencies it brings will allow for a massive and potentially unlimited expansion in first. We do not need to preach enforced equality to believe in widening opportunities or the sermon of improvement, nor do we need to possess any set of political views save those touched by the Enlightenment belief that the world is improvable. Such a belief is not the same as having faith that all will be for the best in the end. An awareness of how badly economic and technological changes can impact on people can fortify our efforts to ensure they don't.

Automation and technology will reshape society but we have a choice in how, which makes it important to want the best. If Ötzi died in the Alps with the best thoughts of his society in his mind as he gazed around him, we would view his life and the culture he lived in differently from if he had been a drudge with no opportunity to be better. That some cultures are worth more than others is demonstrated by demography: not in its headlines of population numbers but certainly in its measurements of life and death, literacy and social mobility and freedom. The kindness, thoughtfulness, freedom and creativity of societies are no less valuable for being hard to measure; life expectancy and survival and health no less so for being so countable. When lives are longer and healthier it is good evidence they have probably been happier and freer. The trends are encouraging. The qualities they should most encourage in us are optimism and effort.

Sleep

High on any list of futurological fantasies is the control of sleep.

We spend a third of our lives asleep. Wasted time: let's do better. So far, we've failed. And there is reason to think we will continue to do so, not only in the near future but for ever – that innovations to reduce or eliminate sleep are not possible.

Activity levels in single-celled organisms often fluctuate predictably but they do not really sleep since they cannot properly be said to be awake. Pretty much every other form of life does and one does not need to rise very far up the tree of life before one can delete this sentence's opening two words. Some worms and flies sleep, and like everything else that needs sleep they suffer without it. Most fish sleep; it may be that all of them do, even those that appear not to and need to keep moving in order to drive water over their gills and survive. Birds, certainly, are able to sleep with half their brain at a time, leaving one eye open and alert. The small number of apparently sleepless fish may be doing something similar.

There has to be a good explanation for sleep. Its costs are too high for there not to be. An organism that sleeps is not resting and conserving energy. It is doing both of those things, but it is doing something more since it is possible to rest and conserve energy without being asleep. When you sleep you withdraw from the world. Animals sleep not only when there is nothing much to do, like a lion after a big meal, but also when there is a very great deal to do, from searching for food to ensuring one does not become a meal. The lack of activity and awareness comes at a price of vulnerability and missed opportunity. The presence of sleep is different from the absence of activity. Something vital is going on.

Apes, ourselves included, sleep more, and sleep better, than monkeys. This may have come about simply because we got bigger while still living among the trees. Being large and arboreal entails the need to create a bed to stop yourself waking up as you fall. Creating those beds put us in a position, literally, to sleep better. Sleeping a lot is not particularly human; other creatures sleep more. Those that graze generally sleep less while those that hunt and gorge take a longer break. But it may still be that evolving to get a better night's sleep was followed the next day by being able to live more brightly. 'Our results', wrote two physical anthropologists of their research, 'suggest that relaxed sleeping postures may have been enabled by sleeping platforms as a behavioural facilitator to sleep, which could have allowed for greater sleep depth and next-day cognitive capacities in both great apes and hominins.'[1]

Odd that a period in which we seem lifeless should be so absolutely vital. Yet it is. A disease called fatal familial insomnia (FFI) illustrates that. Steadily destroying the brain, it destroys sleep, and with sleep gone, life follows. The torture of sleep deprivation makes it an unnerving way to die.

How do we know that the disease kills people by depriving them of sleep, rather than depriving them of sleep as it eats fatally away at their brain? 'It is for the doctors to decide whether sleep is such a necessity that our very life depends on it', wrote Michel Montaigne, 'for we are certainly told that King Perseus of Macedonia, when a prisoner in Rome, was done to death by being prevented from sleeping.'[2]

Neither doctors nor Romans are needed: science stands ready. In 1995 two Chicago researchers took rats and put them on a half-metre disc suspended in a cage. There was as much food and water as the rats wanted. The cage was divided in two with the disc in the middle a couple of centimetres above water. In each experiment, one rat served as the control and the other as the subject. When the subject fell asleep, the disc was rotated: in order to avoid being pushed into the water, the subject rat needed to wake up and walk along the disc. When that happened the control rat, on the other side of the divide, needed to do the same. The difference was that when the subject was awake, the control could sleep. The object was to compare the fate of the two rats. 'All rats subjected to unrelenting total sleep deprivation died, usually after 2–3 weeks', ran the report. 'Evidently sleep and its substages serve vital functions.'[3]

What is so essential? It cannot be rest because one can rest without sleeping. The subject rat was quite at liberty to rest. It might be that we are so used to sleep – meaning we have evolved in its presence for so long – that our rest cannot physiologically now happen without it. But that would not explain why sleep developed, with its enormous costs to evolutionary fitness, or why it persists. If it can be reduced to a need to rest, it would have been. Sleep could gradually be transferred to a state of lazing. It hasn't happened and it doesn't happen, not in us and not in any creature like us. Something other than the need for rest must have driven sleep and must be driving it still.

In FFI one aspect of sleep, when sleep becomes impossible, breaks through into waking life:

this condition of persistent subwakefulness or drowsiness was interspersed with episodes of unresponsiveness during which the patient would be animated by massive twitches and perform complex purposeful gestures that they subsequently referred to dreams. These episodes, which we termed oneiric stupor or enacted dreams, are one of the most characteristic features of FFI.[4]

The aspect of sleep that forced its way through was not restfulness but dreams. People being deprived of sleep to the extent it was killing them, people quite able to rest, experienced breakthrough convulsions of dreams. Might dreams be the essential quality that differentiates sleep from rest, without which we die?

For that to be the case, it would have to be true that the situation was not unique to humans, just as sleep is not. The researchers who killed the rats did not comment on whether their bodies made any last efforts to dream. But we can prove that other species, too, do dream. The term 'oneiric stupor' comes from the Greek for dreams, *oneiros*. Oneiric behaviour was a term used by the late Michel Jouvet, the neurophysiologist who helped explore the phenomenon of rapid eye movement – REM – sleep. He showed that dreaming appeared to be as much a part of the most evolutionarily ancient portions of our brain as it was of the later additions. He also showed that if you destroyed certain small parts of a cat's brain, you eliminated the physical stillness of sleep. During the periods when an observer might expect it to be dreaming, during periods when it was otherwise asleep, the brain damage meant the cat was not still. It moved. It did what we might imagine a cat would do when acting out its dreams. There was no way of asking the cat, Jouvet wrote, but any sensible interpretation 'would lead us to believe that cats do dream'.[5]

Brain imaging with electroencephalographs (EEGs) and functional magnetic resonance imaging (fMRI) scanners can tell you if someone is in REM sleep. We know from experience that people in REM sleep are often dreaming, and so with scanners and electrical recordings we can predict that they are. But the only way of knowing they have been dreaming, the only way in which the electrical and MRI appearances of dreaming were discovered, remains the gold standard for determining if dreaming has been taking place: you poke the person and when they wake up you ask them. Against that standard, the power of brain scans has nothing extra to offer. It is notable that dolphins and whales have no REM sleep. The likely implication is not that, uniquely among mammals, they do not dream. It is more likely that dreaming is not unique to REM sleep, only that REM sleep is the period when we remember our dreams if we are woken. The implication of all of this is that we sleep in order to dream.

It is impressive to say that we can see the activity of dreaming with an fMRI scanner but the impression is overdone if we don't point out how little this tells us, or how limited it is. In a play Molière has a medical student being asked why opium makes people sleep. He is being examined to see if he is worthy of becoming a doctor. He answers that opium makes people sleep because it contains a sleep-inducing virtue.* His examiners applaud. When it comes to talking about sleep, science and medicine have a habit of saying things that do not amount to

---

* '*Mihi a docto doctore / Demandatur causam et rationem quare / Opium facit dormire. / A quoi respondeo, Quia est in eo / Vertus dormitiva.*' Most English translations give the question as 'Why does opium induce sleep?' and the answer, 'Because it has a dormitive virtue'. But the candidate is not even replacing sleep with a synonym: *dormire* merely becomes *dormitiva*. *The Works of Molière*, vol. 10, 'Le Malade Imaginaire', John Watts (London, 1748), p. 362.

much, like highlighting the awesome power of fMRI to reflect what someone tells us when we ask them. Dreaming is often explained on the basis of being the random firing of neurons when the brain is at rest. It's an explanation that doesn't fit with what happens when the firing of neurons is randomly stimulated: dreams are not created. Nor does invoking randomness pass the test of Occam's razor. It introduces a new mystery – how random neural firing can result in dreams – without explaining the existing mystery of the importance of sleep.

We sleep less with age and do not know why. It might be that we have less need of sleep and dreams, or that we are unable to sleep and dream with the youthful vitality we once had. It is likely to be some mix of the two, and likely also to be nothing that medicine, in the form of drugs or surgery or gene alteration, can do anything about. No single pathways or targets seem addressable. Nor should we expect them to be. If easy options with only benefits existed, evolution would have found them. The conclusion has to be that sleep, by virtue of the dreams that come, is an essential part of biological life and cannot be removed.

We complain about lack of sleep and are right to do so. We are right not because our lack of sleep is unique but because it is commonplace. Lives immemorial have been lived on the edge of the line between as much wakefulness as we can get and as little sleep as we need. There is a tension between the two and it is proper to feel the strain of it.

More evidence for the unavoidable position in our lives of sleep, and of futurological fantasies of overcoming it being poor predictors of the future, comes from our history of using drugs. Alcohol and opium are long familiar to us. Temporary sedatives and stimulants have their uses, but they are not the same as interventions that alter the nature of sleep. The host of modern drugs to influence sleep, drugs that have been searched for with all the energy of an industry quite aware of where the billions are, are largely failures. The benzodiazepines – Valium being a successful trade name – were sold and swallowed as drugs that enhanced sleep. Like alcohol and morphine, they are sedatives and in the long term their benefits are small or swallowed up by their harms. If you have long-term problems getting enough sleep, avoid benzodiazepines. Drugs to make us wakeful share similar properties. From coca, cocaine and amphetamines through to caffeine, their temporary effects can be useful to many. None, though, provides profound, lasting and helpful changes to our wakefulness or our need to sleep.

We are built to sleep. People vary in how much they need, but no single biochemical route exists to turn a nine-hour-a-night slugabed into a four-hour powerhouse of wakeful industry. We should not expect one to be discovered. Managing the tension between what sleep brings to life, and needing to be awake to live, has always lain beyond the province of medical technology. It will continue to do so.

Race

Will races homogenise? There has always been interbreeding but for sexual creatures all breeding is interbreeding. Which is another way of pointing out that races, in some respects, don't exist. More precisely, we use the concept of race in such a muddled way that its potential usefulness, as a way of classifying and thinking and human variation, is reduced.

Race means different things to different people. It means different things to the same person at different times and often at the same time. In biological terms a race would be a relatively isolated population, breeding chiefly with itself and different in character from other races, while still capable of fertile reproduction with them – a subspecies. Subspecies reflect not objective demarcations but the conceptual lines it can be useful to draw. The history of biology, particularly from the eighteenth to the mid-twentieth century, is full of efforts to classify subspecies and races, in every context from snails to bacteria to humans. It was part of the great urge to classify that lay behind a great deal of good, but also of many unread encyclopedias and fruitless lives. Classification needs to be useful: it is not a good in itself. One can divide and classify humans by the size and shape of their earlobes, but the world is not enriched by the effort.

Biologists' problems with race are magnified out of all proportion by the well-meaning public-policy attempts to categorise people by 'ethnicity' – understood to be a polite term for the otherwise taboo word 'race'. In the UK, one is routinely asked to classify oneself by a bizarre mixture of skin colour, geographical ancestry and nationality. Categories include White British, Irish, Black British, other European, Asian, African and Mixed. In the USA, people are categorised into, among others, Latino, Hispanic, African or Caucasian. In the USA, 'Asian' means someone from Japan or China, whereas in the UK, it tends to mean someone from the Indian subcontinent. For obscure reasons, 'Caucasian' means White in the West, presumably based on assumptions about Palaeolithic population migrations into Europe from the Caucasus. But, in Russia, people from the Caucasian republics are popularly – and denigratorily – referred to as 'Blacks.' The confusion is complete.[1]

It is not that the concepts and terms are not real, only that they are muddled. What is it that one is trying to think about, the effect of skin colour or country of birth, of culture or of genetics? Any trait will be distributed in a manner that varies geographically. Leclerc, the Comte de Buffon, was one of those early enthusiastic encyclopedists of the eighteenth century. He was alert all the same to the dangers of endless subclassification. Variation could not helpfully be cut up into endless entities, each distinct and unique. That was not the way to understand reality. Hence Leclerc's lastingly influential and very practical definition of a species as consisting of those creatures who could interbreed and produce fertile offspring.

Races, like species, have no Platonic essence – any definition is a working one whose truthfulness is its utility. The geographical isolation of a primitive world, stretched out over the past tens of thousands of years, did not come close to producing the genetic drift necessary for two widely separated human groups to split into different species; Khoisan bushmen can breed with Inuit as easily as those from Oxfordshire can with the Welsh. The barriers are orders of magnitude greater when it comes to the notion of social classes splitting into different species. No obstacles of geography there, nor any cultural fences that come close. The odds are against someone moving from the lowest-earning fifth of society into the highest, but they are not outlandish. With complete mobility – if one's place in the final hierarchy was entirely random – a child born in the bottom fifth would have a one in five chance of ending in each of the divisions. In Britain the barriers of class and culture cut the odds of making it to the top from that 20 per cent down to 11 per cent. Far from perfect, but farther still from the sort of social isolation needed to make nightmares of genetic separation come true. The perception in Britain is that the odds are worse and social mobility is lower than it is. In the USA the perception is that the odds are better and social mobility greater – but it's actually less than it is in Britain.[2] It's not minimising the importance of social mobility, or dismissing concerns about it falling in recent years, to point out that fears of it vanishing are oversold. Americans don't worry enough about their class system, which is what their low level of social mobility represents, but if they worried about class partitions hardening into genetic ones they would be going too far. Concerns about social classes separating into different species may be restricted to science fiction writers and lunatics, but the anxiety that different social classes possess different degrees of genetic potential is more insidious and more widespread. It also isn't the case.

'Science has now made visible to everybody the great and pregnant elements of difference which lie in race', wrote

Matthew Arnold, 'and in how signal a manner they make the genius and history of an Indo-European people vary from those of a Semitic people.'[3] Nothing wrong with pointing out that the spirit of Jewish history has a distinct character but attributing it to genetics makes conclusions less likely to be useful, true or interesting.

Is it unreasonable to speculate that genetic and cultural heritage go together? The intent does not have to be disparaging. The violinist Isaac Stern joked that Cold War cultural exchanges between the USSR and the USA were straightforward: 'They send us their Jews from Odessa and we send them our Jews from Odessa.'[4] But the ease with which disparagement can rear up is plain: Jews, blacks, gypsies, homosexuals, the working classes, the upper classes – pick the group of your choice. Any attempt at genetic analysis will not necessarily be wrong since all those groups, like any others plucked at random, will have some observable pattern of genetic variation. But the variation seen will have little or no bearing on the cultural characteristics, and the attempt at reducing them to genetics offers a long history of being harmful to our understanding and to each other. Weigh up the chance of a genetic approach being the right one – of being the correct way to analyse a difference in culture – and you balance a feather with a lump of lead. Race and ethnicity are not best approached from the presumption that they can be understood on the basis of DNA.

Muddy thinking dirties the water. Brutalise complexity and you produce brutality. The differences between human groups are hard enough to articulate at the best of times. The most one can hope for are tenuous generalisations. Undermine the effort by mistaking its nature, by replacing a discussion of cultures with a false image of biology, and it collapses before it begins. What results is usually as wrong as it is ugly. 'Of all vulgar modes of escaping from the consideration of the effect of social and moral influences on the human mind,' wrote John Stuart Mill, 'the most vulgar is that of attributing the diversities of conduct and character to inherent natural differences.'[5]

Races vary and genetics vary and undoubtedly there is some correlation between the two, however small or uncertain. The many times in which the attempt to identify it has been done badly should make us cautious, but should they make us despair? Are there no insights to be gained?

The answer is that there are not. Not because there is no signal, no information linking genetic to racial variation, but because the mismatch between the signal and the noise is too great. 'Height may be 90 per cent heritable, but a conclusion, in the nineteenth century, that the shorter average height of blacks was due to genes would have been quite wrong.'[6] Culture itself is more subtle than height. The noise outweighs the signal to such a degree that no attempt to differentiate the two can be expected to succeed. It can be expected to fail, and anyone making the attempt puts their understanding or their intent into question. We have moved on from John Stuart Mill's 'inherent natural differences' to talk of specific genes, and the jargon of genetics brings an impressive sense of accuracy. It's misleading. Our ability to use genetics to predict human lives – as opposed to identifying particular genetic diseases – is so poor as to barely be there at all.

With race, as with class and inequality, biology is of limited use and capable of wild misuse. Dislike and fear of others gets too easily transformed into fear of genetic difference. The qualities of different classes, races or religions, or skin colour, cannot be accurately attributed to genes but have to be thought about for what they are. Putting a high or a low value on a cultural property and then defending or attacking it on the basis of it being biological is failing to take it seriously. Some cultural qualities are fictional, the product of prejudice, while others are real, aspects of the variety of human groups. Some attributes are attractive and some repulsive. They need to be seen for what they are, and they are not seen for that if they are intuited as being reducible to genes.

> Is it not, then, a bitter satire on the mode in which opinions are formed on the most important problems of human nature and life, to find public instructors of the greatest pretension, imputing the backwardness of Irish industry, and the want of energy of the Irish people in improving their condition, to a peculiar indolence and insouciance in the Celtic race?[7]

That was written in 1848. It sounds dated, partly because recent Irish social, cultural and economic success means racist fashions now ascribe constitutional laziness elsewhere. But they do it in the same way. Their prose and genetic terminology will be modern but that's a change of dress not of substance.

We can return to the question we started with, the question over whether human races will become more similar, will homogenise. It should be clear that this is not a question over whether blacks and whites will become more similar, or Catholics and Indians, or Caucasians and Aryans. None of these are races – the first two refer to skin colour, the third to a religion, the fourth to a subcontinent (either to those who live there or those who once did; it isn't clear), the fifth and six to euphemisms. But traits from skin colour to earlobe size do vary in a predictable geographical manner. So do genes for arm and leg length, for the skin folds around the eye, for the size and shape of the nose.

All of this will homogenise to some extent. The homogenisation is certain while the extent is not. It will happen because people move more than they did before. The geographical spread of genetic differences between north and south Wales, in which the distributions of some variants get greater in one direction while others follow different and sometimes opposing patterns, will be as affected by the mobility of modern life as will everywhere else. It took 10,000–15,000 years for migrants from south-east Asia, crossing into Alaska and travelling down through the Americas, to take on the skin colour that has begun to match the latitude they settled in. Without modern life the trend would have continued, for skin colour is highly selected by sunshine, and indigenous central Americans are still lighter than those in central Africa. Not only has the selection pressure eased with advances in clothing, suncream and dermatologists, but the geographical isolation that allowed it to express itself has been reduced. Skin colour is likely to homogenise to some extent, as are all other human traits. Variation will always remain and with it there will be geographical and ethnic patterns, for genes as for cultures.

The result of more outbreeding will not be blandness. To whatever extent the qualities we value most in humans are influenced by particular patterns of genes, rather than by the influences of culture and history and upbringing, the result will be new combinations and new possibilities. Even had we an understanding of the links between genes and gene expression beyond that which might ever be possible, such an understanding (explaining what had happened in the past) would fail to predict what will happen in the future. The number of factors and the explosive potential of their permutations are unknowable in advance.

★

To what extent is the superiority of East African distance runners, or black American and Caribbean sprinters, reducible to genetics?

Answering the question has to start with making it more precise. By East African we do not mean people who live there, we mean people whose ancestors have lived there for a large number of generations. We don't even mean East Africa overall but a small area within it. Races reflect no objective divisions within a species so their definitions need to be carefully stated. The origin of humans in Africa means that Africa contains the greatest degree of human genetic variation. Dividing the world by skin colour carries the implication of dividing up variation evenly, of blacks being equivalent to whites in the sense of being a comparable group. In that both possess a skin colour they are, but with regard to any other genetically identifiable trait they are not. Success in distance running or sprinting is not a black trait or an African trait, but a trait of certain groups of black Africans and not others.

The chief interest, in looking ahead to what human lives might become, is in considering the extent to which causes can be understood. Understand the cause of a trait and you can nurture and encourage it. To do that you have to know if your efforts need to aim at a cultural property or a genetic one. The technology and technique for the latter are going to wildly improve.

The vast majority of human genetic variation is common to us all: races, however you define them, contain only small fractions of it. Is there any interest to us in these fractions? Yes, if their distribution helps us understand what they are. When it comes to running, some genes have been identified which correlate – to a small, uncertain but real extent – with outcomes. We have fewer of them for athletic success than for height but that should not surprise us. Although height is profoundly shaped by culture and upbringing, athletic success is even more so. That means that the links between genes and outcomes are weaker, subtler and even less direct. One should always accept the simplest explanation even if it is not very simple and even if it does not explain very much. Better that than an explanation that is clever, satisfying and wrong.

We can glimpse occasional links between genetics and athletic performance but we cannot get very far. There are genes for which variations seem to have a measurable effect.* Their effects are small. They are associated with outcomes rather than determining them. This does not mean that some patterns of genetic inheritance do not set people up to be better for sports than others. Obviously, they do. We don't need any knowledge of the genetic basis of ability to note that some are born with more than others, just as they are with a greater ability to grow tall or study or work. That genes contribute to these things is not in doubt. What is in doubt is our ability to understand genes sufficiently to use them to predict outcomes. Currently, we are not even close. We are not even sure the link can reliably be made. Read a very simple computer program and you can see what it will do. But humans are something else entirely. To what extent will the genetic component of athletic success be analysable much as we would analyse a simple computer program? To what extent will it remain impenetrable, emerging only at the level of organisation of a person growing in the world, just as the effect of a poem is not apparent except from reading it as a whole?

Sport may become amenable to some minor extent to genetic analysis. Quite how much is unknowable, but it does not look like being very much, certainly not in the foreseeable future

---

* ACTN3 in muscle fibres, for example.

and possibly not ever. We have consistently overestimated the degree to which our lives, in their variety, are biologically determined. The consequences of having done so have often been bad. The most we can confidently say about our future is that this habit will continue.

Stress

What could be more important when considering our lives than contemplating the role of stress, and the prospects for it in the future? Perhaps the only thing better would be not contemplating it: or at least considering how poor a reward we get for our rumination.

Are we evolved for stress? Sure we are. The fact doesn't take us very far. A life without stress would be a life unlived. But how much stress is the right amount and how much is too much? Unless the answer aims to consider how to get the best out of ourselves, with a consequent need to consider what the best might look like, the question isn't worth asking. Stress can be measured in a host of ways but it cannot be defined down into a level or a number.

In 1994 the American neuroendocrinologist Robert Sapolsky wrote a best-selling book called *Why Zebras Don't Get Ulcers*. Modern life, he pointed out, was incessantly stressful. Zebras had moments in their lives of abject terror, moments when death literally pursued them across the plain, but those moments were rare. Modern life, in contrast, was fretted with stress. It never stopped. The commute, the battle for a parking space, the uncertainties of employment, the strains of family life, the pressures of needing to compete. Had he written in the era of Facebook and social media, they would have been in the mix too.

It's an immediately recognisable story, soothing in its familiarity. But the heart of it is hollow and false. If you have ever had a pet rabbit, you get a feel for life as a zebra. For prey animals, death may only leap out and give chase from time to time, and only catch them once, but they spend their lives quivering in fear of it. They startle so easily because for them the shadows always have sharp teeth and every noise is an alarm. Like so many prey animals who find safety in numbers, they are social. That adds to the burden, their hierarchies being a continual added source of anxiety.

Humans are not prey animals but we have long lived in a world where death padded behind us on soft feet. Like rabbits and zebra, our death was often violent, even if the main threat was not from a different species but from our own. Beyond that we lived with unique awareness of possibilities no less horrible. Disease and accident have always blindly scattered their gifts and no animals are blind to them in return. Awareness aids survival. Cowards die many times before their deaths but the valiant, who never taste of death but once, meet it sooner. Humans, more capable of apprehending possibilities, more aware of the arbitrary fates ready to be heaped upon them or on those they loved, have long lived in a world pregnant with stress. There is something very odd, whatever the strains of contemporary life, in thinking that the tension of the modern world pulls tighter than the old. Anxiety about commuting and working is real but its prominence comes from what else has slipped away. The steady improvement in mortality rates, the evaporation of infectious illness as a common cause of premature death, the huge reduction in violence: these things are treated too lightly by any story that paints modern life as especially stressful. Crowded roads are infuriating but to hold in your heart the belief that modern life overall is worse or more stressful than life a century ago, when random death stalked us with such greater frequency, is strange. It must be conforming to fantasies because it does not fit with facts. The notion that stress caused ulcers has melted away. It did that when we discovered the bacterium that was actually responsible. The German news magazine *Der Spiegel* has run a column called *Früher war alles schlechter*, 'Everything used to be worse'. They were right. The bacterium can now be killed with antibiotics.

Stress, like ageing, power, class, culture, intellect or happiness, is not a single physical or psychological entity, either in its manifestations or in its causes. That's not to say that the word and the concept of stress are bad, or useless, but it is absolutely to say that there can be no drug 'for' stress in the same way there is no gene 'for' it. The 'for' implies an equivalence, a one-to-one relationship between a cause and an effect.

If stress is not a disease, not in the way of flu or other infections, the door is open to not worrying about it so much. That's not the same as not worrying about it at all. To aim for a life free of stress is to aim for a life free of striving. So long as we have hopes and interests, striving and struggling to pursue them is more stressful than indifferently letting them slip by. It's also better. Which is not to say that stress is always productive, or always the by-product of some attempt to live life fully. Here medical research has at least a small amount that it can contribute. The aspects of stress that seem to come at the highest cost, that convert into shorter lives via raised cardiovascular risk and other mechanisms, appear to be those to do with lack of autonomy.

If we wish to suffer less from unproductive stress, from stress that does nothing to help us pursue our desires, the answer is not going to come from gene therapy or bioprosthetic implants or drugs. It will come from culture, from socioeconomics. Specifically, it will come from shaping the world as much as possible to help make people's struggles those that aid their pursuit of their desires. To try and do a job well that you fervently wish to be good at is stressful but it is a healthier type of stress, both psychologically and physically, than the stress of an indentured servitude that destroys the soul and fibroses the heart. The loss of less skilled jobs to technological change offers the chance of both harm and of benefit. If we fail to raise the standard of education we will be left with an underclass, impoverished in opportunity and belittled in autonomy. Both of those are disadvantages in which stress will shorten lives as well as subtracting from them. If we use the riches that technology creates, if we use them to put a greater portion of our effort into education and into creating a culture and an economy where more individuals can better pursue their interests, the quantity of stress may end up being no less but its quality will be different. Autonomy does not require that every man be a master of others, only that all have the wherewithal to feel master of themselves, as much as any of us ever can be.

Drugs exist and have always existed that obliterate stress, from alcohol and opium to modern mind-numbing equivalents. None works by some magic method of altering one facet of our lives, divisible from the rest. They dial down stress by dialling down life. Better societies will not mean more options available for those who wish to opt out, but a smaller number driven to do so.

Creativity

'Anyone who has mastered the wisdom of the scientific method and therefore knows how to think scientifically undergoes any number of delightful temptations', wrote Chekhov in 1888 to a friend:

Present-day hotheads want to embrace the scientifically unembraceable: they want to discover physical laws for creativity, they want to grasp the general law and the formulae by which the artist, who feels them instinctively, creates... Hence the temptation to write a physiology of creativity... A physiology of creativity probably does exist in nature, but all dreams of it must be abandoned at the outset. No good will come of critics taking a scientific stance: they'll waste ten years, they'll write a lot of ballast and confuse the issue still further – and that's all they'll do. It's always good to think scientifically; the trouble is that thinking scientifically about art will inevitably end up by degenerating into a search for the 'cells' or 'centres' in charge of creative ability, whereupon some dull-witted German will discover them somewhere in the temporal lobes, another will disagree, a third German will agree, and a Russian will skim through an article on cells and dash off a study... and for three years an epidemic of utter nonsense will hover in the Russian air, providing dullards with earnings and popularity and engendering nothing but irritation among intelligent people.[1]

It's a brilliant letter. Chekhov even underplayed it a little: a physiology of creativity definitely exists. We often experience creativity as something we owe to a force outside ourselves – as inspiration, a dream, an idea, a conception coming by grace, some force or spirit giving life to our imagination. The feeling of creativity describes something important and real but not literal. Our creativity is based on our physiology just as all parts of ourselves are.

The physiology of creativity exists in that the physiology underlying our creativity is understood. But all dreams of understanding creativity at the level of physiology must be abandoned at the outset. At the outset of artistic effort, certainly, and at the start of any attempt to understand art. The only way to do that is to understand it as art; rip it apart into the pixels, electrons and neural bursts it is made up of and you lose everything you valued about it to begin with. One could no more learn a foreign language by being given a list of the neuronal changes required. Neuronal changes are certainly needed, but they have to be made as a result of studying the foreign words.

Creativity, imagination, fertility of mind – these qualities must be achieved if artificial intelligence is to be true to its name. Computers are better than people at chess because computers have more computational grunt and chess can be reduced to computations. The day a computer beats a person at chess through gut feeling, through a moment of inspiration, its designers will have achieved something more.

Chekhov was correct, in 1888, to suggest that creativity could not be embraced scientifically. Brain scanners and genome sequences give us more data than Germans poring through the temporal lobes of corpses. But the quantity of data is not what counts. Millions of genomes, details on individual neurons and neurotransmitters: none of these help us locate creativity in any useful way. Pointing to particular genes and particular regions of the brain gets us nowhere: we knew before we started that the biological structures giving life to creativity were in the brain and that the design for the brain was in our genes. Pinning it down further does not equate to lighting it up. Illumination depends on embracing creativity for what it is, a mental and cultural phenomenon. Creativity is a property of a certain level of organisation, a property of a working mind. It is based on lower levels of organisation but does not exist in them. A map of the neurons involved would be as informative as a list of the chemical elements they contain. When it comes to making the most of our own creativity, the study of physiology can only be a rude distraction. The situation would be different if there were any likelihood of a gene for creativity, or a neurotransmitter, or a circuit. There is no possibility of any of those things. They feel likely because the metaphors we use when thinking about the brain lead us to speak sometimes as though such things existed. Creativity is the product of neurophysiology but not analysable at the level of neurophysiology, just as the different characters of dogs and cats cannot be understood on the basis of their atoms, only by observing the living creatures.

We have no way of understanding the physiology of creativity in any way that adds to our appreciation of it. There is no prospect in view of that changing, not even a dim apprehension of one. Our interest in developing creativity through artifice, through computing, is unaffected by that, but our success in that regard is neither close at hand nor likely to be of much use when it comes.

What can be usefully said is negative. Creativity is not predictable. It cannot be read from someone's social class or sex, their skin colour or their genome, nor their background, upbringing and education. Such things have an effect but the effect, even if it is clear in its generalities, is opaque in its specifics. Teach children to read and they are more likely to develop literary genius, but genius cannot be produced by a formula. We cannot design creativity with science. Educational and parental strategies are testable, through formal experiments or normal experience, and testing what works for ourselves and our children will always remain productive of useful improvement. Understanding the limits of our powers is not the same as saying we should limit those powers we possess.

Has genius got more or less common with modern life? What aspects of education are best designed to bring it out? Is a better education for all likely to raise the general standard at the cost of eliminating the best? Might long formal education and a more organised, safer life reduce the chance of another Twain or Dickens, who both left school at twelve? None of the answers are clear and some of them are not relevant but the questions can be helpful. There is something necessarily poetic about creativity, and whatever the word poetic means, it contains the certainty that the quality of value cannot be split into the building blocks of which it is made. 'The Genius of Poetry must work out its own salvation in a man', wrote Keats in 1818. 'It cannot be matured by law and precept, but by sensation and watchfulness in itself – That which is creative must create itself'.[2] He had trained under the greatest surgeon scientist in the country and while working as a surgeon himself had removed a bullet from a woman's head.[3] He knew when the physical substrate for life was the proper scene of attention and he knew when it wasn't.

The future of creativity does not seem amenable to being augmented in any straightforward way by technology, unless it is by technology being used to enrich and widen and encourage our culture and our education and our lives. No precise cultural recipe for creativity exists, but many recipes for diminishing it have been discovered. Authoritarian regimes and ideologies that chop people to size, slicing off their freedoms to fit them to a model, do the trick nicely, as do poverty and disease and lack of opportunity. The fact that stubborn rebellions occur against all of these, from Solzhenitsyn writing in the Gulag to Austen scribbling novels on her portable writing desk, make the generalities no less true. Genius is always an exception, always identifiable by its uniqueness. The genius of a baby is its individuality, and its individuality is always partly unfathomable. It has to be: to an extent, genius always creates itself.

Talent can cluster. Such clusters are evidence, certainly, but it is hard to know what they are evidence of. They might be the result of one intelligence sparking others into life, or of some cultural or historical shift or pressure acting on many. Galton, in his *Hereditary Genius*, took clusters as proof of genes for brilliance – but they are not even proof that anything non-random is going on. Cast seeds at random onto the soil and the plants will come up in clumps, not regularly spaced. Equally, eminence can be transmitted across generations in a non-random way without being genetic:

> Although it has been found nearly everywhere that eminence runs in families, it is just at this point that one must proceed with the greatest caution. The environmental bias in the data is patent – other things being equal, a son may find his way smoothest if he follows the calling in which his father excelled.[4]

Stupidity and dumbing down, thoughtlessness and a failure to value the best of what has been achieved, incivility and violence and intolerance: the threats to creativity are real and recognisable and tend to be the same that threaten other aspects of our lives. Numbered among them, in a minor way, are expectations that creativity can be reduced to cells and physiology or fostered through drugs and implants. Such expectations amount to something, but even at best only ever to wasted time.

The role of passion in creativity is vital and hard to understand and impossible to think about at the level of neurons. Without passion, there is only calculation. Passion can take the form of a reverie as easily as an ode, a caress or even an observing, memorising gaze, but it has to be there. How it gets there is a stumbling block for those contemplating artificial intelligence, and one they can best hope to tackle by observing how nature overleaps it. We are born passionate. The aesthetic impact of life is plain in the sense of wonder babies greet it with. Those looking for a gene for this will be disappointed, those wanting to replicate it with a pill or by activating some brain centre will waste their lives and may waste the lives of others. Neither the gene nor the neuron nor any brain centre holds the key.

As our technology changes our metaphors change, and each time the intoxication of a more sophisticated technology can make people forget that metaphors are metaphorical. Creativity and passion exist at the level of whole people. We may get better at fostering them or we may only learn how to remove some of the obstacles that stand in the way of them creating themselves, but we run up against a paradox. The obstacles are part of the solution. The difficulties count. Free verse can be a vehicle for genius, but it also offers generous demonstrations that a lack of rules does not necessarily lead to an increase in quality. 'Nuns fret not at their convent's narrow room', wrote

Wordsworth: he meant that the form of a sonnet was restrictive but the restrictions sometimes helped. We can take heart from the paradox only being partial. We do not have to embrace every difficulty and hardship. Some of the tedious rote-learning of Shakespeare's minimal education may have given life to his mind, and some may be worth considering, but our schools can aim for better. The global reduction in heartbreak from premature death and disability may have robbed us of some of the great art that broken hearts would have produced but they have granted us more than they have taken. The early death of Shakespeare's only son helped give us his later plays but it robbed us of others, and robbed us entirely of anything the son might have been capable of. By the time he was my age Keats had been dead twenty years. The serious business of wondering what parts of modern life might encourage genius does not need to become a wish that life might once again be corroded by misery and early death. King Edward VI grammar school in Stratford-upon-Avon would not get good results from adopting its methods of four centuries ago. If creativity were that easy to germinate, those looking to neurophysiology, genetics or technology might have a hope.

Eating and drinking

Since history began we have known which diets were good and which bad. The confidence is consistent; all that changes are the beliefs. The confidence is not justified and the knowledge has been fashion. What is called the evidence base has improved but compared with other areas of medicine it's a century behind. The evidence is harder to acquire and strong opinions are too easy to come by. Medical attitudes to alcohol are a good example of the muddle, generally being a reflection of the views of the doctors closest to the microphone. When the British government's guidance on healthy alcohol intake recently changed it was not because of any new evidence, simply because the group with the government's attention had different views from their predecessors.

Noticing what has happened yesterday and the day before is a good guide to what will happen tomorrow, and much of it will continue to be fashion. Like asceticism this has its place but neither should wear the mask of science:

Just as the first advocates of abstinence were undoubtedly maladjusted, the first enthusiasts of moderation were surely people lacking in appetite... It is not the first time that charlatans, misguided and well spoken, have come to consider a virtue, that which is a well-organised vice.[1]

Honoré de Balzac stuck to ground that rightly belongs to opinions. 'An empty stomach makes an empty mind', he argued, adding that 'it could be said, perhaps as accurately as la Rochefoucauld said it, that good thoughts come from the stomach'.[2] He was neither the first nor the last to believe that, psychologically, we are what we eat. 'How many of our joys that we think intellectual are purely physical! This joy of the morning that the poet carols about so cheerfully', wrote David Grayson in his 1907 *Adventures in Contentment*, 'is often nothing more than the exuberance produced by a good hot breakfast.'[3] Jeffrey Steingarten called his second book of food criticism *It Must've Been Something I Ate*, noting how deficient we were in making such a remark when we woke up feeling refreshed and eager. J. H. Kellogg agreed with the connection but hearty food, he believed, heated the desires and disordered the morals. His cereal replaced cooked breakfasts in the confident expectation that a blander diet would dampen libido, reduce masturbation and inhibit the resulting tendency to communism. Your corn flakes have designs on you.

Such attitudes will not go away and nor should they. The only environment in which humans stop battling over how best to live their lives is one authoritarian enough to obliterate humanity. What will change, more prosaically, is that we will get a better idea of what people eat. Big data will see to that. Shops and banks already track what we buy to an unprecedented extent. A part of life that has been hard to see clearly will sharpen into focus. Academics will cotton on to its potential for investigating associations between diet and health: researchers will spot papers to write and companies some useful publicity from supporting them. Not that the results will be of much use, except to research careers and PR departments. Too many other factors play a part, intervening to prevent observers confidently concluding that an association is a causal link. Alcohol in moderation – even in generous moderation – persistently shows a beneficial effect in observational studies. There is reason to think the benefit may be fictional, the result of people who live healthier lives being more inclined to enjoy a drink.

Research that just observes what people do will always be subject to such confounding, to the possibility that the differences are due not to what people do but to the fact that the groups who chose differently were different to begin with. To be reliable, a study needs to randomise, to allocate people to one choice or another. Such trials in diet are difficult – they need to be long and large and they need to get people to stick to whatever they are randomised to. They also lack the support of drug companies willing to fund them. This last is not a minor point. A single recent trial of a new cardiovascular risk-reducing drug cost a billion dollars.[4] What government or charity is going to come up with that sort of money for studies of diet? Easier to pontificate. There's a satisfaction in telling people what to do that can't be found in saying you're unsure about it. The largest reliable trial of a dietary intervention looked at the effect of dishing out free nuts or olive oil.[5] The trial concluded that doing so was beneficial, but it was too small and short to say whether the impact was trivial or important. To arrive at that useless conclusion, the trial had enrolled 7,500 people and followed them for five years. It's possible that the world will embrace randomised trials with an enthusiasm never yet seen, to the extent of large portions of the population submitting to have their diets randomised by eager researchers, but it doesn't seem likely. Governments and charities and those with opinions to sell will continue to push their half-invented lists of good and evil.

Too much food is certainly harmful. Of the deaths caused by being overweight, more than two-thirds come from cardiovascular disease.[6] Obesity will go on becoming more important but not because it will reverse the gains of modern life. Obesity's importance will rise because such gains will continue. The life expectancy of fat people will continue to go up and as their health improves in other ways their obesity will come to account for a bigger proportion of the ill health they suffer.[7] It will continue to be a bigger proportion of an ever smaller total.[8]

Questions over the magnitude of effects will gather a greater share of our attention. That is different from saying they will grow more important. They are already important, but we are stuck too often just with lists of good and bad. And since almost everything can be both, from calories to talcum powder, those lists become more plainly useless as they expand. What magnitude of impact will a dietary choice have? Adding a statin to your diet reduces your risk of a heart attack or stroke by about half.[9] Plant sterols – supplements that also lower cholesterol, and that form a part of various health-oriented margarines and yoghurts – have a smaller effect, about a sixth as powerful, equating to a drop in risk of about a twelfth.[10] They are also significantly more expensive. At what point does something become worth doing? The question is a personal and not a scientific one but it can only be answered if science quantifies the consequences involved. Our freedom to choose is threatened more by lack of information than overly zealous regulation. At the moment we are too often merely free to guess.

The drug ezetimibe illustrates the uncertain value of marginal gains. By blocking the absorption of LDL (bad) cholesterol from the gut, it lowers cardiovascular risk – by a small amount, about a fifth as much as a statin.[11] The finding has not resulted in many people taking it. The gain feels too small to justify a drug. But it also illustrates the extent to which our choices are not rational, either because they are based on mistakes or because they are based on a failure to quantify. The realistic impact of actually trying to eat a healthier diet is likely to be smaller than a 6 per cent per year relative risk reduction, which is what the drug provides. Yet the newspapers are crammed with recommendations for diets and none for ezetimibe. Ezetimibe blocks absorption from the gut but is not itself absorbed. Vitamins, by contrast, are drugs that are absorbed. In the developed world almost half the population take a vitamin supplement.[12] Their benefits for health have been extensively studied. Unlike ezetimibe, the benefits are not small. They are non-existent.[13]

Since a number of people are born without the protein that ezetimibe targets, we can see what the effect might be of taking the drug from the day you were born. The longer term impact is unsurprisingly greater than the shorter. Those without the protein are half as likely to suffer heart disease as those who have it.*[14] As ezetimibe goes off-patent and gets cheaper, use of the drug may change, but it is unlikely to change much. Technology will do more. Imagine ezetimibe no longer being a separate pill but simply folded into whatever pill is individually tailored for us each day: a small benefit now comes at no extra effort whatsoever. A 6 per cent relative risk reduction at the

---

* There is a separate but important question about why so many of us do have the protein, when its only effect appears to be that of making us more likely to die of heart attacks. The question gets more pressing the more our power to manipulate the protein grows.

price of a tablet a day is probably insane for almost all of us. An extra 6 per cent risk reduction from the same tablet we take anyway is not.

No one would consider taking ezetimibe from birth, from childhood or even from young adulthood. But if the drug consisted of a single intervention – a vaccine to knock out the target protein – and if the intervention were part of a nasal spray or injection being given for other reasons anyway, the situation would be different. Other studies support the idea that being born with a natural predisposition to low cholesterol is hugely beneficial.[15] Drugs capable of swapping newborns over into such healthy categories would be immensely more powerful than those we use today. If we took them once and forgot about them they would be less intrusive too. We use statins and ezetimibe to retard the progression of disease once it has bitten into us. In the future we will alter ourselves – with drugs that block biochemical pathways and with drugs that block genes and shade into being gene therapy – with a view to fending off the ageing process to begin with.

Our attitudes will be shaped by evidence showing how much extra health our interventions buy. In 1842 Edwin Chadwick proposed to reform London's sewers. They were open troughs, running down the middle of the streets and dumping their diarrhoea into the Thames. It was known that cholera and typhoid and other diseases resulted, but the extent – the magnitude – of the effect was not. Chadwick wanted a centralised response of a kind alien to Victorian England. The state simply did not intervene in that way, nor did it have the funds to do so without more taxation. 'We prefer to take our chance of cholera and the rest than to be bullied into health', proclaimed an editorial in *The Times*. 'England wants to be clean, but not cleaned by Chadwick.'[16] A huge intrusive change and massive spend for a marginal gain was not acceptable. What altered the attitude was the demonstration that the gains were not marginal, that state intervention to ensure sanitation made a big difference, not a small one. Change became acceptable when we appreciated what it bought.

'Porridge or prunes, sir? These are grim words, and they fell grimly on my ear that bleak October morning', wrote E. M. Forster:

> That cry still rings in my memory. It is an epitome – not, indeed, of English food, but of the forces which drag it into the dirt. It voices the true spirit of gastronomic joylessness. Porridge fills the Englishman up, prunes clear him out, so their functions are opposed. But their spirit is the same: they eschew pleasure and consider delicacy immoral. That morning they looked as like one another as they could. Everything was grey. The porridge was in pallid grey lumps, the prunes swam in grey juice like the wrinkled skulls of old men, grey mist pressed against the grey windows... I paid dumbly, wondering again why such things have to be. They have to be because this is England, and we are English.[17]

It is the sort of England Orwell had in mind when he wrote admiringly of a future in which we all ate in communal canteens. In *1984* his heroine Julia struck out the greyness of the world by taking her clothes off. Orwell felt lucky to have met and married the woman Julia was based on. He would have been luckier still had he been susceptible also to the potential beauty of the table. Within a family or with friends, it's no mean or colourless part of life. Much of the sensation of being hungry or full can be understood and potentially modified with drugs and electrodes and technology. We are already able to put a tube into someone's stomach, or into their veins, and deliver them the calories they need for physical health. We do it as a last resort. Technological props will help curb our excesses and make moderation more satisfying. As aids to a happy life of eating and drinking, interventions to alter how food tastes and how filling we find it are potentially helpful. They will need to be helpful in the wider context of relishing life. For most of us, cooking, eating and sharing are central to the enjoyment of life and of company. We are suspicious of those for whom this is not true. The apostle was right when he said the life was more than meat, and he wasn't drawing attention to vegetables. We enjoy company, and the word has the literal meaning of those we break bread with.

Quantifying the impact of dietary choices is achievable in the future, but we have a track record of failing to see the need of it. An easy confidence about guesses and strong opinion comes too naturally. We can certainly look forward to more soft paternalism, nudging people towards healthier choices, along with technological interventions, like stomach surgery, to reduce our appetites and drugs to soften their effects. Improvements will depend on us being sufficiently dissatisfied with our current state of knowledge to feel the need to improve it. The fact that we are currently not sufficiently dissatisfied is demonstrated by how happy we are to peddle guesses and theories and fads as though they were reliable dietary advice.

As medicine grows more effective it will consume an ever larger portion of our money and our time. The goal is to buy us the riches of health and the delight of them. If eating and drinking ever become completely medical, medicine will have failed.

Beauty

Over the centuries, people have grown more beautiful.
Smallpox ravaged lives and did the same to faces. So
did syphilis and tuberculosis and the thousand traumas whose
breaks and cuts were badly stitched and set. Disfigurement was
more common in the past. It was more common yesterday:
within five years of the Australian papillomavirus vaccine
programme, genital warts, which have been a part of human
history since before it began, went from common to entirely
absent.[1] If genitalia without warts feels too trivial – and it
shouldn't, since it promises lives that will not be cut short by
cancer – consider the future of a baby with a cleft palate. Today
that future is as good as anyone's. Yesterday it would never
have got started and the boy or girl would have grown up
knowing that was the case and seeing it in the eyes of everyone
who looked at them.

Old people, too, benefit. Less crooked and bent double, less
scarred and broken down. The widow's humps that were once
so common have become rare. They are the result of osteo-
porotic collapse of vertebrae, the bones of the spine squashed by
age. The sight of older people stooped forward and shuffling is
rarer than it was, much rarer. Drugs to prevent the weakening of

bones, drugs designed and given chiefly to prevent hip fractures, have been effective, as has the invisible hand of better general health. Fewer bones break. Old people stand more upright. Come to that, they stand more overall – we are better at keeping people mobile. The effects of strokes have also been softened. Less than a generation ago, when I was training, the marks of having had a stroke were obvious and common. The fixed deformities – arm bent at the elbow, leg held straight back at the hip – followed a stroke as the night follows the day. No drug has been responsible for reducing such deformities. Improvements in physiotherapy get the credit. Help people stretch and move their limbs after a stroke and their arms and legs do not tighten and bend in the way that once seemed normal. Technology can consist of technique. People with inoperable cancers of their neck can bleed unstoppably to death as the tumour erodes into a major blood vessel. Opiates ease the way for the patient when surgery has nothing left. For family and friends there are red towels. Packed around the bleeding area, they remove the awful horror of watching white ones turn crimson. Removing some of the horror from the world is also a way of adding to its sum of beauty.

To what extent will we reshape ourselves more deliberately? The plastic surgery designed to reduce the terrible sight of war-related injury has been refashioned. Such aids to looks are newly powerful but are not new. God gives you women one face, said Hamlet to Ophelia, and you give yourself another. At least in part, he meant make-up. It was old back in his day, just as it was in the day of the Sumerians. What will the impact be of the desire for perfection as the technology to manufacture it grows better? What might happen to the fashions that shape our idea of beauty, and will they be shaped by considerations of health or the appearance of it? Will we become ever more intolerant of small differences? The French term *jolie laide* – ugly and pretty – gets used for those whose looks are so unconventional that features which should make them unattractive do the opposite. Behind it is the hopeful notion that what makes the difference is their character, but then we always hope that beauty is a guide to what lies beneath.

Darwin's idea that natural selection was driven not only by the 'law of battle' but also by 'taste for the beautiful'[2] explained how what started as functional could become aesthetic. Coming to see the signs of health as beautiful morphs into admiration of beauty for beauty's sake. We develop an aesthetic sense, meaning our perceptions depend not only on the quotient of beauty in front of us, but also on our ability to apprehend it. But in contemplating how our physical beauty might change in the years to come we need to be sensitive not only to the way surgical tools can copy its outlines, but also to how our capacity to appreciate it might alter. The notion that human beauty is encapsulated by Californian ideas about what youth should look like, and that medical power should strain to preserve it, is as wrong as it is unsavoury. By forty, quipped Martin Amis, everyone has the face they can afford. He meant to highlight how inferior the notion was to Orwell's line that by fifty we have the face we deserve.

Henry James wrote of meeting George Eliot. 'To begin with she is magnificently ugly – deliciously hideous', he told his father. 'She has a low forehead, a dull grey eye, a vast pendulous nose, a huge mouth, full of uneven teeth and a chin and jawbone *qui n'en finessent pas.*' That much had been widely noted by others. 'In this vast ugliness', James continued, resides a most powerful beauty which, in a very few minutes, steals forth and charms the mind, so that you end as I ended, in falling in love with her... a delightful expression, a voice soft and rich as that of a counselling angel – a mingled sagacity and sweetness – a broad hint of a great underlying world of reserve, knowledge, pride and power – a great feminine dignity and character in these massively plain features – a hundred conflicting shades of consciousness and simpleness – shyness and frankness – graciousness and remote indifference.[3]

Darkness makes any woman fair, wrote Ovid, but for darkness he might have written character, so long as the man gazing on her possesses the beauty of character to notice.

There is no cause to worry that people will stop being irrationally ravished by beauty, tormented by the difference to them between one person and all the rest, if our appearances become more similar. They will never get similar enough. Californian plastic surgery has certainly not encouraged a culture in which physical differences, by being minimised, become less important. Facial transplants are currently just about feasible, but no one would want one who was not appallingly disfigured and willing to risk hell to become only moderately so. To scaffold faces with tissue grown from a patient's own flesh, to build them a new face with no need of drugs for rejection and with vastly improved surgical techniques, all will become more feasible as the years go by. It will be a factor which strengthens the gap between rich and poor but there is nothing new in the world possessing such a thing, or even in the power of such gaps to advertise themselves on people's faces and in their bearing.

Wounds are survivable that would once have been fatal. To lose one limb and survive was never rare. The diplomat William

Hamilton wrote to Nelson, down to one arm by then, inviting him to come and stay, with the remark that 'Emma is looking out for the softest pillows to repose the few weary limbs you have left'.*4 To lose three or four limbs and live was practically unheard of. The improvements in care that have saved lives in Iraq and Afghanistan mean it is unheard of no more. Such injuries demonstrate our ability to improve in our perception of beauty. Multiple amputees are so associated with the bravery of war that we have grown better at seeing the injuries not as detracting from the person bearing them but even as adding to them. Some have lost legs but gained stature. Oscar Pistorius is condemned for the ugliness of committing murder; before that he was admired for responding to physical handicap in such a way as was seen to enhance his character.

The moral dimension is what pinches off the possibility of flesh becoming fully as subject to fashion as clothes. Our power to reshape ourselves with technology will always be subservient to our sense of what is sweet and fitting, and that will always be a matter for culture and not science. Technology can be used to rescue those who would otherwise be partially lost, to rectify flaws so serious that they eliminate individuals from having a fighting chance. No improvement, no narrowing of what is normal, will eliminate the need to fight. Sexual selection will always be competitive and the competition will always be based partly on looks since looks are partly based on character. However much the spread of looks is narrowed, the differences will matter. There is reason to be hopeful. The most disadvantaged really do find themselves lifted up; the infectious

---

* The attractions Emma offered to Nelson, Hamilton knew, were not just her pillows. The precise nature of their three-way relationship at this time is uncertain; the lack of jealousy and the goodwill is clear.

diseases and crippling injuries that burnt the less fortunate are reduced almost beyond measure. And even should a narrower normality emerge, it may more easily allow us to focus on those differences in beauty that a scalpel can never produce, those differences that appear in faces as they weather, bodies as they move and minds as they express themselves. Much of what the plastic surgeons of California strive for is based on eliminating the signs of age and individuality. The capacity to do that will grow: whether the appetite does is entirely up to us.

Happiness

L ife, liberty and the pursuit of serious interests would have made a less cheerfully phrased American declaration, but then Jefferson had already taken care to distinguish between happiness and the pursuit of it. That such pursuit consisted of taking a serious interest in the world was obvious to him.

When we say we wish to be happy we mean we wish to successfully pursue those things that will make us happy. Much of the unease over Prozac was the anxiety that it created a state of earthly bliss, mild but unearned: that it did not merely correct a defect in one's mood but improved its background state even where no defect had existed. Fortunately, antidepressants do not work like that.

> Depression has too long been considered as an illness of the soul. Currently, it is viewed as a disorder of the brain. This shift in paradigm began more than 50 years ago, soon after the biogenic amines, notably noradrenaline and serotonin (5-hydroxytryptamine, 5-HT), were discovered as brain transmitters.[1]

The notion that depression and happiness were reflections of the balance of individual neurotransmitters was greeted with hopeful expectation. The hope was reasonable, but the expectation was not. To expect that emotional states and single molecules mapped together in such a simple way should have set our alarm neurotransmitter buzzing. It couldn't because there isn't one, any more than there is one for happiness.

'Biogenic amines', a chemical term for the neurotransmitters like the monoamine serotonin and the catecholamines like adrenaline and dopamine and noradrenaline, show no particular pattern in relation to any mood. As one review put it, half a century after the hypothesis emerged, 'Clinical studies relevant to the catecholamine hypothesis are limited and the findings are inconclusive.'[2] The catecholamine hypothesis held that depression was simply the consequence of having the wrong quantity of these neurotransmitters. Noting that noradrenaline and serotonin were involved in brain signalling was sound; the hope they might lead to insights into health and disease a fair one. The conclusion that doses of them dialled happiness up and down, the way a thermostat does for central heating, was not. Fifty years of searching has revealed no such relationship, only an uncertainty about whether biogenic amines are causally involved in mental illness at all.

Modern medicine had antibiotics, and antibiotics had changed the world. For thrusting young researchers eager to prove their worth and build their career, the conclusion was obvious. Psychiatry wanted to get away from Freud and embrace drugs. To do so it needed to conceive of mental illnesses – and mental states – as capable of responding to pharmacological agents. Why should depression not be a disorder of the brain, rather than one of the soul? The former fitted the pattern of successful modern medicine, the latter did not. Define depression as a disorder of a neurotransmitter, and a drug-based antidepressant pops swiftly into mind.

On such sparkling stuff were careers founded, drugs developed and psychiatry reformed. Dishing out drugs felt modern and helpful, and it was profitable and convenient and everyone could see that the drugs helped. Pills to manipulate the biogenic amines, the catecholamines and serotonin, were worth billions. Their worth came from the fact that they worked. Hope and expectation were fulfilled.

In the last years of the twentieth century, a group of researchers began noticing a strange phenomenon. A host of drugs were effective antidepressants. Selective serotonin reuptake inhibitors had become the most popular – like Prozac – while tricyclic antidepressants were popular also. Not only did all the drugs within each of these two classes have the same effect on depression, but the two classes themselves appeared identical in their impact. A third grouping of drugs, antidepressants working in a variety of other ways, was examined: they too had exactly the same impact. A fourth group, drugs not believed to be antidepressants at all, were looked at. They, too, helped, and curiously they again helped to the same extent. In the most expensive trial of antidepressants ever conducted, those who failed to respond to a first drug were switched to a second, either from the same class or a different one. In each case not only was the second drug as likely to work as the first, but the degree of benefit was entirely unrelated to what the drug was. The situation was even more peculiar given the use of a selective serotonin reuptake *promoter* as an antidepressant. In trials, not only did it help with depression, just as selective serotonin reuptake inhibitors did, but it helped by the same amount.[3] The hypothesis that depression was caused by too little serotonin couldn't explain how pills that reduced serotonin levels had the same effects as those which increased it.

How could it be, for so many different drugs, even for two

drugs doing the opposite thing to each other, that the impacts on depression were the same? The researchers who had noticed the puzzle had been investigating the placebo effect, the way in which investing an intervention with hope can make it effective. When their analysis of the data was complete, it showed the bulk of the effect of an antidepressant tablet – three-quarters of its impact – came from its quality as a placebo, and only the remaining quarter through its specific pharmacological effect on brain neurotransmitters.

Depression being such a subjective experience, the role of the placebo effect was bound to be significant. The extent, however, was unexpected and it caused controversy. Critics of the study pointed out that it had looked at only a sample of the trials of antidepressant medication. So the researchers responded by looking at a larger set. So did others. The sets of trials being re-examined got bigger. Crucially, they began to include not only published studies, but unpublished ones also. Positive studies are more likely to be published. Unpublished studies leave traces, chiefly because they require regulatory approval. In the USA, the regulatory authority is the FDA. One search of what happened to studies showed that 31 per cent were never published. Those that were positive and showed the drugs worked would reach the press; those that were negative rarely did. 'According to the published literature, it appeared that 94 per cent of the trials conducted were positive. By contrast, the FDA analysis showed that 51 per cent were positive.'[4] The public and the medical profession had not been given the whole picture.

When the entirety of the data was put together, the picture of what antidepressants did was altered. For those with mild or moderate depression, they did nothing at all. That is to say that they still worked, but they worked no better than placebos. For those with severe depression there was a difference – placebos were not as good.[5] Irving Kirsch, whose initial interest in the placebo effect had led him into the field, thought that this difference was not best explained by suggesting that the neurotransmitter theory of depression was right overall but only in severe cases. He thought it better explained by those with severe depression being less susceptible to placebos.[6]

I offer my own recipe for happiness. It's morally suspect but financially rewarding.

First, find a drug that has been trialled and found to be safe but ineffective. It needs to be in a setting where subjective responses are as important as possible: ideally where the subjective response *is* what matters, as it is when the drug treats pain, mood or sexual function. Drugs that have been trialled and found to be safe but ineffective mean companies have already poured money into them. The safety has been established at other people's cost. The drug is useless, however, so they will be willing to part with it for a nominal sum.

Next step is to set up your own trial. A few small ones would be ideal, leaving you free to publish whichever comes up with the goods. The technique is tried and tested. Even with just one trial, you might get lucky – and you can sway the play of luck by making the trial small and designed to contain bias. Drug companies have been known to go so far as to have trials designed not by their scientists but by their marketing departments.[7] But to really guarantee success, what you need to do is to make sure you pick an active drug with certain side effects and ensure the placebo has none of them.

The side effects need to be mild but noticeable. Dry mouth, blurred vision, restlessness, nausea – enough to give your participants a feel for whether they have been allocated the active drug or the blank placebo. You'll already have warned them they get a random choice between the two and you will have taken care to specifically warn them of the side effects the drug is likely to cause. They'll be on the lookout. Finally, you need to make sure that when you assess and publish your trial, you don't ask the participants to guess what they'd been taking. If you did and their guesses turned out to be accurate, it might make your trial look suspect.

As it is, you're conducting an experiment you can describe as being blinded and placebo controlled. In reality it's not blinded because the side effects of the active agent clue people in. You're comparing a placebo against nothing, and given you've picked a subjective outcome where expectations are critical, it's a comparison you're bound to win. You, my scientifically illiterate or judiciously immoral friend, are in the money.

The side effects of dry mouth, blurred vision, restlessness and nausea are common with antidepressants. If you wanted to reliably test the effects of the drugs, you would need to compare them against a placebo that had the same side effects. You'd also ask participants to guess what they were taking and publish those results, to demonstrate blinding had been successful. Antidepressant trials tend not to do that, despite studies showing that a majority of participants are capable of figuring out whether they are getting the placebo[8] – a finding which means the trials aren't blinded and the placebo effect isn't being controlled for at all.

The notion that antidepressants work was not the result of any one person setting out to distort the evidence and make money. It came about through the net effect of a great deal of scientific illiteracy and a good sprinkling of spin. 'The use of many small randomised trials with clinically non-relevant outcomes,' wrote one highly respected commentator, 'improper interpretation of statistical significance, manipulated study design, biased selection of study populations, short follow-up, and selective and distorted reporting of results has built and nourished a seemingly evidence-based myth on antidepressant effectiveness.'[9] Even the data that existed, noted the critic, were short term, whereas both depression and the prescription of drugs to treat it were not.

The two overviews of the evidence suggesting that antidepressants might not work were published in 2008.[10,11] Ten years later another overview – whose authors included the critic quoted above – also looked at both published and unpublished evidence. 'Antidepressants are widely used treatments for major depressive disorder, which are available worldwide', it noted. 'However, there is a long-lasting debate and concern about their efficacy and effectiveness.'[12] Antidepressant drugs, it found, did work. They didn't work much – they weren't a lot better than placebos – but they were better. The study looked only at their impact after eight weeks and did not report on whether participants were successfully blinded and able to tell if they were taking a placebo. It did note that the vast majority of the studies it drew on had been designed in such a way as to give them a significant risk of being biased and wrong. Our best evidence says antidepressants have small, short-term effects but the best evidence is not very good and there is room for doubt about whether antidepressants work at all.

Their name gives these drugs a sense of reality they do not merit. The increase in psychiatric drugs, both their number and their use, is interpreted as evidence of our increasing ability to control our minds through science. More often, it's evidence of our credulity. The reason the drugs don't work in the brilliant way once pioneered by antibiotics is that there is no single target for them to hit. The analogy with antibiotics, capable of aiming at parts of bacteria not present in human cells, is a false one. So is the notion that mental states can be reduced to a neurotransmitter. Truth is left behind when one imagines that simple chemical pathways are responsible for emotions, happiness or for stress.

'Two soldiers may find themselves shoulder to shoulder in the same ambush', wrote a recent book:

> One will freeze in terror, lose his wits and suffer from nightmares for years after the event; the other will charge forward courageously and win a medal. The difference is in the soldiers' biochemistry, and if we find ways to control it we will at one stroke produce both happier soldiers and more efficient armies.[13]

True but misleading. Grace under pressure, heroism, bravery, character, fighting spirit, happiness – the qualities are real and important and are not taken seriously by attempting to approach them through chemistry. They are qualities of people and not of atoms, chemicals or physiologies. Any attempt to reduce them to neurotransmitters will lead to confusion at best. Such approaches fail to honour the complexity of life.

Neurotransmitters underlie emotions just as brains underpin creativity, but the emergent properties cannot be usefully understood based on the lower level of organisation. Drugs for treating depression will improve but the improvements will be gradual and, unless we take great care, uncertain. Happiness will not yield in any newly profound way to a biochemical or neurophysiological key, not any more than it has already.

We can already produce or eliminate happiness at will. We can inject people with morphine to set them drifting on a sea of bliss or put bamboo splinters under their fingernails to drown them in misery. Altering human mood through technology is not hard. What is hard is to do it in a way that is useful. To leave someone fully human and make them happier will not have a simple solution. It will not have any full solution at all, only the potential for an ever-increasing and ever more gradually effective means of modulation. The talking therapies are not ones that approach depression as a disorder of the brain. They are also therapies that have evidence showing that they work, at least a little. The index of psychiatric diagnosis, the *DSM-V* (*Diagnostic and Statistical Manual of Mental Disorders*), defines depression in ways that defy sense. To still be mourning one's spouse, once they have died more than six weeks previously, is defined as a psychiatric illness. That takes some believing. It takes incredulity a step further to believe such an illness to be a disorder of the brain and not a pang of the heart.

Medicine's best contribution to human happiness has been its demolition of the tyranny of frequent premature death. Hearts have remained unbroken as a result, hopes unshattered. People have been spared not a brain disorder but an illness of the soul. What can medicine do in the future to promote human happiness? If the answer is 'not much', it is better to search for the little that can be done than to base treatments on fictions. I'd rather a bottle in front of me, goes the old joke, than a frontal lobotomy. Humility based on reality beats a sophisticated fantasy. The man who developed the frontal lobotomy won the Nobel Prize for it in 1949.[14] Depression was one of the problems it was used to treat.[15] A significant number of studies showed that it worked, justifying its use until better quality and longer term ones changed the picture.[16] Conceptualising human emotional states as diseases to be treated via specific molecules or brain centres has a track record, and not of conferring generous benefits. Sometimes it can help but the help is modest and the effort must be made cautiously. The use of drugs to treat depression goes back into prehistory with opium and alcohol. As with the sedating drugs that can help damp mania down, such approaches can help, gingerly and temporarily. When they are taken to be more than they are they are dangerous, and when they are treated as complete solutions they are treacherous. The scope to be helpful is greatest when it is also understood to be limited.

*

The 1960s hopes for a biological psychiatry have faded in the absence of new drugs and there are few new insights. It is increasingly recognised that the phenomenology of the latest version of the psychiatrists' bible, the *Diagnostic and Statistical Manual of Mental Disorders*, can't readily be translated into the molecular language of disordered molecules. Now that the brain can no longer be conceptualised as a sea of neurotransmitters whose abnormalities are the causes of depression, anxiety, or schizophrenia, many big pharmaceutical companies are retreating to the safer terrains of cancer and coronary heart disease.[17]

Moods and characters were once explained in terms of the four humours. Individuals were melancholic, sanguine, phlegmatic or choleric depending on which Hippocratic humor dominated their body fluids. As metaphor the notion has potential value; as literal description it is bankrupt. The same can be said when humours are replaced by hydraulic pressures, evolutionary drives, genes, neurotransmitters or fMRI images. Nothing changes save the metaphor, which shifts with technology. Keep it as a metaphor and one can use the language of science to enrich ways of thinking about human characters and experiences. Think of it literally and thought is impoverished.

We have effective mind-altering drugs but our world is rarely the richer for them. Having cared for hundreds of Heroin addicts, the general opinion of society that the drug is to be avoided except as a treatment for pain seems to me entirely correct. Taken for pleasure, the drug buys an illusion. The fact that Heroin makes people happy no more contradicts the idea that happiness cannot be easily produced by a one-hit approach than asserting the intricacy of a human mind is contradicted by the observation that one can abolish it with a brick. Euphoria beyond the scope of humanity does not count as progress if it comes at the cost of making you so much less human. There are drugs that are mild enough to be occasional aids to a life well lived and coffee, tea and alcohol are the most widely used. The grounds for using them are not medical. Any argument for the enriching effect of wine on an evening has to be made on a different basis. A doctor advising a glass from time to time is not prescribing a medicine but dispensing advice.

'There is no one without suffering', believed Sophocles; 'the happy are those who have the least of it'.[18] He was neither the first nor the last to miss the point through pessimism. Happiness may be sweetest when won from misery but the two do not make up the sides of a scale, the one to be subtracted from the other before tallying a total. The old memory of a wonder-filled baby, long since grown and lost to adulthood, the recollection of a loved friend now dead – the lasting happiness of each exists alongside the loss, not as something to be weighed against it.

Our interests and enjoyments constitute our happiness. It is part of what culture offers that the sources of our interest are increased. In *Sesame and Lilies* Ruskin wrote of how we crowd the streets for a glimpse of someone famous yet pass up the chance to know them intimately. That intimacy, he pointed out, is easily available. Opening a book was what he had in mind and we know that because he wrote one about it. When we read Jane Austen we have the joy of her. She really is interested in opening her mind to us, and making us more interesting as a result, even to ourselves. We may have done nothing to deserve the experience but happiness, as many of her characters discover, stems from realising that fate can be more kind than fair. It was Hamlet who said that if we got the fate we deserved we'd all be whipped. Happiness is a matter of being able to experience ourselves as fortunate. The sense of recognising that they are happier than they deserve is a defining feature of Austen's heroines and heroes. Their decency is its consequence, decency being more interested in fairness softened by generosity than fairness made stern by justice.

If wider culture offers the opportunity for taking more of an interest in the world, for expanding our happiness, it also reminds us that an essential human trait is that of dissatisfaction. If happiness comes from striving, we must have things to strive against. The world is full of them. Thoughtlessness can damp them down, as can opting out from the struggle. Leclerc raged against those preaching,

> that it is sweeter to vegetate than to live, to want nothing rather than satisfy one's appetite, to sleep a listless sleep rather than open one's eyes to see and to sense; [that we should] let us consent to leave our soul in numbness, our mind in darkness, never to use either the one or the other, to put ourselves below the animals, and finally to be only masses of brute matter attached to the earth.[19]

Happiness is often muddled up with contentment, a quality that, to be experienced honourably, needs to be intermittent. The means exist, using a syringe and an ever-increasing supply of opiates, to make a human life entirely content, but only at the cost of preventing it being human. No technological innovation will change that. Technology may add to our happiness in the future, or subtract from it, but it will do little of either directly. It will operate chiefly through shaping our experiences and altering our culture. Both would not exist without our biochemistry, but biochemistry will remain a poor way of approaching them.

Mind and intellect

THE BRAIN is wider than the sky,
    For, put them side by side,
The one the other will include
    With ease, and you beside.

The brain is deeper than the sea,
    For, hold them, blue to blue,
The one the other will absorb,

As sponges, buckets do.[1]

EMILY DICKINSON

We have always wanted to improve our minds, and we have always understood that the effort is hard and the end uncertain. To swallow a pill or inject a drug and to have accomplished for our bodies what a year of successful dieting and exercise would have done is a marvellous prospect. Even better to redesign our genes so that the pill or injection was not needed. The sweetness of the notion makes one inclined to believe it must be possible. Neither will be, not for as far ahead as we have any warrant to speak of. But what about a pill, an injection, an implant or a course of gene therapy targeted at the mind?

When the demand is great enough the interventions will always be available. Two thousand years ago the great Greek doctor Galen prescribed treatments to improve the minds of his patients.[2] It would be going too far to say that they didn't work, but it would not be going far enough to point out that they did not work through any neurologically specific recipe. They may have reduced mental difficulties, if the individual regimen prescribed more sleep or less alcohol, and they may have had useful placebo effects, but there was no pharmacological success hidden in the ancient wisdom. We have always believed in these sorts of interventions and have always been wrong. This is a useful thing to keep in mind when approaching news of recent breakthroughs. Recent studies have found that 20 per cent of surgeons take cognitively enhancing drugs[3] and almost two-thirds of undergraduate students do the same.[4] Could such people mistake something for a cognitively enhancing drug when it was nothing of the kind? Galen's patients had the same neurophysiology as we do today and the same intelligence and the same credulity too, which is why the answer to the question is yes.

An obligation to be sceptical is not a necessity for nihilism. Given the ease with which people have mistakenly believed in cognitive enhancers, we should require high-quality evidence before we are willing to admit their existence, but we should be willing to hear of it. Does that evidence exist? Many believe it does.[5] Many others believe it soon will, and their position is more interesting. The American doctor who coined the term 'cosmetic neurology' believes that such drugs are on the way; that they lie in the realm of the inevitable. He called them 'the nose of a camel that is well on its way into the tent'.[6]

The best studied and most lauded drugs are the mild stimulants modafinil and methylphenidate (Ritalin). They interact with a range of brain chemicals – as do caffeine and amphetamines. Listing the brain chemicals gives an aura of science to the discussion that it would be wise to avoid. The question is not what these drugs do to the brain but what they do to the mind. In reliable studies, are they placebos, are they mild stimulants akin to a cup of coffee, or are they designer drugs taking us one step along the road towards the sunlit uplands of genius?

The best available evidence suggests short-term benefits in wakefulness, memory, learning and decision-making.[7,8] The best available evidence, however, is not very good. Some think it so bad as to be worthless.[9] On the basis that people have fooled themselves over the existence of cognitively enhancing drugs for millennia, what we need before we banish our scepticism is overwhelming proof. This is not it. If we feel in need of a pharmacological stimulant to thinking clearly, we might be better reaching over our packs of modafinil for our cup of coffee. The stuff plainly works. Just as plainly, it is a mild stimulant that can sometimes be welcome, not a biochemical key to unlocking new mental powers. It seems worth noting that while a cognitively enhancing drug would be a golden fountain of riches, no drug company markets one. The chances of methylphenidate and modafinil being general aids to human life seem small to those who make their money from judging such things. The Jason Bourne movies, where drugs and psychological training confer superhuman powers, have many good qualities, but being an accurate guide to reality is not among them. There is as yet no pharmacological shortcut to having the mind, memory or attention of a superman. But is it on the way?

Back to the camel nosing into the tent.

*

Colin Blakemore, while Waynflete Professor of Physiology at Oxford, described the potential impact of the then-current 'Decade of the Brain', an American-inspired drive of the 1990s. Blakemore pointed out that achieving complete understanding of localised brain function could, in many respects, be pointless. Neuroscience lags behind experimental psychology for insights into human character. Neither comes close to art, poetry, philosophy or literature. That hierarchy of utility is likely down to the fact that what interests us in people may never be apparent in their neurons, no matter our technological progress.

Advances in knowledge of neurons and neurotransmitters have revolutionised our knowledge of the brain's basic building blocks. Functional MRI scanners – the term 'functional' means they work quickly, unlike normal MRIs, thereby catching images of brain centres in action – have transformed what we know about the localisation of neural processes. For all the technological sophistication of modern imaging, and for all the insights they give about neurotransmitters and wiring, it is not clear that they tell us much more. They may even mislead us. The neuroscientist Steven Rose compared fMRI brain mapping with the delusions of phrenology.[10]

Phrenology emerged as modern neuroanatomy did. The term comes from the Greek for the study of the mind. Phrenologists noted that the brain was the organ of the mind – the brain was the squishy item in your skull, the mind the phenomenon, the you, which it produced when operating – and that the brain was not homogenous. It was not a uniform blob, each part identical to the other. It had a detailed internal structure that was there because the operations of the brain were not homogenous either. They were not all the same and they were not all founded evenly over the entirety of the brain. Certain bits were responsible for certain functions, and processing power was related to the size of the chunk of brain involved.

Thus far the account of phrenology still seems reasonable. But phrenology was born at the end of the eighteenth century and it added to its assumptions a further one that now seems plainly ridiculous. It noted that the skull was not fully formed at birth. Babies are born with their skull existing only in patches. The contours of the outside of the skull, the phrenologists reckoned, mirrored the development of the parts within. Feel the bumps on someone's head and you got a sense of the relative growth of different parts of their brain. Cautiousness, benevolence, linguistic skill, acquisitiveness, hope, wonder and so forth. Phrenology was the science of finding the mind's construction in the bumps of the head.

The theories that explained depression in terms of serotonin or schizophrenia in the light of dopamine have been almost entirely abandoned: only their dying echoes linger. The excitement now is about location. The pictures that fMRI scanners produce are so detailed – so impressive when inserted into papers and articles – that they are taken as containing riches. To some extent, they do.

The potential of brain localisation is not that it will help us develop drugs but that it will open the way to other technologies. It already has. We have some understanding of the bits of the brain involved in initiating movements, just as we do some of the neurotransmitters. That has helped with Parkinson's disease. Those reliant on anti-Parkinsonian drugs can start to suffer from them triggering unstoppable writhing movements. The brain centre involved is known. Put an electrode in it and the writhing movements can be reduced. The patient can carry on taking the drugs they need.

To what extent will an improving knowledge of brain localisation turn the dreams of phrenologists into palpable reality? The
bumps on the skull are real enough; phrenology failed because
they have no relation with the mental faculties once linked to
them. But if the vices and virtues that make up higher mental
function can be linked to brain centres the way movements can
be, both diagnosis and intervention become possible. We will
be able to read character with a scanner and alter it with an
electrode.

No nose is pushing in through the tent doors here. We might
as well be camping in Norway. The reason for the absence of
camel is the same reason phrenology was always going to be
wrong, even if the contours of the skull did reflect the different
growth of brain parts below. The reason is that the idea of
different centres of the brain being convertible into different
qualities is a metaphor taken too far. The function of the brain
is not homogenous, with each function evenly spread over its
whole substance, but neither is it a computer whose creativity
chip is in one place and its morality chip in another. The same
is true when tracing the sources of qualities back to our genes.
We have found a few genes that influence height to a small
amount, in certain situations. We may hope to find some that
do something similar for intelligence, but our hopes have to be
an order of magnitude smaller, since intelligence is at least that
much more complex a trait than height. In a recent vast study
of 150,000 people, only three gene variants were found that
appeared by themselves to have an influence on intelligence.
The estimated impact of each was 0.3 points on an IQ test,
quite literally more than an order of magnitude smaller than
the genes that influence height.[11] Unimpressive, but perhaps
even less impressive than it seems. 'With effects this small, the
chances that they represent false positives are vastly increased',

commented a neurogeneticist in response to the study. 'While intelligence – and proxy measures such as cognitive test performance or educational attainment – are quite heritable, the idea that this trait is determined by common variants in the population at large is really unproven.'[12]

Phrenology was always going to fail because the attributes it sought are properties not of the brain but of the mind. Cautiousness, benevolence, linguistic skill, acquisitiveness, hope, wonder: these are no more attached to particular brain centres than to particular genes or neurotransmitters. The notion that they are is an error-strewn reduction of a complex phenomenon to a 'thing' that is then given a local habitation and a name. Without being attached to particular places, chemicals or biochemistry, we cannot hope to adjust these qualities with medicines, nor with medically inspired rituals. The mental tricks and techniques sold as 'brain training', made glorious by the window dressing of science, are exercises whose value is transient, shallow and non-transferable.[13]

Brain scans show bumps in the brain rather than in the skull. The step forward means we are learning something rather than nothing, but it does not mean the something amounts to very much. In an fMRI scan a single pixel of colour equates to 50 cubic millimetres, one-hundredth of a teaspoon, which contains 5 million neurons, 50 billion synapses and a quarter of a million kilometres of the connecting fibres by which neurons reach out to each other. We prize modern scanners for being able to catch images in real time. But by real time we mean seconds rather than minutes and the signals themselves occur in milliseconds and arise from intracellular processes occurring at a smaller resolution and over smaller timescales. What fMRI offers is like peering into the reflections in a muddy lake in order to get a glimpse of a person walking nearby. We can see something, and deduce something real, but if we draw our gaze up from the water and look directly at the person, we are likely to do better. Neuroscience will tell us ever more about neurons and neural wiring, and its achievements in that regard will be real and interesting and some will even prove useful. At the same time neuroscience will carry on providing the insights into human character it has offered thus far. They are modest, with much to be modest about.

Some differential development of brains can be linked to mental abilities. How much isn't clear, but extreme examples show that at least some relationship exists. A normal brain has more connections and volume than the brain of someone whose head has been flattened by a collapsing building. The correlation with anatomy holds true with function: the flat brain will be performing at a lower mental level, the person being dead. Much more than that is difficult to say. Careers were made in Victorian anthropology by weighing and measuring brains and correlating the results with intelligence or other qualities. Given an infinity of traits to choose from, it was always possible to find a correlation – just as it is today with an fMRI scanner. Einstein's brain has been much studied and many measurements of it made. Some are different from average. The same would be true of any brain. It lies in the realm of the possible that some anatomical features of Einstein's brain may one day be confidently linked to his mental abilities. The number of links we will be able to reliably make, in the future, between brain anatomy and mental function will rise. But this knowledge will not necessarily amount to anything worth having. Being able to identify a whorl on Einstein's brain that related to his ability would tell us nothing about whether the peculiarity of anatomy shaped who he was or was shaped by it. We can detect differences in brains between those who are depressed and those who are not, or between the sane and the psychotic, but we don't know cause from effect. We may never know. Some of the brain changes become apparent before the symptoms of mental illness do, but that doesn't help. Conditions starting in the mind and affecting the brain might have a period in which abnormalities visible on a scanner were perceivable before others affecting behaviour or reported mood. Much the same can be said for what starts in the brain and affects the mind.

When the human hand develops in the womb it looks initially like a mitten. The nimble fingers do not emerge by sprouting outward from the palm; they come as a result of the cells between the fingers dying away. If the cells fail to die, the fingers remain webbed together. Full function emerges from the death of cells, from the reduction in their number. The assumption that more cells equate to better function is not thoughtful or reliable, yet it drives thinking about brains and it drives attempts to correlate anatomy with ability. Such efforts used to be made on the basis of weighing brains, or measuring their volume, and thousands of papers and hundreds of academic lives were poured into an effort as likely to hold water as a net. That should have been obvious even to someone whose brain was smaller than average, as Einstein's was. The subtlety with which the effort is now being made has grown, since the technology supporting it has developed. More often than not the subtleties mean that its mistaken nature has been clouded over rather than clarified. It is widely known that the number of neurons and the connections between them decline with age. The fact is true but the implications are unclear. To what extent is the loss of neurons either irrelevant to mental function or even essential to it, as helpful in improving mental dexterity as the death of cells is to create fingers? We have no idea. What we have, persistently, is the assumption that more is better. It's not a good enough assumption to bring to bear on something so full-throated in its complexity as the brain and its relations with the mind it produces.

One of the profoundest of Darwin's findings, one he only hinted at initially ('light will be thrown on the origin of man and his history'[14]), was that no special case can be made for humans. We are built of the same stuff and born of the same processes as other animals. Wallace thought otherwise. For him, natural selection was proof of God and of man's divinity.

> A brain one-half larger than that of the gorilla would... fully have sufficed for the limited mental development of the savage; and we must therefore admit that the large brain he actually possesses could never have been solely developed by any of those laws of evolution... Natural selection could only have endowed savage man with a brain a few degrees superior to that of an ape, whereas he actually possesses one very little inferior to that of a philosopher.[15]

Both Wallace and Darwin lived in a world that was racist and they shared many of its views, but Wallace's point does not depend on sharing his belief in a ladder of racial ability. The first anatomically modern humans, the first with brains genetically like our own, did not have minds like our own. We see further because we stand on the shoulders of giants, not on the footstools of better genes, but we do see further. Culture – the accumulated genius and wisdom of generations – gives us more intellectual power than if we had been born into society 100,000 years ago.

So Wallace's point stands. How could evolution have given rise to a mind capable of performing in ways that natural selection could never need? How could it have created mental capabilities – for symphonies, snooker, derivatives trading, philosophy – that our life in the prehistorical wild never required?

Wallace thought the lesson was that the mind had to have been created directly by God. Its potential was so underused in primitive societies that it could not follow that natural selection had created such unfulfilled capacities. In his copy of the article in which Wallace made that argument, Darwin wrote 'No!' and underlined it for emphasis. 'I differ grievously from you,' he wrote to Wallace, 'and I am very sorry for it.'[16] Darwin thought his colleague was mistaken, that natural selection could and did create capacities that were incidental to the trait under selection. Bring something into being for one purpose and it becomes available for others. The Internet was created for academics to communicate about science but serves equally well those wanting to watch film clips about cats. It was Wallace's strict selectionism, his idea that every conceivable trait had to have been brought into being by virtue of having a selective advantage, and not his ideas about race, that let him down. Darwin was right. Evolution really can select for potential.

Improvements in our ability to think do not therefore need to rest on hopes of redesigning the brain, since its capacities are not limited by the requirements made on it in the past. Drugs and electrodes are not only likely to fail but are not needed to succeed. We already have ways of improving our intellect: we do it through education. Such education neither starts nor finishes with hours spent in a classroom. It takes shape there because the habit of learning comes with effort and effort comes by practice and practice does not come easily. Education is the lifelong encounter between our mind and the minds of others, filtered and refined through centuries of culture and thoughtful discrimination. 'There are a number of things, the idea of which is a clear gain to the mind', wrote Hazlitt.[17] Numeracy and literacy are among them, and when we learn to count and to write we learn ways of expanding the power of our thought. Ideas, attitudes, ways of speaking, examples of history and biography, the multitude of language and experience all count. Wallace was right to be struck by the capacity of the human mind and how much it outstripped the evolutionary demands that created it. Darwin was right to see no contradiction. We were selected to have voices to speak with. No limits of genes or design constrain what we say. We have evolved to have capacities and some of those capacities appear infinite.

Charles Spearman (1863–1945) believed that intelligence could helpfully be spoken of as having *some* quantitative aspect, however much its value and properties were not summed up by that. He made measurements and his results showed consistency. As a statistician and psychologist, measuring intelligence was part of what he did. Others argued that intelligence was too incorrigibly plural to be given a quantitative measurement. But did not the consistency he demonstrated show you could do just that? Something about intelligence, he wrote, 'is in the normal course of events determined innately; a person can no more be trained to have it in higher degree than he can be trained to be taller'.[18]

The first part of his statement is better than the second. IQ is a measurement showing some consistent relationship to intelligence, even if it plainly does not capture much of its variety, power and potential. We continually judge the intelligence of ourselves and those around us. We do it when we decide what weight to put on thoughts, what value to give to ideas, what trust to invest in a judgement. Discriminating the insight and reliability of each other's intelligence is part of our daily human relations. It is notable, in doing so, how little we find the knowledge of someone's IQ score useful. Not even when measuring potential in those we've never met does the figure have much value. If it did, schools and universities would be relying on it. Each of us is aware of being surrounded at all times by those who can think better in some way or form* – but the number of times we are aware of people who can think better or worse in *all* ways or forms is rare. It may never be anything but an illusion. The bulk of what we mean and notice by intelligence does not exist on a single continuum.

Spearman was partly correct in saying intelligence was innate. Where he was wrong was in the implication that this made it determined. The most one-sided view would admit that external limitations can flatten its potential; a two-sided one would ask what encouragements can draw it out. Even experimental psychologists, whose profession often depends on reducing traits to single measurements, have noted that intelligence, however you measure it, has been increasing.† People are getting better

---

* Shakespeare wrote of looking around at others and being tormented by 'desiring this man's art, and that man's scope' (Sonnet 29). Human gifts are so various that only by curbing our thoughtfulness can we avoid being assailed by awareness of the many ways in which others are our superiors. The fact Shakespeare felt this so acutely should give us some comfort.

† Peter Medawar, whose Nobel Prize came from his success in appropriately reductionist science, felt IQ to be a treacherous concept. 'The Burt disclosures [Burt had manufactured data about heritability of intelligence] gave rise to the widespread suspicion that IQ psychologists generally were frauds; but this is not a charge that can legitimately be brought against any profession. Anyone who studied their writings deeply would incline to the opinion that their principal disability was not fraudulence but sheer stupidity.' He did not mean to imply they had a low IQ. Peter Medawar, *The Limits Of Science*, OUP (1988), p. 32.

at the tests and the increase is not explicable by practice. They have simply been getting more intelligent. That's no more than we should expect from a world getting physically healthier, or hope for from one capable of accumulating and bequeathing mental steps forward.

In 1944 Erwin Schrödinger published *What Is Life? The Physical Aspect of the Living Cell.*[19] It was an account of science for the lay reader, from the perspective of physics. Just as reductionism is inappropriate in some settings, it was vital in others, and physics could demonstrate both. 'From all we have learnt about the structure of living matter,' wrote Schrödinger,

> we must be prepared to find it working in a manner that cannot be reduced to the ordinary laws of physics. And that not on the ground that there is any 'new force' or what not, directing the behaviour of the single atoms within a living organism, but because the construction is different from anything we have yet tested in the physical laboratory.

If you can't actually reduce something to a lower level, in order to subject it to full experimental analysis, it doesn't help to talk or think as though you can. Our sense organs would become useless if too sensitive, Schrödinger pointed out: they would see the randomness of the small scale rather than the sense and directionality it took on when summed into the large. Fog will sink, but that is obvious only if you stand back and look at fog. If you look instead at the molecules of which it is composed, you will see only that the movement of each is random. A single radioactive atom has no predictable lifespan; a half-life is a property that emerges when you observe a clump of them.

Charles Sherrington, the neurologist who coined the word

synapse and pioneered thinking about how neurons worked, referred to the activities of the brain as 'an enchanted loom'. He doubted it would ever be possible to understand the mind by studying the brain.[20] Rather than centres for this or that, with control neurons deciding the fate of others, Sherrington thought the brain comprehensible only as a synthesis where 'each one of all the millions upon millions [of neurons] finally specialises into something helpful to the whole'.[21] Schrödinger agreed. Neither 'the physicist's description, nor that of the physiologist', he wrote, 'contains any trait of the sensation of sound. Any description of this kind is bound to end with a sentence like: those nerve impulses are conducted to a certain portion of the brain, where they are registered as a sequence of sounds.'[22] The experience of listening cannot be understood through physics or physiology, any more than the operation of intelligence. Insights can be gained from the lower levels of organisation that these phenomena are based on, but the overall approach requires something different. Phenomena entirely reliant upon neurons cannot necessarily be traced back into them.

Such conclusions feel unsatisfying next to brilliant suggestions that we are on the verge of transforming human intelligence through drugs and technology. But it is easy to be brilliant if you are not worried about being right. Fantasies do not always gain in truth by sparkling with sophistication. The questions we most desire to understand do not always match those that scientists try and answer. How has it come about that 'the genetics of behaviour' should still be 'uncharted territory'?[23] Why has the genetics of intelligence not been explored? The answer, Medawar once responded, was because the problems were not approachable. They only seemed so via the mistaken metaphor of there being 'genes for' behaviours (aggression or homosexuality are favourite examples) or 'genes for' general intelligence. All traits rest on genetics but not all have a gene or even a group of them, comprehensible by themselves. We can think of traits that correspond with genes because they are the basic examples by which genetics is taught and they are reliable when exploring aspects of biochemistry and physiology. They are not reliable for all. Grand questions can be phrased which cannot sensibly be answered or even addressed. Medawar called science the 'art of the soluble'. Even when science writing strays beyond that, there is not necessarily a problem. Science fiction is only harmful when mistaken for science fact.

Bad histories look back and see how everything had to happen the way it did. Better ones remember how much was unknowable in advance: enough that a good portion remains unknowable even in retrospect. Contingent fate, irrationality and accident exceed the powers of calculation. The system has randomness built in. It's there at every level from global culture to the subatomic. Any serious study of history fails if it forgets to be sufficiently impressed by life's uncertainties. And what is true of history is true of human history, including individual ones. We cannot presume to trace any life back and show how it had to unfold the way it did. It didn't have to, it could always have been different. Given that the majority of conceptions do not lead to live births, it does not take much to see that it could easily never have begun at all. That doesn't mean there is not much to know and study. But it means that, faced with a new life starting fresh, any scheme of thinking that declares its future to be clear will do nothing but diminish our proper sense of possibility.

The increase of opportunity over generations has been neither universal nor without its reverses, it remains true that opportunities have grown. But even in more limited days the exceptions of genius showed that individual histories were not absolutely constrained by social and economic forces, any more than by genetic ones. Mental potential cannot be predicted, no matter what outlines occasionally become visible. It can certainly not be predicted based on genetics or brain imaging. Too much will always remain unknowable. The only proper response is to do the best we can and to hope. The pursuit of education and culture and the preservation of individual freedom may be unreliable, unsatisfying and potentially disappointing but the alternatives are worse. 'After long reflection,' Darwin wrote, 'I cannot avoid the conviction that no innate tendency to progressive development exists.'[24] He meant that the story of natural history was not of the inevitable transformation from simpler creatures into man. It was the ongoing and perpetual triumph of microbes, with the almost incidental emergence of small numbers of more advanced creatures. It may be true to say that our intelligence, having evolved, comes with its own impulse to develop and improve. What is certainly true is that nothing is guaranteed. Given that, however, we can note that our lives have improved over the centuries and say that optimism is justified and adamantine optimism may be helpful.

It is not natural to educate all children as though they can excel. When we start doing it, it will be. It was not natural to believe the working class should be able to read, but the demands of the market and of decency altered our ideas. Ideas of decency and the nature of the market are subject to change. Even more so is the mind of a child; it is fertile ground. If the mind of an adult is not also, something has gone wrong. Stunted bodies and flabby bellies are easy to spot but the mental equivalents are just as plain. We don't see them because they are ordinary. Machines are on the way to make a host of mundane jobs as rare as the experience of leprosy. The jobs are no disease: they are honourable and often interesting. They are being eliminated by efficiency, not design, but the jobs that will remain will on average be richer in interest. The number of places in the world for people whose jobs are routine will fall. Carry on as we are and the amount of misery will rise. Improve access to high-quality education, an education that begins before we enter school and continues until we lie in our hospital bed too weak to think, and we will progress. It is clear which of the two would better serve the demands of the market as well as those of decency. It is plain that the risks of technological change are also real, and that the prospect of an expanded underclass with few entitlements or opportunities is also close at hand. The possibilities should embolden us, as should the recognition that the benign outcome requires enormous effort and that even if we strive we are not guaranteed escape from the countervailing fate of a society degraded by an expanded class of those condemned to be low paid and miserably unskilled.

Pseudoscientific speculations about intelligence and mentally enhancing drugs and techniques are not harmless simplifications. They obscure reality. Like pseudoscientific racism or sexism or a ranking of social classes according to perceived genetic potential, they have an impact. They shroud the unknown potential of those who do not have access to the finest education. They cover over what we could and should be doing. Reductionist assumptions about intelligence have not merely shadowed thinking about what it is and how to maximise it, they have justified offering less education to those with certain skin colours or certain genitals, or from lower social classes.

Most mental illness cannot be understood in terms of properties of the brain for the same reason that mental health cannot be either, nor the aspects of mind that make up ability and potential. Charles Darwin made no impression on his family or his contemporaries as being a youth of promise. His intelligence was contingent on the myriad coincidences of his tastes, capacities, experiences and society. It could not have been foreseen: and what cannot be predicted cannot be preprogrammed. Darwin's genius can be traced and partly explained in retrospect but it could not have been told in advance. The same is true of all of our characters and all our intelligences. Parents trace predispositions in their children but live in uncertainty about their outcome. The notion that an algorithm can do better, fed with sufficient genetic, physiological and sociological details, does not belong to science fiction nor even to the realm of profitable fantasy. It is a sham, whose quotient of truth is so low as to sap our sense of reality. 'With such moderate abilities as I possess,' Darwin closed his autobiography, 'it is truly surprising that I should have influenced to a considerable extent the belief of scientific men on some important points'. He was right that it was surprising but we should not read into that the implication that anything else was ever to be expected. Real life is always a surprise.

The limited genetic consistency of intelligence and capacity tells us that there will be no single switch, nor ten switches nor a thousand put together, that will turn on a light. It tells us that genius, brilliance and insight worth the adulation of a generation can occur in almost any setting. Our efforts are corrupted if they are put into expectations that CRISPR gene editing will produce the next Mozart or Melville, or even that we can identify as children those who will be worth more than others. What history and science tell us is that the development of the traits we value most, from intelligence to compassion to artistic ability, occur so unpredictably that those in cold pursuit of excellence must behave in the same way as those wishing to care for and encourage all. The kind-hearted and the cruelly efficient must behave the same. No art can find the mind's construction in the genes. 'I am, somehow, less interested in the weight and convolutions of Einstein's brain', wrote Stephen Jay Gould, 'than in the near certainty that people of equal talent have lived and died in cotton fields and sweatshops.'[25] The thought of lost opportunities haunts us, appropriately. 'Perhaps in this neglected spot is laid / Some heart once pregnant with celestial fire', wrote Gray in his *Elegy Written in a Country Church-yard*. A century before that Thomas Browne had asked, 'Who knows whether the best of men be known, or whether there be not more remarkable persons forgot, than any that stand remembered in the known account of time?'* We wish to avoid as much as possible the loss of opportunity. What stands to help is not neuroscience but, such as they are, the sciences of education and economics, sociology and politics. 'I do not claim that intelligence, however defined, has no genetic basis', concluded Gould. 'I regard it as trivially true, uninteresting, and unimportant that it does.'[26]

Fantasies of using technology or genetics to improve the mind take fantastical forms, from an overestimation of the power of psychologists through to a delusion that 'brain training' can consist of mindless computer games,[27] and to the belief that the US military has drugs to turn out human 'assets' with enhanced mental powers. The ludicrousness can get easier to spot if the forms are less clichéd. Imagine a proposal to make

---

* Betjeman's 'The pottery chimneys flare / On lost potential firsts in some less favoured town' says the same thing in a minor key. Ed. Simon Wilkin, *The Works of Sir Thomas Browne*, vol. 3, Henry Bohn, London, p. 44.

adolescence more bearable – to invent a drug that alters it from dangerous chaos into something calm and civil. The idea is nonsense. Yet adolescence is hormonally driven to an extent not true of depression or genius or personality. If we were going to flick a switch and change anything, adolescence would be the easiest. Exiting adolescence involves replacing excitement with interest, yet who would think of helping someone do this through drugs or electrodes or gene therapy? The prospect is immediately ridiculous. That is not because it is more unlikely – in fact it is less so – but because we haven't experienced so many Hollywood and journalistic speculations of it that it has become normal to contemplate.

If human intellect were the end result of an evolutionary drive, the highest rung in a ladder of development, we might hope to extrapolate the steady flow of events by which it occurred. Restart the earth and re-run evolution, though, and there's no guarantee what would emerge. Rather than an end result of an inexorable drive, we're an accidental outpouching of luck. We don't know why we emerged, although we know some of the conditions that, by sheer chance, came into existence to allow us to develop. Our functional nudity and superb sweat glands, both allowing the fine control of temperature necessary to support a large temperature-sensitive brain, were a lucky starting point, not the first step on an evolutionary plan. Given our absence of understanding about how intelligence arose, we cannot claim much knowledge of what selective forces it might be undergoing now. We can make up 'Just So stories' about intelligent people doing better and being more sexually successful, just as we can similar stories about less intelligent people breeding more. Neither story is testable and neither is fundamentally interesting. They lead to no insights. All they give rise to are bad eugenics and anxiety.

★

Do crosswords, the research says, and preserve your mind – putting the words in the boxes fends off Alzheimer's. There may be something to it although as a non-crossword lover I am immune to the appeal. The old people on my wards don't do crosswords; they favour word searches. In order to make the letters swim into focus, the rest of life is dialled out. If you're stuck on a hospital ward, the appeal of doing that is plain. Nobody has done the research to see if word searches fend off Alzheimer's but they probably do, at least compared with doing nothing, just as crosswords are likely to fend it off more than word searches, and poetry more than crosswords.

To what extent is Alzheimer's preventable? More broadly, if we have to give up hope of technological shortcuts to improving our intellect, can medicine at least halt its decline? Can we preserve the health of our brains the way we do our hearts and bones?

Studies showing that crosswords slow down dementia are often poor-quality science showing only the effects of confounding. Healthy people are more active, so if you look at what people do and correlate it with health you can create an impression that swaps effect for cause. These studies, though, consistently find links between mental effort as part of leisure activity and the fending off of dementia.[28,29] Without interventional trials that randomise people to one life or another, there is no way of knowing how much such findings are caused by residual confounding too, by groups of people being different in other important ways no matter how one tries to pick them to be identical. And since interventional trials would need to randomise people to different lifestyles, in a way which no sane group of people would ever accept, they are impossible.

It seems reasonable to guess that confounding is important but it is probably not the whole story. Using your mind is likely to keep it in better shape. As speculations go, that fits with how life seems to work.

There is similar confusion between cause and effect when it comes to the neuroanatomy of dementia. The hallmarks of Alzheimer's when looking at cut-up brain down a microscope, the amyloid plaques and neurofibrillary tangles, might be the cause of the disease or the result. The pharmacology industry and research charities bet huge sums of money on the former and they have not been successful. That doesn't mean they're wrong, and even if they do turn out to be wrong they were still probably right to try. These plaques and tangles are a target and, for all they may turn out to be a false one, there aren't a host of obvious alternatives.

Drugs to treat dementia are of limited use. They will stay that way. Dementia is the end result of damage to the brain and brains do not regrow. Future advances in treating dementia will not come from drugs that restore a missing neurotransmitter or fix a broken circuit. They may come from turning back on some of the processes our cells begin with, some of the abilities by which brains first grow, but that does not seem likely to happen soon. In the decades for which I have been reading the medical journals, not a year has passed without a report of a promising new method for restoring to cells that have lost it the power to divide and regrow. It is usually in the context of the heart, with researchers stimulating muscle cells to divide and replenish areas killed by heart attacks, but often it is in the brain after a stroke. Each breakthrough is promising and none ever leads to anything useful. Eventually one will, but plainly the problem is not an easy one. The challenges and hazards of provoking cell division in a living brain are higher than in a heart, so it will not be solved first within the confines of the skull.

A sizable proportion of dementia is certainly not the result of a particular disease or defect but the end result of the harms of getting older. Those are harms we know how to modulate. All of the great causes of heart disease – the passage of years, masculinity, blood pressure, cholesterol, diabetes – cause cerebrovascular disease as well.

Drugs that slow vascular ageing will extend the years for which our brains are healthy and our minds unclouded. Some of the effects have already been seen but others have not. Treatments that slow ageing sufficiently to reduce heart attack risks within one year or five may take ten or twenty to show a drop in dementia. There is more uncertainty when it comes to quantifying the effects of antiageing drugs – those treating lipids, sugar and blood pressure – on brains than on hearts, yet the treatments for the two are likely to be the same. We are not fighting a disease but fighting back the effects of years. Our power in this regard will grow.

In considering the difference between the brain and the mind, Steven Rose suggested it was useful to imagine an instrument more powerful than any real scanner ever could be. Imagine a 'cerebroscope', capable of reading the state of all parts of our brain at all times with total precision. There is reason to think such a machine impossible, since complete accuracy of measurement could not be done without disturbing the brain it measured. But if it were possible, could such a cerebroscope read the mind from the brain?

Rose thought not, on the grounds that the machine would need to know about more than the brain in front of it to make sense of the context. To misquote Kipling by way of C. L. R. James,* any such machine could not fully know of neurons if it only neurons knew. It would have to have full knowledge of the world in which the brain was living. Only then could it understand what it was seeing. That sort of omniscience is definitely not possible.

There is another reason why such a machine could not work, why even in imagination a full understanding of mind through the analysis of brain would fail. It is not enough for the cerebroscope to observe what is happening both in the brain and in the world outside it. When we have an interesting conversation, our interest is not only in what the other person says but in what we find ourselves saying and thinking in response. An imaginary cerebroscope might have all the data needed to take the step of predicting what you were about to say, but in order to demonstrate that this was the case it would need to take that step and make the prediction. It would need to be not only a scanner but an emulator. The only perfect way to read a mind, in other words, would be to recreate it. And since the cerebroscope would be a cerebroscope and not the person's brain, it might be a perfect recreation at the moment it was switched on but experience would make it imperfect the moment after.

The only way to find out what someone is thinking is to ask them. That may remain the only way because until they tell us, they may not know. A cerebroscope that is actually a complete human emulator is not a scanner but artificial life. It would be an answer, but not to the question of how to read the mind

---

* James's 'What do they know of cricket who only cricket know?' is a reference to Kipling's 'What should they know of England who only England know?' from the latter's poem 'The English Flag'.

from a scan of the brain. We can dream one day of creating a new mind with the tools of technology, but then we can do that in the meantime with the tools of biology; that's what we've been selected to do.

Neither drugs nor genes nor electrodes will help us very much in pursuing the qualities of mind we most value. At least not in any ways fundamentally more powerful than those we possess when we hold a cup of coffee or glass of wine, and less so than when we hold a book. Doing better than we have done so far will rely not on medicine but on culture, education, effort, opportunities and discouragements. Some of those will involve the artifice of technology, but then they always have. There is nothing natural about a book any more than there is about the thoughts it provokes.

As much as the future is foreseeable, how technology will affect our minds is more a question of culture than the technology. We interface with technology with our eyes and hands and thoughts and all the other multitude of our senses.* How such technology might be more literally plugged into our bodies is a related question.

---

* The notion of five senses was a classical one, a conception that at the time might have seemed neurological but in retrospect is either metaphorical or wrong. Senses can be flexibly defined in many ways but are most sensibly defined by the stimulus they respond to. The neurons responding to cold are different in design from those responding to hot; our sense of temperature is an amalgam of their data, not a single sensory mode. Whether we combine those two types together and call them thermosensors is a matter of choice, but they are not sensing touch any more than are those detecting vibration or angular momentum and linear acceleration. Books talking of five human senses combine ignorance of their subject with indifference to looking it up.

Biomodification

There is no stark divide between traditional surgery and the more extravagant forms of biomodification. Putting wings on someone's shoulders or giving them a metal exoskeleton equipped with rocket launchers and a small beer cooler is different in degree but not in kind from replacing their hip. In each case you are adding an ability that wasn't there before, even if in the latter case the ability is to walk without pain despite years of arthritis. One cannot even argue that the beer cooler and rocket launcher are unique in that they add abilities human bodies never had before. Bioprosthetic alterations to make us almost invulnerable to cold come in the form of hats, gloves and clothes. Glasses add new powers too: the human lens loses its elasticity in a predictable way and no one well into middle age has ever been able to focus on a page close to their face without the addition of spectacles. They just happen to be removable (and losable) while attachable beer coolers wouldn't be. But then beer coolers are available to all those who can afford a fridge and they expand your options in life even if you keep them in your kitchen; one can make a good argument that it's the best place for them. Shoulder-mounted rocket launchers are at their most flexibly useful when the connection forged with your shoulders is a temporary one you make yourself by resting them there.*

Nor is foreign material placed inside the human body new. There is a smooth transition from sutures and staples, stents, wires, Dacron grafts, tubing and replacement cartilage through to devices. One could call implantable electronics different but they are also not new. The first successful effort to control a human heart using external electricity came in the nineteenth century. As the twentieth century wore on, pacemakers became better and more reliable, and some of them weighed less than a large horse. It took till the 1960s and 70s before small, implantable devices with no external wires could be slipped under the skin. Nowadays they take twenty minutes to fit and are not reserved for people who need them. As with most medical interventions, drugs or otherwise, they are not life-saving so much as life-helping. We do not reserve them for when they are essential but also offer them whenever they bring a greater chance of benefit than of harm.

The first pacemakers were more clearly bionic. It was not only the power of novelty that marked them out. To be connected to a machine the size of a phone box, the connection protruding in the form of wires through one's chest, was clearly to be partly human and partly machine. That impression is rarely produced by the modern versions. Beneath the skin but making a small bulge over the ribs, their few square centimetres of metal are almost flat but not quite. It's enough to stick out.

---

* It's not stretching the point to mention that young men in possession of a prized car can experience the vehicle as being an extension of themselves and their abilities. Older men who notice only the recklessness perhaps forget how it felt. An infant intoxicated by having learnt to take a few steps exhibits much of the same delight, and experiences some of the hazards.

They are able to record data about our hearts and transmit it wirelessly on command. Many combine an ability to co-ordinate the heart's beating (a technician can alter your heart rate from afar) with the capacity to deliver electric shocks, of the sort so commonly delivered externally in film and television, in the event of certain electrical screw-ups.

As with many medical innovations, the spread of pacemakers and related technology shows a repeating pattern. They were developed for life-threatening problems, for problems that if left untreated meant people were likely to die, or to be severely disabled, and that the devices altered dramatically. They spread from there in search of incremental gains. These became small enough they were soon not reliably detectable through unstructured experience and observation but required randomised blinded trials. In those whose hearts exhibit mild conduction delays, but which also pump less well than they should, such trials found benefit from implanting a pacemaker-like device to make the heart contract in a slightly more orderly fashion. It results in better performance. The performance itself is not the goal – many interventions will improve some measurable part of the body's performance without leaving a person feeling any better or living any longer. But trials showed that these devices, in this setting, did not just improve numbers but meant patients lived longer and avoided hospitals.[1] Once again the relative risk reduction was of the order of 20–30 per cent; important, but small enough to have been invisible to clinical experience unaided by the technique of the trial. There are more people in the world with partly artificial hearts than we realise. That's because as the technology becomes normal it feels that way too. Readers young enough to have first used a mobile phone as an adult may remember how magical they seemed; readers who grew up only knowing a world that already had them will not.

We can grow cartilage and skin and bone or replace them to varying degrees. We can replace some of the functions of skin – but not all, so anything we put in place of skin is temporary. The epidermis, the waterproof outer layer, can be replicated artificially. The other part of skin, the dermis, has a more involved structure and more advanced function. We can't replicate it, not yet.

Bone we frequently replace with metal, particularly when it comes to the larger bones and bigger joints. The data on how many people are bioprosthetic because some part of their skeleton has been replaced with chrome or titanium is limited, but a recent study in the USA found that in 2010 over 11 million American joints were artificial. That's not the total ever implanted, it's the number of people that year whose hip or knee was an implant.[2] Bionic men are among us and many of them use their powers to shuffle around golf courses and nursing homes. Osteoarthritis, the age-related breakdown of joints, and osteoporosis, the age-related weakening of bones, have yielded hugely to medical advances. Both continue to prove problems for many, and neither will cease to be part of our experience. Pain and disability are a frequent part of old age, often to a crippling extent, but we deal with them better than before. Those improvements will continue. The drugs to strengthen bones are another example of what can be viewed narrowly as an intervention to treat a disease, but which more generally are treating something else. The something else is always age.

The French naturalist Cuvier once mocked Lamarck's ideas of evolution, exaggerating them to suggest an animal's structure resulted from its wishes. 'It is the desire and the attempt to swim that produces membranes in the feet of aquatic birds', he scoffed.[3] Human society, though, really is Lamarckian: it is the desire and attempt to swim that has produced wearable flippers for those who want them. Bioprosthetic additions to the human body are at their most sophisticated when they can be added, removed or altered at the whim of an individual. The flippers of wetsuits, like socks and hats, fit that description. Humans have been bioprosthetic for as long as they have been human. Longer: the chimps that pelted me with figs in the Ugandan rainforest a quarter century ago were using the fruits to add to the power of their bodies.

We have had bioprosthetic additions to our brains since culture began. The bioprosthetic additions *are* culture. Their beginnings exist in any animal whose knowledge is not innate. That's not to strong-arm the meaning of any word. Something is prosthetic when it is added on, bioprosthetic when added on to life. A famous example of non-human culture comes from Japanese macaques, some of which possess knowledge of how to wash the sand from sweet potatoes. The example is famous because its birth was witnessed: it was traced to the genius of a single individual whose example expanded the capabilities of her kind.[4] Such innovations make up the exogenetic inheritance we are born into but neither genius nor a specific piece of knowledge is required. When Harry Harlow spent decades showing that monkeys needed stable, loving relationships with their mothers in order to grow up sane and functional, he was showing the extent to which their lives were underpinned by culture. Give them plentiful warmth, nutrition and shelter, and nothing more, and they grow up mad and unable to function. What they learn from the emotional atmosphere they grow up in is as essential as air. They need mothers. Take away the accumulated experience of generations, begin with a monkey born as a blank slate and wiped clean of monkey culture, raised by innate unaided instinct, and the result is catastrophic.[5] Bacteria that require oxygen are termed obligate aerobes. They require an aerobic environment, an oxygen-sodden one, in order to live. The bioprosthesis of culture is obligate to many species; humans are unusual only in being the ones that read about it.

Stories and art were there in human culture from the time of cave paintings and burial practices, and the paintings and burial artefacts were only the earliest records. From Sumeria on appear the great abstractions of writing, maths, bookkeeping, poetry and law. Those were new fuel for human societies and human minds.

Bioprosthetics encompasses everything from air-tight spacesuits through to Wellington boots and the knowledge needed to build and use them both. Clearly a device capable of transmitting information directly to our brains, on demand and about any subject, would be bioprosthetic. We developed those long ago. Books were spotted from the beginning as being dangerous, and Socrates warned that learning to read would allow us to rest on our libraries* and let our memories shrivel: concerns about the effects of technology on us are not new. An encyclopedia, its knowledge passing to our brains through the protuberance of them which makes the retina, enhances our memory and understanding and our ability to learn. When the encyclopedia comes online it gets easier to use: the greatest novelty of Wikipedia is not that it is up to date or flawed but that it gets read. Students rely on it too much because its utility attracts them. The printed *Encyclopaedia Britannica* attracts dust. When Google achieves its aim of delivering search results so directly to our minds as to bypass our senses of sight and hearing, they will have increased the efficiency of our relationship with the

---

* But we know that because Plato wrote it down.

world but not changed its nature. It will be a step forward but the pitter-patter of such steps is ceaseless. When I showed my wife a voice-activated device from Google I had installed in a bedroom, trying to work out if it would make a good Christmas present for the children to listen to music on, she asked how much they cost. I thought about tracking down the email invoice and then remembered to ask the device. Once it replied, we didn't need to know. Biomodification, bringing what was once separate into closer communion with our lives, has been accelerating for centuries. 'Today, when almost every piece ever composed is available at the touch of a button in near-perfect sound from a choice of several superb performances,' wrote the politician Denis Healey,

> it is easy to forget that eighty years ago no one outside the bigger cities knew any orchestral music unless they could read a score, and most music was not even available on printed scores. Similarly, until photographic colour reproductions began to be available at the end of the nineteenth century, most of the world's great paintings were unknown to anyone who could not afford the time or money to visit them on the spot.[6]

He wrote that in 1989, before the Internet made music and painting and everything else more available than he could then have imagined. The power of his imagination was limited but its limitations were external; it was impossible to conceive of what was then still inconceivable. Technology will make available ever more knowledge; what it can't add is understanding. That has to be something we make for ourselves.

Exosomatic evolution, the changes that occur outside our soma, our flesh, mean we dwarves become part of the cultural giant we are standing on. We were to begin with. Like macaques we cannot be any other way and live. We think in manners and with styles and notions developed by the host of those around and those before us, and without them we would not be able to think at all. That is bioprosthetic regardless of not involving wiring or a physical attachment. Machines alter our lives in even the most basic and immediate ways, whether they are attached to us permanently or intermittently, whether they are things we pick up for a moment to vacuum our floors with or implant to regulate our hearts. The key quality is not whether the addition is physical or biological or cultural, nor whether it is implanted or physically separate; the key quality is what it does to us, what it changes and adds and takes away.

None of this stops popular science books declaring the onset of the Era of Technology or the Age of Augmentation. The capital letters and grand phrases are diagnostic of Statements More Sweeping Than True. A cochlear implant is bioprosthetic in an immediate and obvious way but also in another and just as important way: there is no one person alive who could make one. Were the world to undergo a holocaust and start again, even with books and all recorded knowledge preserved, no individual could master the arts of metallurgy and electronics, the building and surgical implantation and care of the device. The continued existence of the cochlear implant is a manifestation of the bioprosthesis made up of the wider set of knowledge, skills, understanding, methods and economies. It is the condensation of other lives added on to ours.

The machinery of technology exists in continuum with the machinery of culture. Both will progress and the progress will add up but the results will be more than arithmetically cumulative. There will be changes of state. Add two atoms of hydrogen to oxygen and you don't get additional gas, you create water. Take grains of rock from the base of a cliff and gradual erosion eventually results in sudden transformation when it falls. When the church educated Christians about the teachings of Catholicism, the slow diffusion of knowledge tipped over into the foundation of Protestantism and the demand for a Bible written in the language people spoke. Some changes are hard to predict. Some are impossible.

The increases in driver-assisting technology make cars more efficient and roads safer but at some point the balance will tip from cars helping us drive them into them driving us. When that happens everything alters. Summoning them on demand means less need for ownership. It means being able to engage in other activities while being driven, it means changes in roads and parking and commuting patterns, changes in how people socialise, changes in mobility for the young and the old. It means a transformation. We can see that it's coming but there's no certainty what form it will take or precisely what it will do to our lives. Such changes cannot always be extrapolated from what comes before them. Any attempt to confidently say what will happen in the future has to remember that we cannot even agree on why things happened in the past. 'Historians, one must admit, were not created by God to search for causes', said the historian Arnaldo Momigliano. 'Any search for causes in history, if it is persistent... becomes comic – such is the abundance of causes discovered.'[7] That was a quote I half remembered, and on double-checking via Google in 2018 found to come from a book written in 1978. My mind, like yours, is bioprosthetic, and through books and through the Internet it is more than it would otherwise be.

The United States' Defense Advanced Research Projects Agency (DARPA) is exploring bioprosthetics, and as with hip replacements much of the goal is to restore what has been lost.[8] For DARPA the losses are often those of combat. The analogy with other fields of medicine is apparent. One begins by attempting to ease or eliminate the harms of a disease, and then the way opens up for using the same tools to improve normality. That was the case with early drugs to fight rare inherited diseases of high cholesterol levels, drugs that are now used to alter ageing through lowering normal levels of cholesterol in people with no such disease.

An artificial hand has been successfully attached to a person who lost their own a quarter century before. Hardware in a backpack connected sensors and controllers in the hand to implants in the upper arm. Sensation and control were partly restored. The recipient, for the six-month period in which they possessed the hand, was able to tell blindfold whether it – they – were grasping something soft or hard.[9] The Italian laboratory responsible has also severed the spinal cord of a rat and used electronics to link the distant portion of the cord back to the rat's brain. It was able to walk.[10] In 2017 *The Lancet* reported the first successful use of technology to allow a tetraplegic man to reach and grasp with his paralysed hand. Eight years after his own spinal cord had been cut, he had electronics inserted into the part of his brain that had previously been responsible for controlling his hand. Motor control and sensory perception, unlike character and mental power, really are precisely localised. The circuits in the brain are reducible to known centres of action to a fine degree. The man first used the implanted circuits to learn how to control a virtual arm on a computer monitor. Months later, he had electrodes inserted into his own arm that connected to the implanted circuits in his brain and let him move it once more. 'It's probably a good thing that I'm making it move without having to really concentrate hard at it', he told the researchers, when asked what it felt like. 'I just think "out" and it just goes.'[11] *The Lancet* noted the study was 'groundbreaking as the first report of a person executing functional, multijoint movements of a paralysed limb with a motor neuroprosthesis'.[12] DARPA had got most of the way to doing something similar[13] and the journal had previously reported on three people whose nerves to their arms had been accidentally destroyed at the shoulder. They had mechanical hands attached – not in place of their own but in addition – and then, when they had learnt to use these additions, their own hands were amputated and the mechanical ones moved into their place. The results were limited but promising.[14]

Cochlear implants contain microphones connected to electrodes implanted into the auditory nerve. The brain is wired to interpret signals from that nerve as sound. Where the process of neural processing is clear and understood, as for parts of sensation and movement, the technology lies firmly in the realm of the possible. Electronics for connecting to such bits are already here. Electronics connecting us to new extensions of our body, not matching any existing parts, will follow. Reconnecting the sensory and motor parts of the brain, after a spinal cord injury, to the sensory and motor parts of limbs will re-enable people to move. When the technology gets slick it will enable them to dance. It will not turn them, though, from a bad dancer to a prima ballerina. Movement patterns are codeable but the creative expression of grace and beauty through physical genius is not.

One can imagine 'maths' chips operated mentally. But then we have those and to operate them mentally is no huge step forward from operating them with our fingers or our voices. Giving us a new way of working a calculator is different from augmenting the power of our minds so that we think like gifted mathematicians. So long as the signals coming from and to the brain are simple enough to piggyback onto the existing set of labelled lines it uses, the communication should be as straightforward as getting bionic hands to work better. The possibilities are limited by the channels of communication evolution has left the brain in possession of. Put electrodes randomly into the brain and you won't communicate with new hidden parts of it any more than if you stopped speaking to the voice-activated device in your room and started thumping it.

What is not conceivable is something more fundamental to the mind, some basic alteration and enhancement of its structure. We have no knowledge of what its structure is. We know the structure of the brain. Our neuroanatomy has improved and will continue to, as will our neurogenetics. Neither verges onto revealing mind. For profundities about how human beings think, the liberal arts beat neuroscience and probably they always will. It's no coincidence that attempts at predicting the future argue on the basis of history and our understanding of science and society. No one can look at an fMRI scanner and divine a thought or a dream, let alone the dreams that will shape our future.

The list of body parts we can regrow or rebuild is long and lengthening. It goes back millennia, to the techniques for restoring a nose ravaged by syphilis or trimmed by a sword. The use of foreign material has gradually risen, accelerating ever since a young surgeon called DeBakey popped into a department store to buy some nylon to see if he could use it to graft blood vessels. Nylon would not have worked but the store was out of it and DeBakey left with Dacron.[15] It was the making of him by virtue of becoming the making of many others: it's a material that works well when sewn into the body to create or repair blood vessels.

We can take part of someone's nose and grow it into new cartilage for their knees.[16] We can rebuild the oesophagus.[17] Using tissue taken from the vulva people have successfully received vaginas constructed from their own cells grown to shape over biodegradable scaffolding.[18] Bone marrow stem cells seeded into a stripped cell-free trachea from a corpse were subjected to growth factors to encourage them to flourish: the result was an immunologically matching new trachea for a boy who lacked his own.[19] Similar techniques have been used to build new veins.[20] Bioprosthetic techniques have been used for centuries to grow new blood vessels, ever since surgeons noted that you could harness the body's own tendency to do so. If a major blood vessel was diseased there was the chance to tie it closed and encourage the growth of collateral circulation.[21] When one ties an artery to a vein, the vein expands and strengthens to cope with the flow – it arterialises – and the resulting vessels are used to create the high-throughput sites into which haemodialysis needles can be attached. If the ravages of the technique leave a person shorn of sites where such fistulae can be constructed, it is now becoming possible to grow new vessels for the purpose using steel combined with cow serum seeded with the patient's own connective tissue cells.[22]

That cardiac pacemakers were once vast machines, much larger than people, is a source of hope for those making artificial hearts. We already have the latter, at least in the form of something bulky and partly outside the body, and we have had for some time. Cardiac bypass machines are in common use to provide circulation during heart surgery. Extracorporeal membrane oxygenation systems can be used as external lungs. More fully implantable artificial hearts have been less successful. They can be helpful in the short term but are not dependable in the long. They are in use as temporary fixes, for when a transplant or a recovery is soon possible. Hearts, lungs and kidney replacements cannot be miniaturised as easily as pacemakers. Engineering can and will improve, but our inability to manufacture artificial organs seems far less likely to be solved by breakthroughs in manufacturing than from advances in xenotransplantation.

The ability to connect more directly to our thoughts will improve. That's not likely to turn us into superheroes, only to mean that we will control the same devices we control now but this time without lifting a finger. This camel is definitely nosing into the tent: sitting here I can turn the lights off by speaking, or do anything else that a voice-connected Internet allows. The threshold at which I resort to a calculator probably will not change much if it alters from one I speak or type into and becomes one I think at. I grew up with a computer from the age of nine; when I type my fingers move the way the man described moving his bionic arm, without conscious effort. When will the accumulated changes of ever more connected life tip over from a life that's ever more efficient into a life that's powerfully different? The tipping point is unpredictable and what comes afterward unknowable.

Of all the power we possess presently for biomodification, the two types that could most powerfully alter our lives are not those of science fiction but instead are ones we are already using. The first is surgery for obesity. If we were to take it seriously, we would provide it for a staggering number. No technological fantasy could have an impact that would come close. It wouldn't just mean keeping those in charge of public health happy, or pandering to the tastes of puritans who disapprove of appetite and flesh. It would mean transforming people's lives: lengthening them, flooding them with health, making them happier and more physically capable. There's speculation, though, in all that sentence because we have never done the trials of obesity surgery required to properly understand its impact. The observational studies suggest the benefits but we aren't sure. Hence the proof that we have not yet taken it seriously.

The second type of intervention is so closely related that it almost certainly includes weight-reduction surgery. The second type is cardiovascular risk reduction. Thus far we have not moved a long way from the days when drugs for blood pressure and lipids were given to treat diseases. We have not followed through on conceptualising them as ways of promoting health, extending longevity and modulating ageing. Our treatments focus on those at high risk and over the term of a few years. When we stop thinking of them as treatments we will have moved on. We don't think of tetanus vaccines that way.

What will change our approach in this regard will be persuasive evidence and improved technology. The evidence is out there but we are not looking for it. There are no trials of these drugs in the young and healthy to see if they add two decades of healthy life to middle age, nor is anyone talking seriously of conducting any. But as the technology for intervening in the ageing process improves, the talk will change. As we shift from pills taken daily to drugs taken monthly, then yearly, and then to single interventions to alter genes or gene expression, our approach will alter. We will embrace the notion that we are not treating disease but altering the course of life. We will properly search for the evidence required to know what we buy for any given intervention, and at what costs. The results will be no less powerful for being partly predictable. We will extend healthy life and cut back on premature death.

The utility of better education – and of lifelong self-education – will rise not only because the number of useful roles for unskilled workers will shrink but also because we will live longer. We will invest more in ourselves and our long-term prospects. As biomodification possibilities go, it's a happy prospect. To be able to summon a car with our thoughts will alter patterns of commuting and travel. To have more places to go to when it arrives, and more interesting things to do when we get there, will be better. As we sit in the car and make use of the travel time, the effects and the power of the devices we interact with will be important for what they do to the thoughts in our head.

Genetics

Medicine changes the impact of traits and genes and of behaviours and choices. That alters the context in which natural selection operates, it does not shut it down. All that is needed is variation. As those who have worried about the higher fertility rates in lower social classes have recognised, you don't even need differential death if you have differential breeding. Their mistake was to express cultural worries as though they were genetic. Social classes are not genetically distinct. There is no gene for fox-hunting or pigeon-fancying. Cultural traits have a life of their own and the battle over them cannot be fought by focusing on chromosomes.

Most concerns over the effects of social or class differences on human evolution are cultural anxieties in the trappings of bad science. Even traits that are comprehensible in genetic terms are made irrelevant by operating over timescales it is unproductive to consider. Inequality and freedom are worth worrying about, but not in terms of genetics. One might as well base one's approach to global warming on the knowledge the sun will eventually cool. It would be a mistake of relevance, not fact.

Which is not to say that genetic changes are not occurring,

or even that all are occurring so slowly as to be undetectable or irrelevant. Delivery by caesarean section is a modern innovation. The driver for it is echoed in the fact that until recently obstetricians did not speak of delivering the baby. Labour was dangerous and the goal of the birth attendant was to deliver the mother, meaning to deliver her from deadly peril.[1] One of the reasons mothers died was that the head of their baby was too big for their birth canal. It was possible to save the mother's life even if the baby was too big, but the possibility was rarely achieved in practice. In order to do it you needed a birth attendant capable of using obstetric tools to pull the baby out in bits. By the time anyone was sufficiently desperate to try that, it was often too late.

Maternal mortality has declined across the world[2] for a host of welcome reasons. Among them is the use of caesarean section. Has the widespread use of the technique, against a background of previously high rates of death when there was a mismatch between mother and baby, resulted in detectable evolutionary change, in babies now having larger heads? Some argue it has.[3] Others argue it has not, and that rising caesarean rates – and especially the high rates in the offspring of those themselves born by caesarean – are entirely due to other factors, like the cultural inclination to operate among modern obstetricians and the effects of obesity.[4] Both of those are passed down through the generations too, but via norms, not genes.

What is certain is that such evolutionary change is possible. The danger comes from misreading the importance of biology. We have evidence showing that the larger the head at birth, the brighter the baby.[5] So if caesarean sections have allowed a measurable increase in human head size at birth, or if they stand ready to do so, does that have implications for intelligence? Almost certainly not. Head size at birth is influenced by a host of factors and most are not genetic. The health of the mother is key. The link between head size at birth and future intelligence is likely a marker of the mother's health and wealth, and the way that sets the baby up for a brighter future. Too many have already tried and failed to measure intelligence by measuring skulls or fingering their bumps.

What will the effects be of miscegenation, of a blending of races? Outbreeding can have beneficial effects, as plant and horse breeders are aware. Some studies looking at the outcomes for children with parents from disparate geographical and racial backgrounds show benefits.[6] Others show no difference.[7] That there is no clear answer suggests that whatever the answer is, it tends towards neutrality. Will more interracial marriage result in a modulation of patterns of skin colour? It might. The question is interesting in its relation to social mobility and geographical mobility and to how people's lives are determined by skin tones. Skin colour has mattered because of limitations imposed by vitamin D production and risk of sunburn. As a biologically important part of future human evolution, though it has been made largely irrelevant by food transport, vitamin tablets and sunscreen. Trying to notice and think about and describe the cultural differences we come across is an essential part of paying attention to the world. Generalisations about human groups, whether they be the group in the corner in the pub or the political class of a foreign country, are difficult enough. Their accuracy is only diminished when you describe society under the belief you are studying genes. 'Man is gifted with pity and other kindly feelings; he has also the power of preventing many kinds of suffering. I conceive it to fall well within his province to replace Natural Selection by other processes that are more merciful and not less effective,' wrote Francis Galton in 1908. 'This is precisely', he added, 'the aim of eugenics.'[8]

Earlier, in 1873, he had written more plainly:

I do not see why any insolence of caste should prevent the gifted class, when they had the power, from treating their compatriots with all kindness, so long as they maintained celibacy. But if these continued to procreate children inferior in moral, intellectual and physical qualities, it is easy to believe the time may come when such persons would be considered as enemies to the State, and to have forfeited all claims to kindness.[9]

It was, pointed out Medawar, the morality of the gas chamber. It was also just as stupid. Neither the traits Galton wished to encourage nor those he felt entitled to eliminate were genetic to begin with. The gifts he sought and the characteristics he feared were those produced by culture, operating on the endless variety of genes and of nature and nurture combined. Except for in a few extreme cases, which carried no implication for the others, inferiority of intellectual and physical qualities could not then be understood by virtue of genes.* It still can't be done today and it won't be done tomorrow. Galton, for all his genius, was faulty in his imagination and his grasp of genetics. That natural selection operated in subtler ways was apparent to others even then. A few years later Thomas Hunt Morgan, whose study of genetics meant that units of genetic distance on a chromosome are today called Morgans, noted that:

There are, then, in man two processes of inheritance: one through the physical continuity of the germ-cells; and the

---

* By extreme cases, I mean major genetic abnormalities such as Down's syndrome, where triplication of genes on chromosome 21 reduces intellectual and physical ability.

other through the transmission of the experiences of one generation to the next by means of example and by spoken and written language. It is his ability to communicate with his fellows and train his offspring that has probably been the chief agency in the rapid social evolution of man.[10]

One did not need to look to eugenics for the hope of human improvement.

There is a partial exception. The perpetuation and increase of major genetic diseases genuinely is a question of genes and their frequencies. Some of those genes are lethal if untreated and there is no doubt that modern medicine, by making them survivable, is making them more numerous.

As examples of major genetic diseases go, haemophilia offers a neat sketch, currently being coloured in, for what the future holds.

Both haemophilia A and B are rare 'X-linked' recessive disorders of the blood-clotting cascade. With one copy of the gene an individual is fine. Because the genes are on the X chromosome, women tend to have a matching and unaffected gene. The Y chromosome providing no backup copies, men are more vulnerable: they only have one edition of the gene to begin with so if it's faulty then so are they. Each type of haemophilia is a cluster of different genetic problems, the typing relating to the clotting factor involved. The severity of the bleeding tendency varies with each mutation. The existence of the disease in different human populations does not seem to be because it has a corresponding advantage in other settings or other forms, as is true for sickle-cell anaemia or cystic fibrosis, but because it represents a range of ever-occurring new mutations. Genes that would formerly have been snuffed out by virtue of their own disadvantages are no longer being so swiftly removed.

If we were a few paragraphs ago, thinking in the long term about human evolution, we would view a gene that cut life expectancy by a decade as a gene on the way out. Over the long term, it would be, if that was all there was to it. But some areas of the genome are more subject to mutation than others. That evolution has not left haemophilia much rarer than it is today says something about the rate at which new mutations occur in the relevant genes. Without technology, haemophilia would continue at its traditional frequency, and it would not be snuffed out by natural selection.

If we increase the longevity of those who carry the genes, by helping them survive and have children themselves, we increase the number of copies of the faulty genes in circulation. An increase in the survival of individuals with haemophilia will lead to a rise in their numbers. But we judge medicine for its overall impact. If it helps people live longer, the fact that it makes the gene pool worse relative to an environment that no longer exists – an environment without modern medicine – is irrelevant. It's not even a disadvantage, only a potential one in a fantasy scenario of global catastrophe.

The only argument for relevancy is the economic one. As medicine gets more effective, the demand for it goes up. The blood-clotting products that treat haemophilia are expensive partly because they are expensive to produce. If medicine allows the propagation of harmful mutations as they become treatable, the cumulative costs of treatment will rise. Treating someone with severe haemophilia runs to about £200,000 pounds per person per year.[11] Sometimes we decide that some benefits are not worth the price but the benefits of treating haemophilia are substantial. The rise in its frequency might eventually cause an economic problem but it would likely be solvable through technology, both by making the production of clotting factors cheaper and, more finally, by allowing us to edit the faulty genes.

Gene therapy has been a concept for fifty years and a reality for twenty-five. The reality has been in research, not practice. It has been difficult to make it work. Our technology for inserting genes at a particular point has changed from being that of a blunderbuss to that of a shotgun. Insert them at the wrong place and they can do something different, or make whatever was there before do so. As an ever higher percentage of genes get slotted into roughly where we want them, our improvement has been greeted with appropriate triumph. But shotguns are not known for their pinpoint accuracy and nor is our gene therapy. Popular science books are full of accounts of the surgical precision of CRISPR technology. This latest technique for gene insertion is exciting, and a step forward from the technology it replaced. Surgical precision, however, is itself often overrated, particularly when used as a cliché. Scalpels are sharp but surgery itself is usually a blunt instrument, packed with hazards and side effects. Part of the point of a scalpel is that it gashes in healthy structures in order to reach the unhealthy.

In a non-traditional sense, gene therapy has been useful for some time. We have used human genes in bacteria to manufacture proteins – an unqualified success. When we take an organ from one person and put it in another, we move genes. The movement is incidental to the main event but it occurs all the same. In people with cancers of the blood, deleting their bone marrow with drugs and radiation can be used as a precursor to replacing it with marrow from someone else: again, a transplant in which gene transfer takes place.

In 2009 this incidental transfer was recognised as an opportunity. A man with HIV required a marrow transplant. It wasn't to treat his HIV, it was to treat his leukaemia. But his doctors looked through the matching donors for one who also had the mutation protecting against HIV. Antiretroviral therapy was stopped the day the man received the bone marrow and two years later there was still no sign of HIV.[12] Effectively, the procedure dodged the need to make sure the gene got into the right place. The bone marrow transplant worked by inserting cells, not inserting genes into them. Recently, a related strategy has been used where bone marrow has been removed, genetically altered, then put back, the better to help the individual fight leukaemia.

We are not at the stage of altering multiple genes to create new constellations of physiological attributes. We're not close. What we are mainly trying to do is to add a working copy of a gene when people don't have one. The effort is more achievable because success can be partial. If a gene is churning out something harmful in place of something needed, treatment needs not only to add the new gene, but also to get rid of the old one and often get rid of it entirely. With a gene that is merely missing or non-functional, getting a working alternative into even a small proportion of cells can produce enough of an effect to make a person better. In 2017 a gene was successfully introduced into children suffering from a rapidly fatal disease called adrenoleukodystrophy. Lacking a gene, those affected lose the essential cellular covering that allows brain neurons to work. It's the sort of treatment that responds already to the gene transfer resulting from bone marrow transplants, but not very well. Stem cells from the marrow grow into more than just blood and such transplants can alter the genes of faulty cells in the recipient's brain. It can help but it can also fail, and either way bone marrow transplants are major procedures fraught with hazard – they can easily kill.

So seventeen boys instead received a virus altered to introduce into their own DNA the gene that they were missing. After the treatment it was being expressed in a fifth of the cells tested, enough to account for the good results seen.[13] Whether the approach is better than a bone marrow transplant is not yet clear; the long-term effects are not well known enough. 'For many years,' said the editorial accompanying the publication of the research, 'gene therapy has shown great promise, but clinical applications have always seemed just beyond the horizon.'[14] The editorialist made clear their hopes, but also their conviction. This was another example of great promise, not a demonstration the promise had been fulfilled.

At any point in the last fifty years, predictions about the future of medicine could safely have included the hope that gene therapy would soon be here. It soon will, but how soon isn't clear. The steps forward are full of promise but then they've been that way for decades. Gene therapy of acceptable safety and effectiveness seems like it will come into regular clinical use within the next decade, albeit on a small scale, but it has seemed that way for some time.

Improving technology has led to promising results in human embryos, like the correction of a gene predisposing to sudden cardiac death.[15] Those results are preclinical: they are done in laboratories, not in people, and the embryos are not implanted and allowed to develop. Calling them embryos is technically correct but does not convey the reality. These were fertilised eggs, not fetuses. They were allowed to develop until they consisted of four or eight cells only. In other experiments the correction of faulty genes was done in model eggs that are barely even that – for example, connective tissue cells fused with human eggs that had had their own DNA-containing nucleus removed.[16] In that study, a defective gene involved in making red blood cells was corrected with moderate success – enough to mean that about a fifth of the cells were converted. That doesn't imply that one in five embryos would be cured but that in each embryo one in five cells was successfully infected with the new gene. That's almost certainly enough to make a helpful difference to an adult's experience of their disease, possibly enough to get rid of it altogether. It also highlights how far away we are from being able to design genomes at will. Getting a gene to change is only part of the problem: you also have to ensure you do not have effects on any of the others. We can tolerate the risk of failure better when dealing with fatal diseases that are otherwise almost impossible to treat; hence these are the settings in which they will first be used.

This sort of technology is moving firmly into the realm of the possible. But 'this sort of technology' means the correction of single-gene defects. There are not so many ineffable ethical dangers here, just the normal cautions of medicine. Correcting single-gene defects offers the power to fix inborn errors of metabolism, not the potential to design supermen. There are no single-gene changes to turn Bart Simpson into Albert Einstein. If single-gene editing has any profound ethical danger, it lies in the tyranny of the normal. But given the state of our genetic understanding, the only normality we can expect to lord it over is the normality of freedom from catastrophic genetic error. The dangers of mad scientists, demanding we are built the same to think the same and be the same, are illusory. Not only do we have no idea how to do that, we also have a reasonable suspicion it may not be possible, the steps by which genes produce thoughtful people being what they are. Our poor understanding of something so genetically and physiologically simple as height – a quality that is linear and measurable beyond the dreams of an experimental psychologist wishing to reduce human mental capacity to an IQ number – makes even a tyranny of the tall look impossible. A totalitarian nightmare of uniformity is not so bad if it consists only of the absence of the most life-sapping single-gene defects. Such defects are terrible for those affected, but the number of those affected is small. Such gene therapy will changes lives but it will not change the world.

The Human Genome Project was launched with great fanfare almost thirty years ago. The project has finished but the fanfare continues. 'The Human Genome Project (HGP) was one of the great feats of exploration in history – an inward voyage of discovery rather than an outward exploration of the planet or the cosmos', as the US National Institutes of Health puts it today.[17] They were chiefly responsible, so the trumpet they are blowing is their own. But the chorus of others has been deafening with its celebratory predictions of benefits and breakthroughs. What have they amounted to, and to what will they add up to in the future? To what extent have life and medicine been revolutionised by our exploration of our genome?

The use of stem cells to replenish and regrow failing bits of body has obvious appeal. Using them to create solid organs, which like the heart or the kidneys need to grow slowly and in response to their living context (especially the circulation of blood), seems so far off as to be presently incredible. A liver might be feasible, not least because even segments of liver are usable: a single donor organ can already be split for multiple recipients, not through using clever gene technology but simply by cutting it up. Technology would not need to create a whole organ from a single cell. Just being able to portion one up and make it go further would be terrific. The liver, which unlike the brain and the heart and muscle maintains its power to re-generate, is a good target.

Also promising is the use of stem cells to add a little bit to tissue that has failed, worn out or been damaged. No other solution seems so promising for the problem of what to do with gristle – with the decay of bone, cartilage, joints and muscle. Of the four, muscle might prove the hardest to deal with. Its decay over the years of our lives is not well understood. To what extent does its atrophy – an atrophy that exercise can reduce but not prevent – result from causes external to the muscle? We don't know how much of its slow death is down to the fading of the nerves that supply it.

Getting nerves to rebuild themselves has eluded us. In 2016 *The Lancet* reported on eleven men whose brains had been injected with immortalised human neural stem cells. The injections had been into areas of their brains killed off by strokes. The results were promising but no breakthrough.[18] The trial was not designed to see if the treatment could offer real and lasting benefits: it was exploratory, to test the feasibility of better trials. 'Despite consistent efficacy in animal studies, functional benefits after transplantation of stem cells remain to be shown unequivocally in stroke patients.'[19]

Our hope should be nourished but it should be small. Stem cells to rejuvenate the brain are a wonderful idea but stem cells to rejuvenate simpler tissues have a long record of failure. Decades of studies amount to nothing useful whatsoever.[20] It cannot be technically impossible to reprogramme differentiated muscle cells to divide, however ferociously difficult it might be to get them to do it, and do it in a controlled manner. But decades of failure tell us that the arrival of success is impossible to predict. Some day – that's all we know. Not soon, though, at least if past performance is any guide to future earnings.

And what of the Human Genome Project? It was published in 2003. One of its most surprising findings was that we had overestimated the number of genes it takes to build us. Rather than over 100,000, there were only a fifth of that.[21] Our lives are not the result of a host of genes for a host of traits but 20,000 of them combining in endlessly intricate ways. That should change our expectations when it comes to altering them.

It took over a decade of work to complete the Human Genome Project, and it was done at a cost of $3 billion. In 2007 a whole sequence was published taken from one individual[22] and it cost only $100 million and took a fraction of the time.[23] In 2008 another individual's genome was published, this time at a cost of $1.5 million and after only five months. A prize of $10 million for the first team to sequence genomes for less than $10,000 was cancelled in 2013 on the grounds the prize was not needed as the technology was advancing so fast anyway; the cost was already below $5,000.[24] Today the price is $1,000 and projected to soon be $100.[25] The result of all this, in terms of knowledge and research publications, has been immense. In terms of clinical benefits, not so much.

That gap is not surprising but it is rarely mentioned, and seemingly never mentioned at all by those who talked about the project in such a way that the lack of these benefits should have come as a surprise to them. The fanfare trumpeted so loudly was that of clinical benefit. The incredible steps forward in sequencing were beyond what we imagined and they were commented on widely. Rapid steps forward in therapeutics were predicted and their absence goes unremarked.

Rather than a sober reassessment of the gap between genetic knowledge and therapeutic power, discussions today stay packed with expectations of powerful clinical benefit just around the corner. 'Individualised analysis based on each person's genome will lead to a powerful form of preventive, personalised and pre-emptive medicine. By tailoring recommendations to each person's DNA,' says the US National Institutes of Health, 'health-care professionals will be able to work with individuals to focus efforts on the specific strategies – from diet to high-tech medical surveillance – that are most likely to maintain health for that particular individual.'[26]

They've said it before and they'll say it again and they'll keep saying it. One day they'll even be correct, but not soon. Some of the reason why not is lurking there in that mention of diet. A vast number of tools and models and tests exist to detect those people for whom a good diet is particularly important. They exceed what we need by a long way, yet we are still adding to them. We don't need tools to work out who would benefit from a good diet for the straightforward reason that we all would. Genetics cannot add to that. It might identify a subset of people who can get away with eating badly. That would be of benefit but it's not the sort of innovation the National Institutes of Health has in mind. Equally, genetics is likely to increase our stock of risk factors relating to common disease. That's helpful but only barely. Common diseases are common: if there's a behaviour or diet or drug that helps avoid them, it's helpful for almost everyone. When the common diseases are reflections of ageing – cancer, high blood pressure, diabetes – one can delete 'almost'. Discovering ever more risk factors won't help the world, only the careers of those who publish them.

What genetics will do over the next decades is to uncover drug targets. Since the number of diseases that can be eliminated with a single treatment is small, and most have been discovered, these targets will not be for individual illnesses but for risk factors, and again the risks they will deal with will chiefly be those of ageing. 23andMe is an American company that will sequence large parts of your genome for a small price. They were stopped by regulatory authorities from selling their services as having any medical benefits, although the implication they will help you predict your risk of certain diseases is still palpable in their descriptions of their product. What the company chiefly offers you is the interest and entertainment of learning a bit about your genes. What you offer the company is more valuable. By sending 23andMe your money and your DNA, you subsidise their accumulation of the world's largest bank of genetic information. The most valuable part of that will lie in the form of data that can seek targets for developing drugs to reduce the harms of ageing and the risks of its common diseases.

Ever more sophisticated genetic knowledge has had other benefits, and will continue to have, but the search for drug targets will remain the most valuable prize. We occasionally use genotyping to select one drug or treatment over another for an individual. The frequency with which that happens will rise – gradually, and with real but minor results. The excitement of gene-powered individualised medicine has been greatly oversold. It will continue to be. Too many of the ills that flesh is heir to, and too much of our genomes, are common to us all. Genetically individualised medicine will not alter the fact that the knowledge that matters most will continue to be that which can be applied most broadly.

Oversimplification will continue to be one of the fruits we pluck most often from our study of genetics. Optimism, depression, intelligence, morality – characteristics that need to be carefully approached from psychological, sociological and cultural perspectives – will go on being discussed as though they were traits like 'blue eyes' or 'brown eyes' and open to illumination through genetics. The arts and social sciences are tentative and full of error but for certain problems they will remain the best tools we have. Scientific confidence is not superior to the humanities when its science is bad and its confidence misplaced. The mistaken eugenicists of the twentieth century were not all motivated by racism or self-interest. Some of the most dangerous were sincere and well intentioned, their sincerity and their compassion just happening to be based on a fundamental failure to grasp what it was that they were talking about. A lot of those who have poured years into the study of genes for criminality have been thoroughly well meaning. Their time has been wasted all the same. It has been more than wasted, since their genetic delusions have led to harmful changes in practice and policy. There is no gene for criminality. One may as well imagine genes that make you support a particular political party or football team. Some people do.[27] The fact that some are professional geneticists is a heartening demonstration of scientific freedom, which is nothing if it does not include the freedom to be heartbreakingly wrong. Perhaps it is a mistake to blame those who produce science that retards rather than propels our understanding. They may have been born with the gene for doing so.

We like ascribing genetic causes to things. There is something reassuring about it, something satisfyingly scientific and technological. The satisfaction explains the endless books and articles on genes for homosexuality or creativity, criminality or happiness. The satisfaction comes from feeling we have been scientific and from the relief of having moved a topic out of an endlessly complicated arena – caught in the crosswinds of psychology, sociology, culture and the ineffable typhoon of human life – and pinned it neatly like a butterfly on the board of scientific classification. But there is no gene for homosexuality. As mentioned before, there isn't even a gene for height. There isn't even a genetic explanation for height. Not so much as the prospect of one lies before us.

We understand the genetic basis of single-gene disorders that manifest overwhelming and predictable effects. We are building up rafts of known polymorphisms that contribute small amounts to the risk of more common conditions, but understanding predispositions is an ocean away from explaining events. Some known variations make people more or less likely to get a cold – but no scientific constellation of genes can predict someone will catch a cold in particular circumstances on a certain day. The convolutions are too dazzling. Ditto for flu or pneumonia or almost all the other perils we are born to face. With height we shall steadily get better at generalisations, but specific predictions would need to encompass not only understanding how our genes gave rise to stature in every environment in which every human has ever lived, but also how they would respond to every conceivable different environment in the future, and in combination with every other possible gene we might then possess. Our generalisations will improve, and the technical sophistication underlying them will get more impressive, but when it comes to speaking meaningfully about a person's predisposition to homosexuality, or their sense of duty or love of football, genetics will continue to offer nothing but distraction and confusion. To fathom someone's character is helpful only if you remember that the effort is metaphorical.

The Human Genome Project and its excitements have slightly damped down our long-standing fondness for dividing traits into being x per cent environmental and y per cent genetic, but the tendency remains. It should be resisted, and not only because a knowledge of heritability is often useless or harmful when trying to make decisions about the world. Water does not have two-thirds the properties of hydrogen and one-third of oxygen. As molecules get bigger it gets ever harder to predict their properties from knowing their components, and humans are

more than their sum of molecules. The heritability of a trait, even
when very high, does nothing to tell us that it cannot be changed
best through environment. A simple genetic condition called
phenylketonuria results in severe developmental abnormalities.
In the past, everyone who had the mutation suffered the effects:
its heritability was 100 per cent. The problem was that the body
could not cope with a particular nutrient. Remove the nutrient
from the diet and life becomes normal: the heritability of the
condition drops to zero. Intelligence will respond in radically
different ways to the endless permutations of genome and environment. In any but the simplest of examples, investigating the
heritability of a trait can be to pursue a non-problem when
nothing rests on the answer, when the result can have no benefits. As with intelligence, it can only harm, by distracting from
ways in which investigation of the same trait can be more
helpfully pursued. Not one researcher into the heritability of
happiness or intelligence has added to either and more than
one has deducted from both.

We cannot predict what gene therapy – gene alteration – will
allow us to do but we can predict how it will start. It will start
by tackling simple mutations that leave people dying or appallingly disabled. Risks of new technology are more acceptable in
those with most to gain and least to lose. Initially, we will gain
success in correcting loss of function mutations: already we are
beginning to. Omissions are easiest to find solutions for. Next
will come simple mutations where the errors are commissions
– slightly harder, since it is more difficult to delete or alter a
gene than to add one, but still relatively simple because the
link between genetic mistake and its physical effect is relatively
straightforward too. Again, the initial steps forward will be
taken in people whose defects are so extremely damaging as to
be life-limiting.

As we grow in confidence, the indications for gene alteration will spread. We'll know the costs and we'll be able to better insert the genes we wish in the places we want. Off-target effects, where genes are inserted in the wrong place or in ways that alter coding elsewhere in the genome, will be acceptably minimised. But the chain from gene to protein to person will always contain unpredictable elements. Even with simple problems our mutations will have unpredictable consequences. We will grow confident of knowing how an intervention will alter DNA and the proteins it codes for, but except in the simplest of biochemical settings we will never eliminate the unpredictability of how they go on to interact with all the others, and how the whole combines or, once combined, interacts with the wider world.

Gaining confidence with particular simple mutations, we will gradually lower the amount of disability required to merit intervention. From altering aberrant pathways in those with extreme variants, we will move towards changing normal ones in order to decrease risk and decelerate ageing.

Drugs for cardiovascular risk are already changing from pills we take each evening to injections we take every few months. Rather than a drug that fights the effect of a molecule in our bodies, we are beginning to inject ourselves with agents that block their production, that interfere with the expression of our genes. The next step will just be to alter those genes. Taking a statin every day is too much trouble to be worth it when our chance of benefiting from them any time over the next decade is vanishingly small. When we need just one pill to benefit for the rest of our lives, the situation changes. We already have injections that silence genes for months.[28] This is the manner in which gene therapy will first transform most human lives. Rather than adjusting our physiology with daily pills we will alter the expression of the genes themselves. That form of gene therapy, in a manner that is common, reliable and effective, will be here within a decade. In 2016 haemophilia was corrected in a mouse.[29] In 2017 both haemophilia A and B were corrected, at least to a preliminary extent, in people.[30,31] Only a small degree of correction is needed to make a difference. If the body produces even 1 or 2 per cent of the missing clotting factor, people benefit, and only a fraction more is needed to rid them of the disease entirely.[32] Haemophilia will yield to gene therapy. The genetic error is simple and precise and well understood, the disease relatively common (as severe genetic diseases go) and so hugely expensive to treat and live with that research offers the chance to save not only lives, but also money.

Our success will be only a beginning. Restoring as little as 5 per cent of a missing clotting factor is enough to cure haemophilia. So what difference does it make having 5 per cent as opposed to 100 per cent? We have evolved for an environment in which trauma was common but trauma surgeons were not. Might it be that we clot a little bit more than suits our modern world? Many of the drugs used to treat cardiovascular ageing are drugs that damp down clotting. From aspirin to warfarin, the use of these agents is getting more common. Once we prove our ability to genetically adjust the clotting cascade, by taking the risks needed to cure people of haemophilia, we will move on to working out the effects of smaller adjustments. Some of those treated with gene therapy for haemophilia respond more than others. From the variation in response we will examine what part of the normal range in human clotting tendencies gives us the greatest advantage. Once we understand that optimum range everything beyond it will get defined as a disease. If it turns out we do clot more than suits our modern lives, our normal evolutionary inheritance will get classified as a disease too. That's what we've done with hypertension. The rise in blood pressure with age is called a disease, despite being normal in every sense of the word and even when causing no symptoms. Our language could do with refurbishment to reflect the fact we are moving away from curing afflictions and towards endless adjustments that preserve health and the loss of it as we grow long in the tooth, yellow in the leaf.

Experiments on embryos will continue and so will clinical trials of interventions in children and adults. The two approaches will fade into one another. So will the battle against disease blend into the alteration of normality. A recent editorial in the *New England Journal of Medicine* reviewed why we might want to alter the genes we are born with. Among the 'compelling reasons to repair human DNA' were, it noted, 'infirmity of our embryos, infertility in adults, and cognitive decline in our oldest citizens'. But its next sentence was the greatest indication of where medicine is going. 'When people aim to restore health, they might justifiably aim slightly higher than average.'[33] It sounds startling but it is only stating where medicine has got to already. In trying to ensure that no one dies early, we have changed the average age of death. We did it by changing the course of life.

It is bad science and not good analogy which concludes that since haemophilia and intelligence are both based on genes, and we are gaining the ability to adjust haemophilia, the capacity to alter intelligence will shortly follow. What will come instead will be a continuation of the trends that medicine has shown so strongly already: the minimisation of ill health and premature death and the pursuit of health and human capacity. We will continue to aim for a life better than average. The result will be that the average will rise and life improve.

The book of life

As a medical student I was aware that the teaching of anatomy was in decline. An angry letter from an elderly surgeon in *The Lancet* bemoaned the poor state of knowledge possessed by younger doctors and those still at medical school. A few weeks later the journal printed a response from an old classmate of the surgeon's. When they were students, it said, they learnt a lot of anatomy, but that was because there was little else to learn. As an example they summarised what they had been taught of immunology in their student days: that the blood had white cells in it and that they were somehow relevant.

In the decades since, anatomy teaching has changed sufficiently to further chill the hearts of those who fondly remember it being taken more seriously. Rather than laboriously dissecting their own corpses, as even I did, students now barely dissect at all, relying on models or on dissections done by others. The loss has been deliberate. Archie Cochrane, a twentieth-century pioneer who did much to improve the state of knowledge in medicine, had won the prize for anatomy when he trained at Cambridge. Years later he found he could hardly recall anything about it. It was not worth arguing about whether the training had been useful, he said, it was worth an experiment.

Students should be randomised to being taught detailed anatomy or not, and their effectiveness as doctors measured. Not a bad proposal but one overtaken by fate. Those fighting the battle for detailed anatomy teaching have lost.

They have lost because there is so much else to learn. The statistical tools that underlie clinical trials, and the trials themselves and the reasons for doing them, take up swathes of the curriculum. What is it that doctors now need to learn? What should be in the books they study? The questions relate to asking what it is they do. Behind that is the question to what extent they can be helped by technology. Or replaced. We are right to worry about getting the answers to those questions wrong, but not to hanker for the fine old days, when doctors were caring and compassionate and looked at their patients rather than computer screens. It is not the artifice of technology we should fear. 'All things are artificial, for nature is the Art of God', wrote the physician Sir Thomas Browne in his *Religio Medici*. The amount of time doctors spend with their hospital patients has not changed in the fifty years over which we have been measuring it, and technology can be used to aid the human relationships good medicine requires.[1]

Evidence exists about what computers do well and what doctors do well.[2] More is needed but it always will be. That's the nature of evidence even when it relates to nothing of any practical use – even more so when the utility is real. Our ability to acquire evidence about what works and what doesn't, and our improvements in understanding what that evidence needs to consist of in order to be reliable, has driven the transformation of medicine over the past seventy-five years. As much as technology, the technique of the randomised controlled trial has created medicine's effectiveness: it's just that the technology is more impressive.[3] 'Knowing why is more important than

learning what', said James Watson.⁴ In many settings, clinical
medicine included, the reverse is true. Knowing why something has its effect may help you plot your next experiment but
the experiment is what tells you what the effect is; knowledge
by itself cannot predict that. The techniques of acquiring good
evidence are not going to appear in a film drama about the
future. They should. They were key in medicine changing from
a profession that did more harm than good from the beginnings
of history through to the 1930s,⁵ and into one partly responsible
for our modern improvements in life and health. Most medical
decisions today are taken on the basis of good evidence but
about a fifth remain guesses, and even those based on decent
evidence could often helpfully be based on better.⁶ Finessing our
knowledge matters as much as improving our technology. The
single greatest change that would most improve human health
over the coming century would be if randomised trials, rather
than being separated from the practice of daily medicine by a
bureaucracy that discouraged them, were embedded within it.
To call that the single greatest possible change is to say that
it would do more than the elimination of tobacco, which is to
say a very great deal.

If we need no more evidence about the harms of tobacco,
we need it about almost everything else. We need it because the
results of a medical intervention are unpredictable. No matter
our understanding of the theory and the underlying science,
reality can be relied upon to wrong-foot us. Drug trials go
through a number of formal stages. By the time they get to phase
3, we are confident they are going to work. Phase 1 happens
only after theory and expert opinion and animal experiment
all justify a new treatment. Only if the results are good does
the drug then proceed to phase 2, in which its physical effect is
measured to check it meets expectations. Only if those results

are good does it go to phase 3, in which its actual impact on clinical practice is tested. Given the high degree of confidence everyone possessed even before phase 1, phase 3 should be a formality. Such was our certainty that these final obstacles were unnecessary that, up until a few decades ago, we didn't routinely do such phase 3 trials. Many still feel that these hurdles are formalised bureaucracy which stifle innovation and cost lives. Why hold the experts back, why not trust them? 'I think that both with regards to AIDS and cancer and any other life-threatening disease,' the US Congressman in charge of health said in 1995, 'we ought to make available to people as quickly as possible drugs and other therapies that may extend their lives and not wait until we know with certainty that something is going to be effective.'[7] Many doctors feel the same. All are wrong. By the time a new intervention gets to a phase 3 study, it does not face a final bureaucratic hoop but a vital test. Results from phase 3 trials, when you look at them as a series stretching back decades, are fifty–fifty. The new interventions are as likely to harm as to help.[8] With regard to AIDS and cancer and all life-threatening diseases we ought to make available to people as quickly as possible drugs and other therapies that will extend or improve their lives. But first we need to know with certainty, or as much as life allows, that they really do help rather than harm.

The physical world and the human body are so tangled and intricate that predictions are unreliable and tests are needed. If one makes a change at a more basic level of organisation than that of an enzyme or neurotransmitter – at the level, say, of a gene responsible for them – then the convolutions are greater. Recall how few genes we have. With 20,000 proving responsible for all that makes us, each gene is almost always going to be doing more than one thing and the permutations and combinations with which they interact will be astronomical.

Predictability goes down, not up. Hence the certainty that gene therapy will not proceed by a gene-programmer conjuring a blueprint for a new human being. It will get going by learning how to make small changes to dreadful diseases, where the consequences of doing nothing are so awful they justify the hazards of doing anything at all. From there it will edge forward by aiming, each time, a little higher than before and eventually a little higher than average.

The repeated lesson of the twentieth century is of the refrain running through this book: that a host of small changes accumulate into something big, and that at some stage they result not only in a quantitative accumulation of improvements – a steadily increasing life expectancy – but a qualitative change. A different sort of life. Writing in 1898, in a book about the 1800s called *The Wonderful Century: Its Successes and Failures*, Alfred Russel Wallace thought the technological achievements of the previous hundred years were best compared not with the hundred years before that but with the entirety of previous human history. Change will continue to accelerate. All attempts will fail to accurately predict even what will seem, in retrospect, to have been obvious. 'One of the most prominent features of our century has been the enormous and continuous growth of wealth', wrote Wallace in 1898, 'without any corresponding increase in the well-being of the whole people; while there is ample evidence to show that the number of the very poor... has enormously increased.'[9] Our power at predicting the future is not up to our ability to explain the past and Wallace was getting both wrong. Wealth had already increased the well-being of the whole people and has continued to do so. It is likely to go on doing so, however much rises in inequality make that progress stutter and however many stories tell truthfully of the exceptions.

Medawar called science the art of the possible. Through experiments on cows and mice, he showed how the immune system learnt self from non-self. That led to the conclusion that it must, in theory, be possible to conduct a successful organ transplantation. If the system for differentiating self from non-self could be understood, it could be altered. The eventual success did not come from techniques Medawar developed. His effect on the emergence of organ transplantation was to encourage the people who brought it about to believe that they could. The notion that the germ warfare of microorganisms could be harnessed therapeutically had been around for some time but had never been taken seriously. Pasteur mentioned it, noting how fungi killed bacteria, and speculated in passing that it might be medically useful. But the idea did not seem to belong to the realm of the possible. Fifty years passed before Ehrlich, excited by the emergence of organic dyes that stained particular cells and tissues in unique ways, noted that some of these dyes were toxic. If one could find a dye that was taken up only by bacteria, and was toxic to them, the discovery would amount to a 'magic bullet' that would harm the invading microbe and leave the host untouched. Ehrlich took the term from German folklore and used it so persuasively that he put into the realm of the possible a new idea. Doing so triggered a serious search to track down the antibiotics he had predicted were out there. It was a matter of time and the time was only ever going to be short.

Sweeping fantasies and bold predictions are rarely helpful. But sometimes, if they are based closely enough on a sense of how the world actually is, they are. They open up a window onto new views of life. Some willingness to risk making a fool of oneself by being imaginative is necessary, lest the realm of the possible be narrowed down to the scope of what is already there. Ehrlich's idea that dyes could kill microbes was ludicrous – even in retrospect, his idea that they needed to be dyes was a ridiculous muddle – but it was an idea of enough imaginative genius to lead to the prevention of millions and millions of premature deaths. His prediction could have been made decades earlier. It was the insight that was lacking, not the technology.

There is no profit in routine and banal predictions that we will soon rebuild, redesign and improve all bits of the human body and mind: their effect is to demean the incorrigible intricacy of the world. But the future is uncertain and hence its excitement. The uncertainty is not only due to the importance of imagination and genius but because tiny incremental gains will continue to add up to profound changes and these are unpredictable. Water gradually evaporates as the temperature rises in a kettle, but at a certain point everything changes and it boils. Each passenger pigeon or dodo that was killed subtracted only a small amount from the sum of life except when the final deaths, of birds no different from the others, meant the extinction of their species. These phenomena are predictable because we know them; when they first happened, they weren't. The computers I use today are incrementally faster than those I used yesterday but the difference does not mean they are doing the same things faster. They are doing different things entirely. 'Often quoted is the saying attributed to the architect Ludwig Mies van der Rohe, "Less is more"', wrote the physicist John Archibald Wheeler, adding an alternative:

'More is different'. When you put enough elementary units together, you get something that is more than the sum of these units. A substance made of a great number of molecules, for instance, has properties such as pressure and temperature that no one molecule possessed. It may be a solid or a liquid or

a gas, although no single molecule is solid or liquid or gas...
When enough simple elements are stirred together, there is no
limit to what can result.[10]

In sleeve notes written to accompany a recording of Mozart's
Requiem, Stephen Jay Gould – in his capacity as a student of
history and evolution – remarked that 'Unpredictable contin-
gency, not lawlike order, rules the pathways of history.'[11] How
easily, he pointed out, Mozart might have survived as long as
Händel. The collision of microorganisms with a single immune
system had consequences we still feel. But then so did the good
luck of Mozart surviving smallpox, typhoid and rheumatic fever
as a child – and of having existed at all. As it was in the past so
shall it be in the future. The trends of technology show some
predictability. If Florey, Chain and Heatley had not discovered
penicillin, someone else would have.* Computers would have
been interconnected through a worldwide web had Tim Berners
Lee never been born. But human culture is less easy to prophesy.
Science has not changed that and shows no sign of being able
to. In the discussion after a talk given by Gould, Peter Medawar
asked the audience whether anyone present could give a single
example of a successful prediction about human societies made
on the basis of biology. None could.[12] Genetics and evolution
and biology are full of interest, but their insights cannot be
applied to all problems. Sociologists, psychologists, economists,
political scientists and historians have precious little to offer.
It is precious because it is the best going. 'Say not, let there be

---

* Fleming discovered a property of a broth of penicillin mould. It
was Florey, Chain and Heatley who isolated the specific molecule. Had
they given it a new name, as is normal when a drug is discovered, their
role would have been clearer. Bayer, when they discovered Aspirin and
Heroin, would never have dreamt of calling them Willow Bark or Poppy.

light,' wrote Hazlitt, 'but darkness visible'.[13] It was the same thought which Keats put so famously:

> Several things dove-tailed in my mind, and at once it struck me what quality went to form a Man of Achievement, especially in Literature, and which Shakespeare possessed so enormously – I mean Negative Capability, that is, when a man is capable of being in uncertainties, mysteries, doubts, without any irritable reaching after fact and reason.[14]

'Science lives in a perpetual present, and must always discard its own past as it advances', wrote Clive James.[15] Bewitchingly put and entirely wrong. Science is a historical project. 'Poetry comprehends all science', Shelley said, which was better.[16] He meant that science was necessarily imaginative. Its processes can be automated but not its creativity. 'A man cannot say I will write poetry', he asserted; 'the greatest poet even cannot say it'. Imagination comes with no guarantees. 'An art of discovery is not possible', noted William Whewell, the man who coined the term 'scientist'. One can write down words or perform an experiment but that is no guarantee of producing either poetry or science. What is true of individuals is not true of societies. At a higher level of organisation, results cease being random and become at least partly predictable. In the right cultural environments, science and poetry prosper.

'A scientist can revisit scientific history at his choice', wrote James; 'a humanist has no choice: he must revisit the history of the humanities all the time, because it is always alive, and can't be superseded'. That was wrong too. A man doing a scientific experiment has to be basing it on history, and the better his judging of history the more likely he is to have sensed the future possibilities he hopes his experiment will reveal. A man who wishes to be a scientist must live in the past, or at least with an acute awareness of how the past influences the present and how the two together determine the future. 'Fashion is something barbarous,' wrote Santayana, 'for it produces innovation without reason and imitation without benefit.'[17] Without a feel for history, there is no distinguishing the weak touch of fashion from the grip of reality. The difference is vital. 'The certainty that life cannot be long, and the probability that it will be much shorter than nature allows,' said Samuel Johnson, 'ought to awaken every man.'[18] Ehrlich's insight about the existence of antibiotics carried weight with his audience for the same reason that it turned out to be so broadly and usefully correct. It was based on a sense of the possible. It was a piece of imagination, of poetic inspiration. Such moments – in science as in all else – come by grace, and grace comes by art, and art does not come easy.[19] Ehrlich had spent his life putting in the work that gained him such a feel for the history and progress of science that he could sense its possibilities. What seems obvious in retrospect was obvious at the time to nobody but him, and not even to him until he thought of it.

Over a century ago Osler pointed out that anaesthesia was a miracle not anticipated even in the Bible. Today we can add that neither were antibiotics, nor the progress the world has seen in mortality and morbidity, in social mobility, in racial and sexual equality, in freedom of behaviour, in the open access technology offers to the best of culture. Riches for all have been preached by religions, but the riches were of the afterlife or they were spiritual; they were never the worldly ones we have achieved. It is easy to overlook that Christ told the rich man to give his money to the poor in order to help the rich man's soul, not the poor man's life. Even the New Testament's message of love focused on the benefits of being a better person, not of making a better world. To aid and ease the poor and the diseased has been a common aspiration of religions since religions began. The elimination of absolute poverty and the annihilation of premature disease has not. We have gone some way to managing what our greatest prophets never conceived was possible.

Miseries that were once common have become less so. The achievement is no less precious for being incomplete. In his memoir of the First World War, the tank commander Wilfred Bion recalled the noises of a quiet night on the Western Front, sounds that he remembered ever after in 'the watch fires of a thousand sleepless nights'.[20] The sounds had struck him when he first heard them as being the cries of bitterns, of marsh birds. In fact they were the cries of the men stuck in mud of no-man's-land, sinking and dying. 'Do you mean no stretcher bearer gets them?', he asked, on the night he first understood what they were. 'No stretcher bearer would be such a fool', he was told. Those who left the tracks and paths in order to try sank into the mud themselves, and were never found.

Many have been lost and many will continue to be, their lives and their hopes sucked down without a trace. Everyone reading this will be able to think of a hundred counter-examples to progress, a hundred reasons not to give in to cheerfulness and optimism. But everything is disappointing in practice. Counter-examples do not outweigh what has happened in human history and what is set to continue happening, which, for all its flaws, is justly called progress. So many people have drowned in the mud of war and in the metaphorical mud of disease, lack of opportunity and life's other hazards, the hazards in which lives that could be well lived are swamped and sunk. It matters that the fate befalls fewer than ever before, and knowing that this is so matters also. It matters because fortifying our sense that the world is improvable helps our efforts to improve it. The world has never been so beautiful. Those born into the most miserable and bleak of today's countries face a brighter future than those born into the richest and best of two centuries ago. The fact that these are generalisations means they have exceptions. It also means that in general they are true. The improvements are likely to keep coming, so long as climate change or nuclear war or the toxic effects of autocracy and mob rule do not eliminate their ability to do so. Science has proven its worth as a way of making life better. To think the world will continue to be improved by science is an act of optimism that has to be shakily advanced, but to think it will be put right without science is not even good enough to be shaky. Today few of us have first-hand experience of the loss of one of our children, let alone several. First-hand experience of death before old age is still normal, in the statistical sense. It is shocking when a friend dies in middle age. It will become more so. Generations of children will grow up for whom losing a parent prematurely shall be as rare an experience as for a parent to lose a child is now.

Ötzi

Ötzi the ice-man fell into the Alpine ice 2,000 years before the Pharaoh Tutankhamun walked the earth. He emerged in 1991.

When Ötzi was alive civilisation was flourishing. We have the poetry and laws and medical knowledge of Sumer, and much of it feels modern. From concerns that publicans might take advantage of consumers by serving them small measures,[21] through to its curses ('may your columns… fall to the ground like tall young men drunk on wine'[22]), it is a culture we can recognise. A teacher tells a student about to begin his adult education, 'you will never return to your blinkered vision'. Eyes once opened to ideas cannot be easily closed on them, nor, he explains, should they be – 'that would be greatly to demean due deference, the decency of mankind'.[23]

How much of this cultural knowledge reached Ötzi, with his flint knife, copper-headed axe and clothing of grass and leather, we cannot know. Some fraction. The clothes he wore and the equipment he carried are recognisable to us; so too would have been the thoughts in his mind. Both are less than they would be today. The tools his hand and his mind could grasp were the tools of his age. Our capacities have expanded. The bioprosthetics available to Alpinists are beyond what he could have dreamt of – and so are their dreams.

Free of a modern diet, Ötzi's teeth showed no signs of decay but the roughness of his diet had ground his molars flat. His incisors were worn too, probably the result of needing to use them as tools, biting down to work the leather his life depended on. He might have been twenty when he died or he might have been sixty; we can't tell. He was arthritic in his back and in his right hip. He had broken his ribs long enough beforehand that they had had enough time to heal. He had the calcified blood vessels of atherosclerosis. He had survived frostbite, but incompletely – his left little toe bore the scars. The bones of his legs were thickened from hard use.

Away from the great civilisations of his day, Ötzi lived and died at the shadowy edge of the world. Even for the luckiest, life was shorter and more run through with violence and uncertainty and random death. The scope of human imagination was not so broad, nor were lives buoyed up or made rich by thousands of years of written culture. It was not only teeth and bones that were worn down. Ötzi was about 1.65 metres (5 ft 5 in), but modern times would have changed his thoughts more fundamentally than his measurements. The real difference it would have made would have been to the life of his mind. When life was wilder and more inexplicable, when the horrors of fate that were common could not even be understood, Ötzi would have lived in fear. He was right to. His fate was to die from being shot in the back.[24]

Darwin was thought of by many as a lucky plodder. He still is, the verdict of those who notice that alongside *On the Origin of Species* and *The Descent of Man* he wrote chiefly on the details of worms, barnacles, orchids and corals. Medicine is often felt to consist of advances like penicillin – of discoveries where the word 'breakthrough' must always be applied. Both views are wrong. It was absorption in detail that meant Darwin produced grand sweeps of view that were not grandiose. His study of worms and corals and natural selection showed how small changes could create landscapes and create species. Medawar wrote of how often the public assumed biology institutes were full of people arguing about the definition of life, when actually the question was of no interest there because it inspired no experiments. Detail and uncertainty are hallmarks of seriousness. The effortful interest in truth is supported by the habit of always reaching for explanations whose conceptions match the phenomena one is trying to explain. The length of the coastline of Maine is measurable with a ruler on a map but not with one on a beach. 'At each stage, entirely new laws, concepts and generalisations are necessary... Psychology is not applied biology nor is biology applied chemistry.'[25]

Most of the time we sense there is something wrong with any explanation that makes out life is simple. Much about the world is too muddled to be systematic. From the crooked timber of humanity, nothing straight was ever made.[26] When even physics serves as an imperfect model for the world, biology and social science cannot hope to do better. Knowledge and information too easily accumulate enough to impress but not sufficiently to help. 'She had a great many opinions,' said V. S. Naipaul of a character he disliked, 'but taken together they did not add up to a point of view.'[27] Life can never be seen clearly, but having a point of view allows one a position to occupy when peering at it. Collections of facts and opinions are not substantial enough to ward off ideology, and ideology subtracts from what one can see of life.* Such thoughts are not out of place in a book about medicine and medical science. Famine and war count when it comes to avoidable mortality. They counted in the twentieth century and they count today. Liberal democracies are deeply, profoundly and permanently flawed, packed full of compromise and dishonesty, self-interest and fudge. 'The worst government is often the most moral', wrote H. L. Mencken. 'One composed of cynics is often very tolerant and humane. But when fanatics are on top there is no limit to oppression.'[28] Liberal democracies remain the fundamental drivers of human improvement. They have been since they started and they started a long time ago. When the Romans invaded Britain and health improved sufficiently for human height to rise, the improvement came because Roman society

---

* 'As Darwin discovered the law of evolution in organic nature,' said Engels, 'so Marx discovered the law of evolution in human history.' Cited in Terrence Ball, 'Marx and Darwin: A Reconsideration', *Political Theory* (1979) 7(4):469–483. To describe the socioeconomic structures he saw in society, and to point out who benefited and who did not, was one thing. To claim human society had to be seen in the light of the model, rather than the model in the light of observations of society, was another. It was consistent with his false analogy between biology and social history.

was better than that of the Britons. To say that is just saying the same thing twice. What's not tautological is to point out that it is evidence that Roman society, for all it was far from being liberal or democratic in a modern sense, allowed more human freedom and fairness, more tolerance and liberality, than had been managed by pre-Roman Britons. When freedoms and opportunities are balanced and compromised in a more civil way than before, people get healthier. One does not need to wait for perfection in order to look for improvement.

Science and ideology are mutual antagonists. Being empirical – experimental – science opposes the idea that the world can be understood in advance, through theory, which itself is the bedrock of ideology. 'There is a mask of theory over the whole face of nature', said William Whewell in the nineteenth century.[29] It was science that was capable of seeing past the mask, and it still is, because science is the methodical prioritising of experience over expectations. Science strengthens our ability to learn from experience just as ideology weakens it. Science flourishes best in societies whose beliefs are incomplete and inconsistent. It is blighted by orthodoxy, as Soviet agriculture was by Lysenkoism, a system of beliefs about biology and genetics that fitted well with communist ideals and badly with reality. Scientists who objected were killed and their objections proven correct when crop yields fell. Many more then died too, and they died from starvation. Compared with that, measles outbreaks among 'anti-vaxxers' in the southern USA feel like lessons in progress.

Progress in medicine equates to expansion. Two hundred years ago Britain's 11 million inhabitants were served by a few hundred physicians. Now there are 65 million people living here and if the number of doctors had gone up in proportion there would be a couple of thousand, not many more than staff my own hospital. Instead, there are a quarter of a million.

Will medicine just get ever bigger, occupying more and more of our lives? Potentially, yes, and let us hope so. Not only will it get bigger as it gets more effective, it will get bigger as we need to spend less of our time on other occupations. It's no coincidence that medical activity is increasing as other forms of employment are shrinking. It's one of the luxuries progress buys us. As we develop we get better at doing many things with fewer people. Mechanisation reduces some opportunities but by making the world more efficient it creates others. That could leave us with greater inequality, and a large underclass of long-term unemployed, or it could make us strive to ensure that entry into the professions that remain is never limited by lack of education. It's certainly not limited by genes. Societies with fewer menial jobs will need to direct ever more investment into education. Increasing wealth should mean a rising number of people employed in education and in health care. More is not necessarily better when it comes to health and education but a better world certainly has more. There are no limits to education. Whether results are worth the expense and the effort depends on how much we have to spend and on how wisely we spend it. The same applies to medicine. The notion that health-care services will shrink as we get better at health prevention was a fond fantasy and a bad mistake. Age shall always weary us, and the years condemn, and staving off premature death ever more effectively will only make the problems of old age weigh more heavily. As we cope with those problems we have to remember to celebrate the fact we have them.

Health promotion and healthy living do not catch the idea of what medicine is now about. The notion that we ought to live well, physically speaking, has a moral edge to it, an edge sharp enough to cut. Its puritanism contains more than a seed – more even than a sapling – of the notion that the proper way forward is not to swallow pills or submit to surgery but to eat little, drink less, exercise heartily (preferably out of doors and in bracing weather while wearing shorts) and fend off illness through strength of self-denying spirit. One sees this in the policies that health promotion and healthy living lead to and in the way they are pushed. It accounts for the absence of clarity about the evidence, and the absence of quantification when it comes to what we buy ourselves through brisk walks and small meals. The lack of evidence and lack of clarity result from the policies being based on puritanism, not science. Puritanism believes healthy living is a moral good, and moral goods need not be justified by measurement or assessment. 'The Puritan hated bear-baiting,' wrote Macaulay, 'not because it gave pain to the bear but because it gave pleasure to the spectators.' That spirit still lives.

The prolongation of healthy life is what medicine is now about, but this is obscured by its overlap with the tradition of good advice and puritanism. The overlap is harmful. Critics of medicine's increasing tendency to intrude into our healthy lives take it for being puritanism. The extra days of health that pills buy us are not worth their costs, these critics point out. They should be encouraged: encouraged and answered, for sometimes they might be right. Health prolongation is no more something that should be sold on the basis of moral superiority than is healthy living. The precise costs and benefits of pills need measuring. Only on the basis of good measurements, of what they have to offer and what burden they bring, can anyone decide whether to take them. There should be no obligation on anyone to accept or deny any therapeutic arsenal. But there should be an obligation on everyone to be clear what they are about. Rejecting the proven benefit of a drug in the full understanding of what it is will always be a reasonable response, but if the person doing the rejecting is simultaneously swallowing a pill proven to have no benefits and some harms, as with many vitamins, they are not thinking clearly enough to be reasonable. To defend a choice as being a thoughtful one is always a good defence except when the thoughtfulness is a fraud.

'Wait thirty years and then look out over the earth. You shall see marvel upon marvels, added to those whose nativity you have witnessed; and conspicuous above them you shall see their formidable Result – Man at almost his full stature at last! – and still growing, visibly growing, while you look.' That was Mark Twain's prediction in 1889.[30] There is no reason not to aim for that prediction always being true, save that the notion of a full stature is a false one. Neither evolution nor our genes have placed limits we need bump our heads on. Physical height will not extend indefinitely but culture and intelligence and thoughtfulness offer gardens for cultivation that have no boundaries.

Twain wrote that as part of Walt Whitman's seventieth birthday celebrations. The hazards of reductionism, the way they damped down the fires of imagination and froze the human face divine into a mask of theory, were as palpable to Whitman as they had been to Blake and Wordsworth.

Of physiology from top to toe, I sing;
Not physiognomy alone, nor brain alone, is worthy for the
    Muse
I say the Form complete is worthier far.[31]

Reducing phenomena to their constituents is a hazard only when taken too far. In some situations it works, and works marvellously. Science depends on it, just as it depends on not stretching it beyond the bounds of what is likely to add to understanding. History gives us a guide to where those bounds are, and where they are likely to be tomorrow. Much of what most fascinates us will remain enthralling rather than explicable. Science will never pluck out the heart of our mystery. When it gets close to trying it ceases to function and it ceases being science.

Beware of trying to say too much. In his diary the ageing Whitman wrote of adjusting himself to the half-paralysis that followed a stroke. 'The trick is, I find, to tone your wants and tastes low down enough, and make much of negatives, and of mere daylight and the skies.'[32] Predictions need to be good enough to be wrong. The grandest aren't. Modest successes come from modest efforts. We should all properly be half paralysed in the face of the world's complexity, and nowhere more than when we prophesy. I have made much of negatives, of what does not seem possible or likely or predictable. But the daylight and the skies of history – the brave o'erhanging firmament, the majestical roof fretted with golden fire – make for a fine view of what we have achieved and what is stretched ahead of us. What a piece of work is man. The beauty of the world, the paragon of animals: and a work in progress.

Of Life immense in passion, pulse, and power,
Cheerful, for freest action form'd under the laws divine,
The Modern Man I sing.

Notes

The shape of things to come

1 Richard Lovelace, 'To Lucasta, Going to the Warres', *Lucasta* (1649).
2 Raphael Lemkin, 'Axis Rule in Occupied Europe', in *The Lawbook Exchange* (New Jersey, 2005), p. 79.
3 Found in Trevor Levere, 'A letter to Humphry Davy', *Poetry Realized in Nature*, Cambridge University Press (1981), p. 21.

Death

1 Lewis Carroll, *Alice's Adventures in Wonderland and Through the Looking-glass*, Dell (1992), p. 182.
2 Yuval Noah Harari, *Homo Deus*, Harvill Secker (2016), p. 23.
3 Kim Beernaert, Tinne Smets, Joachim Cohen, et al., 'Improving comfort around dying in elderly people: A cluster randomised controlled trial', *The Lancet* (8 Jul 2017) 390(10090):125–134, https://DOI.org/10.1016/S0140-6736(17)31265-5.
4 Marcus Tullius Cicero, '*How to Grow Old*', transl. Philip Freeman, Princeton University Press (2016), p. 17.
5 Yuval Noah Harari, *Homo Deus*, Harvill Secker (2016), p. 65.

Age

1 George C. Patton, C. Coffey, S. M. Sawyer, et al., 'Global patterns of mortality in young people: A systematic analysis of population health data', *The Lancet* 374(9693):881–892.
2 Simon C. Griffith, Ian P. F. Owens, Katherine A. Thuman, 'Extra pair paternity in birds: A review of interspecific variation and adaptive

function', 9 Oct 2008, https://DOI.org/10.1046/j.1365-294X.2002. 01613.x.

3   Darren P. Croft, Lauren J. N. Brent, Daniel W. Franks, Michael A. Cant, 'The evolution of prolonged life after reproduction', *Trends in Ecology & Evolution*, (2015) 30(7):407–416,

4   https://www.nytimes.com/2012/03/18/automobiles/as-cars-are-kept-longer-200000-is-new-100000.html.

5   Alexander Pope, *Epistle to Dr. Arbuthnot* (London, 1734).

6   J. P. A. Ioannidis, 'Inconsistent guideline recommendations for cardiovascular prevention and the debate about zeroing in on and zeroing LDL-C levels with PCSK9 inhibitors', *JAMA*, (2017) 318(5):419–420, DOI:10.1001/jama.2017.6765.

7   B. A. Ference, F. Majeed, R. Penumetcha, et al., 'Effect of naturally random allocation to lower low-density lipoprotein cholesterol on the risk of coronary heart disease mediated by polymorphisms in NPC1L1, HMGCR, or both: A 2 × 2 factorial Mendelian randomization study', *J Am Coll Cardiol* (21 Apr 2015) 65(15):1552–61, DOI: 10.1016/j.jacc.2015.02.020, Epub 11 Mar 2015.

8   Sadiya S. Khan, Sanjiv J. Shah, Ekaterina Klyachko, et al., 'A null mutation in SERPINE1 protects against biological aging in humans', *Science Advances* (15 Nov 2017):eaao1617.

9   Maurice Cross (ed.), *Selections from the Edinburgh Review*, vol 3, Baudry's European Library (Paris, 1835), p. 91.

10 S. J. Gould, 'The Power of Narrative', in *The Urchin in the Storm*, W. W. Norton (1988).

11 http://ec.europa.eu/health/archive/ph_projects/2003/action1/docs/2003_1_08_rep2_en.pdf.

Early childhood

1   Simon Wilson, *Tate Gallery: An Illustrated Companion* (London, 1997), p. 90.

2   https://ourworldindata.org/child-mortality/.

3   Taken from the transcript of a lecture given by Richard Peto at the Royal College of Physicians, Harveian Oration 2012, 'Halving premature death', *Clin Med* (Dec 2014) 14:643–657, DOI:10.7861/clinmedicine.14-6-643.

Youth

1   https://ourworldindata.org/war-and-peace.

2   P. Sheehan, K. Sweeney, B. Rasmussen, et al., 'Building the founda-

tions for sustainable development: A case for global investment in the capabilities of adolescents', *The Lancet* 390(10104):1792–1806.

3   Kwang Sung Kim et al., 'Current status of human papillomavirus vaccines', *Clinical And Experimental Vaccine Research* 3(2):168–175.

4   https://www.nobelprize.org/nobel_prizes/medicine/laureates/1966/press.html.

5   https://www.cdc.gov/cancer/hpv/statistics/cases.htm.

6   J. Olsen, T. R. Jørgensen, 'Revisiting the cost-effectiveness of universal HPV-vaccination in Denmark accounting for all potentially vaccine preventable HPV-related diseases in males and females', *Cost Eff Resour Alloc* (11 Feb 2015) 13:4, DOI: 10.1186/s12962-015-0029-9, eCollection 2015.

7   Ali Hammad, Donovan Basil, Wand Handan, et al., 'Genital warts in young Australians five years into national human papillomavirus vaccination programme: National surveillance data', *BMJ* (2013) 346:f2032.

8   Robert E. Wittes, 'Therapies for cancer in children – past successes, future challenges', *N Engl J Med* (20 Feb 2003) 348:747–749, DOI: 10.1056/NEJMe020181.

9   Robert E. Wittes, 'Therapies for cancer in children – past successes, future challenges', *N Engl J Med* (20 Feb 2003) 348:747–749, DOI: 10.1056/NEJMe020181.

10 Kumar Ambuj, Soares Heloisa, Wells Robert, Clarke Mike, Hozo Iztok, Bleyer Archie, et al., 'Are experimental treatments for cancer in children superior to established treatments?' Observational study of randomised controlled trials by the Children's Oncology Group, *BMJ* (2005) 331:1295.

11 John Stuart Mill, *A System of Logic*, vol. 2, John Parker (London, 1843), p. 537.

12 https://www.cdc.gov/mmwr/preview/mmwrhtml/mm5811a1.htm.

13 'Nonfatal fall-related injuries associated with dogs and cats – United States, 2001–2006', *JAMA* (2009) 301(23):2436–2437.

14 Stephen Gwilym, Dominic P. J. Howard, Nev Davies, et al., 'Harry Potter casts a spell on accident prone children', *BMJ* (2005) 331:1505.

15 C. C. Branas, A. E. Kastanaki, M. Michalodimitrakis, et al., 'The impact of economic austerity and prosperity events on suicide in Greece: A 30-year interrupted time-series analysis', *BMJ, Open* (2015) 5:e005619, DOI: 10.1136/bmjopen-2014-005619.

16 G. Chapman, N. Talbot, D. McCartney, et al., 'Evidence based medicine – older, but no better educated?' *The Lancet* 382(9903):1484.

17 O. W. Morgan, C. Griffiths, A. Majeed, 'Interrupted time-series analysis of regulations to reduce paracetamol (acetaminophen) poisoning', *PLoS Med* (2017) 4(4):e105, http://journals.plos.org/plosmedicine/article?id=10.1371/journal.pmed.0040105#pmed-0040105-b005.

18 Ambui Kumar, Heloisa Soares, Robert Wells, et al., 'Are experimental treatments for cancer in children superior to established treatments? Observational study of randomised controlled trials by the Children's Oncology Group', *BMJ* (2005) bmj;bmj.38628.561123.7Cv1.

19 Footnote 3 from the essay 'The Limits of Science', in *The Limits of Science*, OUP (1984).

20 A. L. Jones, P. C. Hayes, A. T. Proudfoot, et al., 'Controversies in management: Should methionine be added to every paracetamol tablet? No: The risks are not well enough known', *BMJ* (1997) 315: 301.

21 O. Bennewith, M. Nowers, D. Gunnell, 'Effect of barriers on the Clifton suspension bridge, England, on local patterns of suicide: Implications for prevention', *British Journal of Psychiatry* (2007) 190(3):266–267, DOI:10.1192/bjp.bp.106.027136.

22 Mark Sinyor, Anthony J. Levitt, 'Effect of a barrier at Bloor Street Viaduct on suicide rates in Toronto: Natural experiment', *BMJ* (2010) 341:c2884.

Middle age

1 See the two biographies of Osler by Harvey Cushing and Michael Bliss.

2 'He believed that the climax of his public career was the honorary doctorate of letters which Oxford University awarded him in 1907.' Justin Kaplan, 'Introduction', in *Connecticut Yankee At King Arthur's Court*, Penguin Classics (1986).

3 Mark Twain, *Autobiography of Mark Twain*, vol. 3, University of California Press (2015).

4 Data from https://ourworldindata.org/child-mortality/ for the USA and for year of birth of the three women.

5 Harvey Cushing, *The Life of Sir William Osler*, Oxford University Press (1925).

6 http://www.westernfrontassociation.com/great-war-people/brothers-arms/2245-obviously-all-was-lost-the-life-and-death-of-edward-revere-osler.html#sthash.Wo8slo9H.cbLQ4RKv.dpbs.

7 R. L. Golden, 'Paul Revere Osler: The other child', *Proceedings* (Baylor University Medical Center) (Jan 2015) 28(1):21–24.

8 A. B. Paine, *A Short Life of Mark Twain*, Doubleday (New York, 1920).

9 M. Thun, R. Peto, J. Boreham, et al., 'Stages of the cigarette epidemic on entering its second century', *Tobacco Control* (2012) 21:96–101.

10 R. Doll, A. B. Hill, 'Smoking and carcinoma of the lung: Preliminary report', *British Medical Journal* (1950) 2(4682):739–748.

11 R. Doll, A. B. Hill, (1954), 'The mortality of doctors in relation to their smoking habits: A preliminary report', *British Medical Journal* (1954) 1(4877):1451–1455.

12 R. Doll, R. Peto, J. Boreham, et al., 'Mortality in relation to smoking: 50 years' observations on male British doctors', *BMJ* (2004) 328: 1519.

13 All figures in this paragraph taken from the transcript of a lecture given by Richard Peto at the Royal College of Physicians, Harveian Oration 2012, 'Halving premature death', *Clin Med* (Dec 2014) 14: 643–657, DOI:10.7861/clinmedicine.14-6-643.

14 http://www.tobaccoatlas.org/topic/smokings-death-toll/.

15 http://visual.ons.gov.uk/what-are-the-top-causes-of-death-by-age-and-gender/.

16 http://visual.ons.gov.uk/what-are-the-top-causes-of-death-by-age-and-gender/.

17 With thanks to Rupert Yardley for the literal translation.

18 K. Britt, R. Short, 'The plight of nuns: Hazards of nulliparity', *The Lancet* 379(9834):2322–2323.

19 C. D. Williams, 'The story of kwashiorkor*', *Nutrition Reviews* (1973) 31:334–340, DOI:10.1111/j.1753-4887.1973.tb07041.x.

20 S. B. Eaton, M. C. Pike, R. V. Short, et al., 'Women's reproductive cancers in evolutionary context', *Q Rev Biol* (Sep 1994) 69(3):353–367, Review.

21 K. Britt, R. Short, 'The plight of nuns: Hazards of nulliparity', *The Lancet* (2012) 379(9834):2322–2323.

22 Pope Paul VI, *Humanae Vitae: On the Regulation of Birth*, Catholic Truth Society (London, 1968), cited in K. Britt, R. Short, 'The plight of nuns: Hazards of nulliparity', *The Lancet* (2012) 379(9834):2322–2323.

23 A. Kent, 'Nuns and contraceptives', *Reviews in Obstetrics & Gynecology* (2012) 5(3–4):e166–167.

Old age

1   John Jowett, William Montgomery, Gary Taylor, et al. (eds), *The Oxford Shakespeare: The Complete Works*, 2nd edition, OUP (2005), p. lxxii.

2   Andrew Kingston, E. Green, et al., 'Is late-life dependency increasing or not? A comparison of the Cognitive Function and Ageing Studies (CFAS)', *The Lancet* (2017) 390(10103):1676–1684.

3   http://www.weeklystandard.com/hitting-eighty/article/2006010.

4   T. Wolfe, *Hooking Up*, Farrar, Strauss & Giroux (2000).

5   http://www.mortality.org/hmd/GBR_NP/STATS/bltper_5x10.txt.

6   http://ec.europa.eu/eurostat/tgm/table.do?tab=table&init=1&language=en&pcode=tsdph220&plugin=1.

7   J. F. Fries, B. Bruce, E. Chakravarty, 'Compression of morbidity 1980–2011: A focused review of paradigms and progress', *Journal of Aging Research* (2011) 261702.

8   V. Mor, 'The compression of morbidity hypothesis: A review of research and prospects for the future, *Journal of the American Geriatrics Society* (2005) 53:S308–S309, DOI:10.1111/j.1532-5415.2005.53496.x.

9   Eileen M. Crimmins, Hiram Beltrán-Sánchez, 'Mortality and morbidity trends: Is there compression of morbidity?', *The Journals of Gerontology: Series B* (1 Jan 2011) 66B(1):75–86, https://DOI.org/10.1093/geronb/gbq088.

10 Edna St Vincent Millay, 'Spring', *Collected Poems*, Harper Perennial (2011).

11 Paul M. Ridker, Brendan M. Everett, Tom Thuren, et al., for the CANTOS Trial Group*, 'Antiinflammatory therapy with canakinumab for atherosclerotic disease', *N Engl J Med* (21 Sep 2017) 377:1119–1131, DOI: 10.1056/NEJMoa1707914.

12 Chris Mullin's *A Very British Coup*, as portrayed on Channel 4 (1988).

13 Mark Ellen, John Fisher (eds), *The Complete Prose and Poetry of Geoffrey Chaucer*, Wadsworth (2012), p. 562.

14 http://visual.ons.gov.uk/what-are-the-top-causes-of-death-by-age-and-gender.

15 G. P. Morris, I. A. Clark, B. Vissel, 'Inconsistencies and controversies surrounding the amyloid hypothesis of Alzheimer's disease', *Acta Neuropathologica* communications (2014) 2:135, DOI:10.1186/s40478-014-0135-5.

16 James Boswell, *Life of Samuel Johnson*, vol. 1, Harper & Brothers (New York, 1846), p. 268.

17 Michel de Montaigne, *The Essays of Michel de Montaigne*, Allen Lane (1991), p. 88.

18 Henry Buxton Forman (ed.), *The Complete Works of John Keats*, vol. 5, Gowers & Gray (Glasgow, 1900), p. 168.

19 Henry Buxton Forman (ed.), *The Complete Works of John Keats*, vol. 5, Gowers & Gray (Glasgow, 1900), p. 204.

Diseases

1 Yuval Noah Harari, *Homo Deus*, Harvill Secker (2016), p. 1.

2 Jane Austen, *Sense and Sensibility*, Chapman & Hall (1870), p. 32.

3 Tim Crayford, Richard Hooper, Sarah Evans, 'Death rates of characters in soap operas on British television: Is a government health warning required?', *BMJ* (1997) 315:1649.

4 Jane Austen, *Sense and Sensibility*, Chapman & Hall (1870), p. 264.

5 Jane Austen, *Sense and Sensibility*, Chapman & Hall (1870), p. 272.

6 http://www.who.int/mediacentre/factsheets/fs310/en/index1.html.

7 M. Quinn, et al., *Cancer trends in England and Wales 1950–1999*, Studies on Medical and Population Subjects, No. 66, National Statistics, Stationery Office (London, 2001).

8 R. L. Siegel, K. D. Miller, A. Jemal, 'Cancer statistics, 2015', *A Cancer Journal for Clinicians* (2015) 65:5–29, DOI:10.3322/caac.21254.

9 C. La Vecchia, M. Rota, M. Malvezzi, et al., 'Potential for improvement in cancer management: Reducing mortality in the European Union', *Oncologist* (May 2015) 20(5):495–498, DOI: 10.1634/theoncologist.2015-0011, Epub 17 Apr 2015.

10 R. Doll, R. Peto, J. Boreham, et al., 'Mortality in relation to smoking: 50 years' observations on male British doctors', *BMJ* (2004) 328:1519.

11 Prabhat Jha, Richard Peto, 'Global effects of smoking, of quitting, and of taxing tobacco', *N Engl J Med* (2 Jan 2014) 370:60–68, DOI: 10.1056/NEJMra1308383.

12 Prabhat Jha, Richard Peto, 'Global effects of smoking, of quitting, and of taxing tobacco', *N Engl J Med* (2 Jan 2014) 370:60–68, DOI: 10.1056/NEJMra1308383.

13 http://www.mortality.org/hmd/GBR_NP/STATS/bltper_5x10.txt.

14 Prabhat Jha, Richard Peto, 'Global effects of smoking, of quitting, and of taxing tobacco', *N Engl J Med* (2 Jan 2014) 370:60–68, DOI: 10.1056/NEJMra1308383.

15 Anna Wagstaff, Richard Doll, 'Science will always win in the end', *Cancer World* (Dec 2004):28–34.

16 Anna Wagstaff, Richard Doll, 'Science will always win in the end', *Cancer World* (Dec 2004):28–34.

17 Prabhat Jha, Richard Peto, 'Global effects of smoking, of quitting, and of taxing tobacco', *N Engl J Med* (2 Jan 2014) 370:60–68, DOI: 10.1056/NEJMra1308383.

18 V. Bouvard, D. Loomis, K. Z. Guyton, et al., 'Carcinogenicity of consumption of red and processed meat', *The Lancet Oncology* 16(16): 1599–1600.

19 D. S. M. Chan, R. Lau, D. Aune, et al., 'Red and processed meat and colorectal cancer incidence: Meta-analysis of prospective studies', *PLoS ONE* (2011) 6(6):e20456, https://DOI.org/10.1371/journal.pone.0020456.

20 R. West, A. McNeill, M. Raw, 'Smoking cessation guidelines for health professionals: An update', *Thorax* (2000) 55:987–999.

21 Jeffrey D. Stanaway, Abraham D. Flaxman, Mohsen Naghavi, et al., 'The global burden of viral hepatitis from 1990 to 2013: Findings from the Global Burden of Disease Study 2013', *The Lancet* (2016) 388(10049):1081–1088.

22 Global Burden of Disease Cancer Collaboration, C. Fitzmaurice, D. Dicker, et al., 'The global burden of cancer 2013', *JAMoncology* (2015) 1(4):505–527.

23 S. Iyengar, K. Tay-Teo, S. Vogler, et al., 'Prices, costs, and affordability of new medicines for hepatitis C in 30 countries: An economic analysis', *PLoS Med* (2016) 13(5):e1002032, https://DOI.org/10.1371/journal.pmed.1002032.

24 A. Elgharably, A. I. Gomaa, M. M. Crossey, et al., 'Hepatitis C in Egypt – past, present, and future', *International Journal of General Medicine* (2016) 10:1–6, DOI:10.2147/IJGM.S119301.

25 Cited in G. M. Oppenheimer, 'Becoming the Framingham study 1947–1950', *American Journal of Public Health* (2005) 95(4):602–610.

26 G. M. Oppenheimer, 'Becoming the Framingham study 1947–1950', *American Journal of Public Health* (2005) 95(4):602–610.

27 Cited in Christopher Hitchens, *Arguably*, Atlantic Books (2012).

28 H. K. Li, A. Agweyu, M. English, et al., An unsupported preference for intravenous antibiotics, *PLoS Med* (2015) 12(5):e1001825, https://DOI.org/10.1371/journal.pmed.1001825.

29 W. F. Enos, R. H. Holmes, J. Beyer, 'Coronary disease among United States soldiers killed in action in Korea: Preliminary report', *JAMA* (1953) 152(12):1090–1093, DOI:10.1001/jama.1953.03690120006002.

30 J. P. Strong, G. T. Malcom, C. A. McMahan, et al., 'Prevalence and

extent of atherosclerosis in adolescents and young adults: Implications for prevention from the pathobiological determinants of atherosclerosis in youth study, *JAMA* (1999) 281(8):727–735, DOI: 10.1001/jama.281.8.727.

31 J. H. O'Keefe Jr, L. Cordain, 'Cardiovascular disease resulting from a diet and lifestyle at odds with our paleolithic genome: How to become a 21st-century hunter-gatherer', *Mayo Clinic Proceedings* (Jan 2004) 79(1):101–108.

32 R. C. Thompson, A. H. Allam, G. P. Lombardi, et al., 'Atherosclerosis across 4000 years of human history: The Horus study of four ancient populations', *The Lancet* (6 Apr 2013) 381(9873):1211–1222.

33 S. Lewington, R. Clarke, N. Qizilbash, et al., Prospective Studies Collaboration, 'Age-specific relevance of usual blood pressure to vascular mortality a meta-analysis of individual data for one million adults in 61 prospective studies', *The Lancet* (2002) 360(9349): 1903–13.

34 Cholesterol Treatment Trialists' (CTT) Collaboration, 'Efficacy and safety of more intensive lowering of LDL cholesterol: A meta-analysis of data from 170 000 participants in 26 randomised trials', *The Lancet* (13 Nov 2010) 376(9753):1670–1681.

35 Albert Smyth (ed.), *The Writings of Benjamin Franklin*, vol. 9, Haskell House (New York, 1970), p. 273.

36 M. Kimura, *The Neutral Theory of Molecular Evolution*, Cambridge University Press (1983).

37 Christopher P. Cannon, Michael A. Blazing, Robert P. Giugliano, et al., for the IMPROVE-IT Investigators*, 'Ezetimibe added to statin therapy after acute coronary syndromes', *N Engl J Med* (18 Jun 2015) 372:2387–2397, DOI: 10.1056/NEJMoa1410489.

38 Figures are available from a wide range of sources, since each come from different trials, but this paper collates some handily together: Earl S. Ford, Umed A. Ajani, Janet B. Croft, et al., 'Explaining the decrease in U.S. deaths from coronary disease, 1980–2000', *N Engl J Med* (7 Jun 2007) 356:2388–2398, DOI: 10.1056/NEJMsa053935.

39 N. J. Wald, M. R. Law, 'A strategy to reduce cardiovascular disease by more than 80%', *BMJ* (2003) 326:1419.

40 Victor Medvei, *A History of Endocrinology*, MTP Press (1982), p. 61.

41 Cited in E. A. M. Gale, 'Historical aspects of type 2 diabetes' [internet], *Diapedia* (13 Aug 2014) 3104287134 rev. no. 28, available from: https://DOI.org/10.14496/dia.3104287134.28.

42 C. M. Lawes, V. Parag, D. A. Bennett, et al., 'Blood glucose and risk of

cardiovascular disease in the Asia Pacific region', Asia Pacific Cohort Studies Collaboration, *Diabetes Care* (Dec 2004) 27(12):2836–2842.

43 G. Danaei, C. M. Lawes, S. Vander Hoorn, et al., 'Global and regional mortality from ischaemic heart disease and stroke attributable to higher-than-optimum blood glucose concentration: Comparative risk assessment', *The Lancet* (Nov 2016) 368(9548):1651–1659.

44 K. Outterson, U. Gopinathan, C. Clift, 'Delinking investment in antibiotic research and development from sales revenues: The challenges of transforming a promising idea into reality', *PLoS Med* (2016) 13(6):e1002043, https://DOI.org/10.1371/journal.pmed.1002043.

45 https://www.who.int/malaria/media/world-malaria-report-2017/en/#Global%20and%20regional%20malaria%20trends%20in%20numbers.

46 Arjen M. Dondorp, François Nosten, Poravuth Yi, et al., 'Artemisinin resistance in *Plasmodium falciparum* malaria', *N Engl J Med* (30 Jul 2009) 361(5):455–467.

47 https://www.ons.gov.uk/employmentandlabourmarket/peopleinwork/labourproductivity/articles/sicknessabsenceinthelabourmarket/2016. Within my own hospital, too, doctors get sick less often than other workers.

Transplantation

1 Gkikas Magiorkinis, Daniel Blanco-Melo, Robert Belshaw, 'The decline of human endogenous retroviruses: Extinction and survival', *Retrovirology* (2015) 12:8, https://DOI.org/10.1186/s12977-015-0136-x.

2 F. Maggioni, G. Maggioni, 'A closer look at depictions of Cosmas and Damian', *American Journal of Transplantation* (2014) 14:494–495, DOI:10.1111/ajt.12573.

3 David Hamilton, *A History of Organ Transplantation*, University of Pittsburgh Press (2012), p. 134.

4 https://www.nobelprize.org/nobel_prizes/medicine/laureates/1960/burnet-lecture.pdf.

5 David Hamilton, *A History of Organ Transplantation*, University of Pittsburgh Press (2012), p. 212.

6 https://www.nobelprize.org/prizes/medicine/2018/summary/.

7 Laurent Lantieri, Philippe Grimbert, Nicolas Ortonne, et al., 'Face transplant: Long-term follow-up and results of a prospective open study', *The Lancet* (Oct 2016) 388(10052):1398–1407.

8 Sandra Amaral, Sudha Kilaru Kessler, Todd J. Levy, et al., '18-month

outcomes of heterologous bilateral hand transplantation in a child: A case report', *The Lancet Child & Adolescent Health* (July 2017) 1(1):35–44.

9 Mats Brännström, Liza Johannesson, Hans Bokström, et al., 'Live-birth after uterus transplantation', *The Lancet* 385(9968):607–616.

10 Pierre Delaere, Jan Vranckx, Geert Verleden, for the Leuven Tracheal Transplant Group*, 'Tracheal allotransplantation after withdrawal of immunosuppressive therapy', *N Engl J Med* (14 Jan 2010) 362: 138–145, DOI: 10.1056/NEJMoa0810653.

11 André van der Merwe, Frank Graewe, Alexander Zühlke, et al., 'Penile allotransplantation for penis amputation following ritual circumcision: A case report with 24 months of follow-up', *The Lancet* (Sept 2017) 390(10099):1038–1047.

12 J. A. A. C. Heuberger, J. I. Rotmans, P. Gal, et al., 'Effects of erythropoietin on cycling performance of well trained cyclists: A double-blind, randomised, placebo-controlled trial', *The Lancet Haematology* (Oct 2017) 4(8):e374–e386.

13 Janet Fricker, 'Cartilage transplantation: An end to creaky knees?', *The Lancet* (Oct 1998) 352(9135):1202.

14 I. Fulco, S. Miot, M. D. Haug, et al., 'Engineered autologous cartilage tissue for nasal reconstruction after tumour resection: An observational first-in-human trial', *The Lancet* (July 2014) 384(9940):337–346.

15 Martin A. Birchall, Alexander M. Seifalian, 'Tissue engineering's green shoots of disruptive innovation', *The Lancet* (July 2014) 384 (9940):288–290.

16 Paolo Macchiarini, Philipp Jungebluth, Tetsuhiko Go, et al., 'Clinical transplantation of a tissue-engineered airway', *The Lancet* (Dec 2008) 372(9655):2023–2030.

17 Retracted: Philipp Jungebluth, Evren Alici, Silvia Baiguera, et al., 'Tracheobronchial transplantation with a stem-cell-seeded bioartificial nanocomposite: A proof-of-concept study', *The Lancet* (Dec 2011) 378(9808):1997–2004.

18 The Lancet Editors, 'Expression of concern – Tracheobronchial transplantation with a stem-cell-seeded bioartificial nanocomposite: A proof-of-concept study', *The Lancet* (April 2016) 387(10026):1359.

19 H. Hara, D. K. Cooper, 'The immunology of corneal xenotransplantation: A review of the literature', *Xenotransplantation* (2010) 17: 338–349, DOI:10.1111/j.1399-3089.2010.00608.x.

20 H. Hara, D. K. Cooper, 'The immunology of corneal xenotransplantation: A review of the literature', *Xenotransplantation* (2010) 17: 338–349, DOI:10.1111/j.1399-3089.2010.00608.x.

21 C. N. Barnard, A. Wolpowitz, J. G. Losman, 'Heterotopic cardiac transplantation with a xenograft for assistance of the left heart in cardiogenic shock after cardiopulmonary bypass', *South African Medical Journal* (17 Dec 1977) 52(26):1035–1038.

22 C. N. Barnard, A. Wolpowitz, J. G. Losman, 'Heterotopic cardiac transplantation with a xenograft for assistance of the left heart in cardiogenic shock after cardiopulmonary bypass', *South African Medical Journal* (17 Dec 1977) 52(26):1035–1038.

23 Cited in D. K. Cooper, (2012), 'A brief history of cross-species organ transplantation', *Proceedings* (Baylor University Medical Center) (2012) 25(1):49–57.

24 Dong Niu, Hong-Jiang Wei, Lin Lin, et al., 'Inactivation of porcine endogenous retrovirus in pigs using CRISPR-Cas9', *Science* (22 Sep 2017):1303–1307.

25 P. J. Cowan, A. J. Tector, 'The resurgence of xenotransplantation', *American Journal of Transplantation* (2017) XX:1–6.

26 A. L. Komaroff, 'Gene editing using CRISPR: Why the excitement?' *JAMA* (2017) 318(8):699–700, DOI:10.1001/jama.2017.10159.

Transportation

1 http://www.who.int/mediacentre/factsheets/fs310/en/.

2 World Health Organization, *Global Status Report on Road Safety* (2015), see http://www.who.int/violence_injury_prevention/road_safety_status/2015/en/.

3 http://www.who.int/violence_injury_prevention/road_safety_status/key_data/en/.

4 D. A. Redelmeier, B. A. McLellan, 'Modern medicine is neglecting road traffic crashes', *PLoS Med* (2013) 10(6):e1001463, https://DOI.org/10.1371/journal.pmed.1001463.

5 http://www.economist.com/news/letters/21596494-car-safety-cyprus-nhs-pete-seeger-climate-change-beauty-food-trains-congress.

6 http://www.economist.com/news/international/21595031-rich-countries-have-cut-deaths-and-injuries-caused-crashes-toll-growing.

Sex

1 See, for example, W. H. James, 'Coital rates and sex ratios', *Human Reproduction* (1 Sep 1997) 12(9):2083–2085, https://DOI.org/10.1093/oxfordjournals.humrep.a019608.

2 Anthony Trollope, *Anthony Trollope: An Autobiography*, vol. 1, Cambridge University Press (2014), p. 94.

3   http://avalon.law.yale.edu/ancient/hamframe.asp.

4   See D. Burch, *Taking the Medicine* (in the chapter 'Book of Life'); see also Thomas Dormandy, *History of Pain*, Yale University Press (2006).

5   G. Hart, *The Routledge Dictionary of Egyptian Gods and Goddesses*, Routledge (2005).

6   P. Taberner, *Aphrodisiacs*, Croom Helm (1985).

7   R. Shamloul, 'Natural aphrodisiacs', *J Sex Med* (2010) 7:39–49, DOI: 10.1111/j.1743-6109.2009.01521.x.

8   D. K. Cooper, 'A brief history of cross-species organ transplantation', *Proceedings* (Baylor University Medical Center) (2012) 25(1), 49–57.

9   Ian H. Osterloh, 'The discovery and development of Viagra', in *Sildenafil, Milestones in Drug Therapy*, U. Dunzendorfer (ed.), Springer (Basel, 2004).

10 F. Korkes, A. Costa-Matos, R. Gasperini, et al., 'Recreational use of PDE5 inhibitors by young healthy men: Recognizing this issue among medical students', *The Journal of Sexual Medicine* (2008) 5:2414–2418, DOI:10.1111/j.1743-6109.2008.00792.x.

11 A. Bechara, A. Casabé, W. De Bonis, et al., 'Recreational use of phosphodiesterase type 5 inhibitors by healthy young men', *The Journal of Sexual Medicine* (2010) 7:3736–3742, DOI:10.1111/j.1743-6109.2010.01965.x.

12 N. Mondaini, R. Ponchietti, G. H. Muir, 'Sildenafil does not improve sexual function in men without erectile dysfunction but does reduce the postorgasmic refractory time', *International Journal of Impotence Research* (2003) 15:225–228.

13 Hermann van Ahlen, Sabine Kliesch, 'Disorders of Erection, Cohabitation, and Ejaculation', in *Andrology: Male Reproductive Health and Dysfunction*, E. Nieschlag, H. M. Behre, S. Nieschlag (eds), Springer (2010).

14 R. Shamloul, 'Natural aphrodisiacs', *J Sex Med* (Jan 2010) 7(1 Pt 1):39–49, DOI: 10.1111/j.1743-6109.2009.01521.x, Epub 30 Sep 2009, Review, PubMed PMID: 19796015.

15 R. Shamloul, 'Natural aphrodisiacs', *J Sex Med* (Jan 2010) 7(1 Pt 1):39–49, DOI: 10.1111/j.1743-6109.2009.01521.x, Epub 30 Sep 2009, Review, PubMed PMID: 19796015.

16 H. A. Fink, R. Mac Donald, I. R. Rutks, et al., 'Sildenafil for male erectile dysfunction: A systematic review and meta-analysis', *Arch Intern Med* (24 Jun 2002) 162(12):1349–1360.

17 A. Burls, L. Gold, W. Clark, 'Systematic review of randomised controlled trials of sildenafil (Viagra) in the treatment of male erectile

dysfunction', *The British Journal of General Practice* (*The Journal of the Royal College of General Practitioners*) (2001) 51(473):1004–1012.

18 J. Podhorna, R. E. Brown, 'Flibanserin has anxiolytic effects without locomotor side effects in the infant rat ultrasonic vocalization model of anxiety', *British Journal of Pharmacology* (2000) 130:739–746, DOI:10.1038/sj.bjp.0703364.

19 S. Woloshin, L. M. Schwartz, 'US Food and Drug Administration approval of flibanserin: Even the score does not add up', *JAMA Intern Med* (2016) 176(4):439–442, DOI:10.1001/jamainternmed.2016.0073.

20 http://www.slate.com/articles/double_x/doublex/2014/04/female_viagra_and_the_fda_the_agency_s_rejection_of_flibanserin_has_nothing.html.

21 http://www.slate.com/articles/double_x/doublex/2014/04/female_viagra_and_the_fda_the_agency_s_rejection_of_flibanserin_has_nothing.html.

22 M. McCartney, 'Flibanserin for low sexual desire is not feminism', *BMJ* (2015) 351:h5650.

23 L. Jaspers, F. Feys, W. M. Bramer, et al., 'Efficacy and safety of flibanserin for the treatment of hypoactive sexual desire disorder in women: A systematic review and meta-analysis', *JAMA Intern Med* (2016) 176(4):453–462, DOI:10.1001/jamainternmed.2015.8565.

24 S. Woloshin, L. M. Schwartz, 'US Food and Drug Administration approval of flibanserin: Even the score does not add up', *JAMA Intern Med* (2016) 176(4):439–442, DOI:10.1001/jamainternmed.2016.0073.

25 For example, https://www.ipsos.com/sites/default/files/ct/news/documents/2017-10/bbc-newsbeat-survey-tables-2017.pdf.

26 M. Pierce, R. Hardy, 'Commentary: The decreasing age of puberty – as much a psychosocial as biological problem?' *International Journal of Epidemiology* (2012) 41(1):300–302.

27 Jonathan N. Tinsley, Maxim I. Molodtsov, Robert Prevedel, et al., 'Direct detection of a single photon by humans', *Nature Communications* (19 Jul 2016) 7, art. no.: 12172.

28 M. H. D. Larmuseau, K. Matthijs, T. Wenseleers, 'Long-term trends in human extra-pair paternity: Increased infidelity or adaptive strategy? A Reply to Harris', *Trends in Ecology & Evolution* (July 2016) 31(9):663–665.

29 P. Hartman, D. Wetzel, P. H. Crowley, et al., 'The impact of extra-pair mating behavior on hybridization and genetic introgression', *Theor Ecol* (2012) 5:219–229, 10.1007/s12080-011-0117-1.

30 Charles Darwin, *The Descent of Man*, John Murray (London, 1871).

31 Richard O. Prum, Beauty Happens, *Natural History* (Apr 2017).

32 A. R. Wallace, 'The colors of animals and plants', part 1, *Am Nat* (1877) 11:641–662.

33 Letter from John Adams to Abigail Adams, post 12 May 1780 [electronic edition], Adams Family Papers: An Electronic Archive, Massachusetts Historical Society, http://www.masshist.org/digitaladams/.

34 http://www.pewsocialtrends.org/2015/05/07/childlessness/.

35 L. Ammon Avalos, C. Galindo, D. K. Li, 'A systematic review to calculate background miscarriage rates using life table analysis', *Birth Defects Res A, Clin Mol Teratol* (Jun 2012) 94(6):417–23, DOI: 10.1002/bdra.23014, Epub 18 Apr 2012; and A. J. Wilcox, A. E. Treloar, D. P. Sandler, 'Spontaneous abortion over time: Comparing occurrence in two cohorts of women a generation apart', *Am J Epidemiol* (Oct 1981) 114(4):548–53.

36 C. James, *Cultural Amnesia*, Picador (2012), p. 187.

37 Billy Bragg, *The Short Answer*, from the album Workers Playtime, 1988, Go! Discs.

Height

1 Samuel Johnson, *The Rambler*, Alex Chalmers (ed.), vol. 3, J. J. Woodward (Philadelphia, 1827), p. 95.

2 https://www.economics.ox.ac.uk/Oxford-Economic-and-Social-History-Working-Papers/heights-across-the-last-2000-years-in-england.

3 https://ourworldindata.org/human-height/#global-perspective-of-increase-of-human-height.

4 See G. Stulp, A. P. Buunk, S. Verhulst, et al., 'Tall claims? Sense and nonsense about the importance of height of US presidents', *The Leadership Quarterly* (2012), http://dx.DOI.org/10.1016/j.leaqua.2012.09.; https://www.researchgate.net/publication/232274709_Tall_claims_Sense_and_nonsense_about_the_importance_of_height_of_US_presidents; accessed 4 Jul 2017.

5 Nicola Persico, Andrew Postlewaite, Dan Silverman, 'The effect of adolescent experience on labor market outcomes: The case of height', *Journal of Political Economy* (2004) 112(5):1019–1053.

6 For example, R. A. Fisher, 'The correlation between relatives on the supposition of Mendelian inheritance', *Transactions of the Royal Society of Edinburgh* (1918) 52:399–433.

7 Andrew R. Wood, Tonu Esko, Jian Yang, et al., 'Defining the role

of common variation in the genomic and biological architecture of adult human height', *Nature Genetics* (2014) 46:1173–1186.

8   Andrew R. Wood, Tonu Esko, Jian Yang, et al., 'Defining the role of common variation in the genomic and biological architecture of adult human height', *Nature Genetics* (2014) 46:1173–1186.

9   Eirini Marouli, Mariaelisa Graff, Carolina Medina-Gomez, et al., 'Rare and low-frequency coding variants alter human adult height', *Nature* (9 Feb 2017) 542:186–190.

10 Jian Yang, Beben Benyamin, Brian P. McEvoy, et al., 'Common SNPs explain a large proportion of the heritability for human height', *Nature Genetics* (2010) 42:565–569.

11 Andrew R. Wood, Tonu Esko, Jian Yang, et al., 'Defining the role of common variation in the genomic and biological architecture of adult human height', *Nature Genetics* (2014) 46:1173–1186.

12 C. Langenberg, M. J. Shipley, G. D. Batty, et al., 'Adult socioeconomic position and the association between height and coronary heart disease mortality: Findings from 33 years of follow-up in the Whitehall Study', *American Journal of Public Health* (2005) 95(4):628–632.

13 A. Deaton, R. Arora, 'Life at the top: The benefits of height', *Economics and Human Biology* (2009) 7(2):133–136.

14 C. Langenberg, M. J. Shipley, G. D. Batty, et al., 'Adult socioeconomic position and the association between height and coronary heart disease mortality: Findings from 33 years of follow-up in the Whitehall Study', *American Journal of Public Health* (2005) 95(4):628–632.

15 Emerging Risk Factors Collaboration, 'Adult height and the risk of cause-specific death and vascular morbidity in 1 million people: Individual participant meta-analysis', *International Journal of Epidemiology* (2012) 41(5):1419–1433.

16 A. Adler, *The Individual Psychology of Alfred Adler*, Basic Books (New York, 1956).

17 Emerging Risk Factors Collaboration, 'Adult height and the risk of cause-specific death and vascular morbidity in 1 million people: Individual participant meta-analysis', *International Journal of Epidemiology* (2012) 41(5):1419–1433.

18 Nicola Persico, Andrew Postlewaite, Dan Silverman, 'The effect of adolescent experience on labor market outcomes: The case of height', *Journal of Political Economy* (2004) 112(5):1019–1053.

19 http://www.tennisabstract.com/blog/2017/09/04/how-much-does-height-matter-in-mens-tennis/.

20 Matthew 6:27, King James' Bible.

21 T. Dobzhansky, *Mankind Evolving: The Evolution of the Human Species*, Yale University Press (1962).

Breadth

1 See https://books.google.com/ngrams/graph?content=gritty+realism &year_start=1800&year_end=2000&corpus=15&smoothing=3& share=&direct_url=t1%3B%2Cgritty%20realism%3B%2Cco.

2 https://DOI.org/10.1016/S2213-8587(18)30050-0.

3 S. Austin (ed.), *A Memoir of the Reverend Sydney Smith*, vol. 1, Longman (1855), p. 396.

4 B. Rokholm, J. L. Baker, T. I. Sørensen, 'The levelling off of the obesity epidemic since the year 1999 – a review of evidence and perspectives', *Obesity Reviews* (2010) 11:835–846, DOI:10.1111/j.1467-789X.2010.00810.x.

5 B. Rokholm, J. L. Baker, T. I. Sørensen, 'The levelling off of the obesity epidemic since the year 1999 – a review of evidence and perspectives', *Obesity Reviews* (2010) 11:835–846, DOI:10.1111/j.1467-789X.2010.00810.x.

6 K. M. Flegal, M. D. Carroll, B. K. Kit, et al., 'Prevalence of obesity and trends in the distribution of body mass index among US adults, 1999–2010', *JAMA* (2012) 307(5):491–497, DOI:10.1001/jama.2012.39.

7 D. King, 'The future challenge of obesity', *The Lancet* (Aug 2011) 378(9793):743–744.

8 B. C. Johnston, S. Kanters, K. Bandayrel, et al., 'Comparison of weight loss among named diet programs in overweight and obese adults: A meta-analysis', *JAMA* (2014) 312(9):923–933, DOI:10.1001/jama.2014.10397.

9 Krista Casazza, Kevin R. Fontaine, Arne Astrup, et al., 'Myths, presumptions, and facts about obesity', *N Engl J Med* (31 Jan 2013) 368:446–454, DOI: 10.1056/NEJMsa1208051.

10 K. A. Shaw, H. C. Gennat, P. O'Rourke, et al., 'Exercise for overweight or obesity', *Cochrane Database of Systematic Reviews* (2006) 4, art. no.: CD003817, DOI: 10.1002/14651858.CD003817.pub3.

11 S. L. Norris, X. Zhang, A. Avenell, et al., 'Pharmacotherapy for weight loss in adults with type 2 diabetes mellitus', *Cochrane Database of Systematic Reviews* (2005) 1, art. no.: CD004096, DOI: 10.1002/14651858.CD004096.pub2.

12 Viktoria L. Gloy, Matthias Briel, Deepak L. Bhatt, et al., 'Bariatric surgery versus non-surgical treatment for obesity: A systematic review and meta-analysis of randomised controlled trials', *BMJ* (2013) 347:f5934.

13 L. T. DeWind, J. H. Payne, 'Intestinal bypass surgery for morbid obesity: Long-term results', *JAMA* (2014) 312(9):966, DOI:10.1001/jama.2014.10853.

14 H. Buchwald, S. E. Williams, 'Bariatric surgery worldwide, 2003', *Obes Surg* (Oct 2004) 14(9):1157–1164, PubMed PMID: 15527627.

15 H. Buchwald, D. M. Oien, 'Metabolic/bariatric surgery worldwide 2008', *Obes Surg* (Dec 2009) 19(12):1605–1611, DOI: 10.1007/s11695-009-0014-5, PubMed PMID: 19885707.

16 H. Buchwald, S. E. Williams, 'Bariatric surgery worldwide, 2003', *Obes Surg* (Oct 2004) 14(9):1157–1164, PubMed PMID: 15527627.

17 H. Buchwald, D. M. Oien, 'Metabolic/bariatric surgery worldwide 2008', *Obes Surg* (Dec 2009) 19(12):1605–1611, DOI: 10.1007/s11695-009-0014-5, PubMed PMID: 19885707.

18 H. Buchwald, D. M. Oien, 'Metabolic/bariatric surgery worldwide 2011', *Obes Surg* (Apr 2013) 23(4):427–436, DOI: 10.1007/s11695-012-0864-0, PubMed PMID: 23338049.

19 The Look AHEAD Research Group*, 'Cardiovascular effects of intensive lifestyle intervention in type 2 diabetes', *N Engl J Med* (11 Jul 2013) 369:145–154, DOI: 10.1056/NEJMoa1212914.

20 R. S. Padwal, D. Rucker, S. K. Li, et al., 'Long-term pharmacotherapy for obesity and overweight', *Cochrane Database of Systematic Reviews* (2003) 4, art. no.: CD004094, DOI: 10.1002/14651858.CD004094.pub2.

21 R. J. Rodgers, M. H. Tschöp, J. P. Wilding, 'Anti-obesity drugs: Past, present and future', *Disease models & mechanisms* (2012) 5(5):621–626.

22 N. Puzziferri, T. B. Roshek, H. G. Mayo, et al., 'Long-term follow-up after bariatric surgery: A systematic review', *JAMA* (2014) 312(9): 934–942, DOI:10.1001/jama.2014.10706.

23 The Longitudinal Assessment of Bariatric Surgery (LABS) Consortium, 'Perioperative safety in the longitudinal assessment of bariatric surgery', *N Engl J Med* (30 Jul 2009) 361:445–454, DOI: 10.1056/NEJMoa0901836.

24 The Longitudinal Assessment of Bariatric Surgery (LABS) Consortium, 'Perioperative safety in the longitudinal assessment of bariatric surgery', *N Engl J Med* (30 Jul 2009) 361:445–454, DOI: 10.1056/NEJMoa0901836.

25 N. Puzziferri, T. B. Roshek, H. G. Mayo, et al., 'Long-term follow-up after bariatric surgery: A systematic review', *JAMA* (2014) 312(9): 934–942, DOI:10.1001/jama.2014.10706.

26 M. Neovius, K. Narbro, C. Keating, et al., 'Health care use during 20 years following bariatric surgery', *JAMA* (2012) 308(11):1132–1141, DOI:10.1001/2012.jama.11792.

27 G. R. Faria, J. R. Preto, J. Costa-Maia, *Obes Surg* (2013) 23:460, https://DOI.org/10.1007/s11695-012-0816-8.

28 D. E. Arterburn, D. P. Fisher, 'The current state of the evidence for bariatric surgery', *JAMA* (2014) 312(9):898–899, DOI:10.1001/jama.2014.10940.

29 N. Puzziferri, T. B. Roshek, H. G. Mayo, et al., 'Long-term follow-up after bariatric surgery: A systematic review', *JAMA* (2014) 312(9):934–942, DOI:10.1001/jama.2014.10706.

30 Christopher B. Granger, John H. Alexander, John J. V. McMurray, et al., for the ARISTOTLE Committees and Investigators*, 'Apixaban versus warfarin in patients with atrial fibrillation', *N Engl J Med* (15 Sep 2011) 365:981–992, DOI: 10.1056/NEJMoa1107039.

31 L. T. DeWind, J. H. Payne, 'Intestinal bypass surgery for morbid obesity: Long-term results', *JAMA* (2014) 312(9):966, DOI:10.1001/jama.2014.10853.

32 Lukas Schwingshackl, Georg Hoffmann, 'Long-term effects of low-fat diets either low or high in protein on cardiovascular and metabolic risk factors: A systematic review and meta-analysis', *Nutrition Journal* (2013) 12:48, https://DOI.org/10.1186/1475-2891-12-48.

33 A. G. Tsai, T. A. Wadden, 'Systematic review: An evaluation of major commercial weight loss programs in the United States', *Ann Intern Med* (Jan 2005) 142:56–66, DOI: 10.7326/0003-4819-142-1-200501040-00012.

34 L. Te Morenga, S. Mallard, J. Mann, 'Dietary sugars and body weight: Systematic review and meta-analyses of randomised controlled trials and cohort studies', *BMJ* (2013) 346:e7492.

35 Steven L. Gortmaker, Boyd A. Swinburn, David Levy, et al., 'Changing the future of obesity: Science, policy, and action', *The Lancet* (Aug 2011) 378(9793):838–847.

36 Nicholas A. Christakis, James H. Fowler, 'The spread of obesity in a large social network over 32 years', *N Engl J Med* (26 Jul 2007) 357:370–379 DOI: 10.1056/NEJMsa066082.

Gristle

1 T. Towheed, L. Maxwell, T. P. Anastassiades, et al., 'Glucosamine therapy for treating osteoarthritis', *Cochrane Database of Systematic Reviews* (2005) 2, art. no.: CD002946, DOI: 10.1002/14651858.CD002946.pub2.

2 A. W. S. Rutjes, E. Nüesch, S. Reichenbach, et al., 'S-Adenosylmethionine for osteoarthritis of the knee or hip', *Cochrane Database of Systematic Reviews* (7 Oct 2009) 4, art. no.: CD007321, DOI: 10.1002/14651858.CD007321.pub2.

3 J. A. Singh, S. Noorbaloochi, R. MacDonald, et al., 'Chondroitin for

osteoarthritis', *Cochrane Database of Systematic Reviews* (2015) 1, art. no.: CD005614, DOI: 10.1002/14651858.CD005614.pub2.

4 J. Dequeker, F. P. Luyten, 'The history of osteoarthritis-osteoarthrosis', *Annals of the Rheumatic Diseases* (2008) 67:5–10.

5 Ian J. Wallace, Steven Worthington, David T. Felson, et al., 'Knee osteoarthritis levels have recently doubled', *Proceedings of the National Academy of Sciences* (Aug 2017) 114(35):9332–9336, DOI: 10.1073/pnas.1703856114.

Power

1 http://www.nytimes.com/2008/03/27/health/nutrition/27best.html.

2 'The penalty for talking about poets in universal terms before, or instead of, talking about their particular achievements is to devalue what they do while fetishising what they are.' C. James, 'Camille Paglia Burns for Poetry', in *The Revolt of the Pendulum*.

3 J. A. A. C. Heuberger, J. I. Rotmans, P. Gal, et al., 'Effects of erythropoietin on cycling performance of well trained cyclists: A double-blind, randomised, placebo-controlled trial', *The Lancet Haematology* (Oct 2017) 4(8):e374–e386.

4 Ibid., p. e375.

5 See Clive James, *Cultural Amnesia*, on Hitler being cultured and on culture being no redoubt against violence: 'The lessons of history don't suit our wishes: if they did, they would not be lessons, and history would be a fairy story.'

6 The latter is arguable but probably real, and there is some objective evidence – see, for example, https://www.washingtonpost.com/news/monkey-cage/wp/2017/06/01/theres-little-evidence-that-dictators-are-toppling-democracies/?noredirect=on&utm_term=.2fa0238d6534.

7 Patrick Sharman, Alastair J. Wilson, 'Racehorses are getting faster', *Biology Letters* (1 June 2015) 11(6).

8 Myriam R. Hirt, Walter Jetz, Björn C. Rall, et al., 'A general scaling law reveals why the largest animals are not the fastest', *Nature Ecology & Evolution* (2017) 1:1116–1122.

9 Mark W. Denny, 'Limits to running speed in dogs, horses and humans', *Journal of Experimental Biology* (2008) 211:3836–3849, DOI: 10.1242/jeb.024968.

10 http://www.spiegel.de/spiegel/warum-ein-uwe-seeler-im-modernen-fussball-keine-chance-haette-a-1163547.html.

11 A. M. Nevill, G. Whyte, 'Are there limits to running world records?'

Med Sci Sports Exerc (Oct 2005) 37(10):1785–1788, DOI:10.1249/
01.mss.0000181676.62054.79, PubMed PMID: 16260981.

Culture

1   G. Simmel, 'How is society possible?' *American Journal of Sociology* (1910) 16(3):372–391, JSTOR, www.jstor.org/stable/2763090.

2   Thomas Browne, *Religio Medici* (1643).

3   R. Peto, Harveian Oration 2012, 'Halving premature death', *Clin Med* (Lond) (Dec 2014) 14(6):643–657, DOI: 10.7861/clinmedicine. 14-6-643, PubMed PMID: 25468852; PubMed Central PMCID: PMC4954139.

4   Three Worlds, Karl Popper, The Tanner Lecture on Human Values delivered at The University of Michigan April 7 1978, https:// tannerlectures.utah.edu/_documents/a-to-z/p/popper80.pdf, p. 4.

5   Letter to Asa Gray, 22 May 1860, see https://www.darwinproject. ac.uk/letter/DCP-LETT-2814.xml.

6   Anthony Trollope, *Can You Forgive Her?* Chapman & Hall (London, 1864).

7   Niccolò Machiavelli, *Discourses on Livy*.

8   https://www.economist.com/blogs/graphicdetail/2018/01/daily-chart-8.

9   S. J. Gould, 'Nurturing Nature', in *Urchin in a Storm*, p. 79.

10   S. Brenner, 'Theoretical biology in the third millennium', *Philosophical Transactions of the Royal Society B* (1999) 354:1963–1965, Royal Society Publishing, London.

11   D. Wootton, *Bad Medicine*, OUP (2007).

12   E. Shils, *A Fragment of a Sociological Autobiography*, Routledge (2017), p. 131.

13   Thomas Browne, *Urn Burial* (1658).

14   Willa Cather, 'Death Comes for the Archbishop', ReadHowYouWant (2008), p. 32.

15   http://www.weeklystandard.com/the-cultured-life/article/2007147.

16   http://holocaustmusic.ort.org/places/camps/death-camps/auschwitz/camp-orchestras/.

17   S. J. Gould, 'Ghost of Protagoras', in *Urchin in the Storm*, W. W. Norton (New York, 1988), p. 67.

18   *Urchin in the Storm*, W. W. Norton (New York, 1988), p. 69.

19   E. van de Wetering, *Rembrandt: The Painter at Work*, University of California Press (2000).

20   William Shakespeare, *Troilus and Cressida*, Act 1, Scene 2.

21 http://www.weeklystandard.com/churchills-greatness/article/11653.

22 Matthew Arnold, *Culture and Anarchy*, OUP (Oxford, 2006), p. 39.

23 *The Collected Works of William Hazlitt: Fugitive Writings*, volume 12 of the *Collected Works of William Hazlitt*, edited by Alfred Rayney Waller and Arnold Glover, J. M. Dent (publisher), the University of Michigan (1904), p. 171.

24 Cited in S. J. Gould, *The Lying Stones of Marrakech*, Three Rivers Press (New York, 2000).

25 Matthew Arnold, *Culture and Anarchy*.

26 Cited in J. G. Gould, 'A biological homage to Mickey Mouse', *Natural History Magazine* (1978) 88(5):30–36.

27 https://www.thenation.com/article/noble-and-base-poland-and-holocaust/.

28 http://www.thenation.com/article/171262/noble-and-base-poland-and-holocaust?page=full#.

29 *The Collected Works of William Hazlitt*, J. M. Dent & Co. (1904), p. 399.

30 See the wonderful *The Great War and Modern Memory* by Paul Fussell, OUP (Oxford, 1975).

Class and inequality

1 Robert M. Sapolsky, 'Social status and health in humans and other animals', *Annual Review of Anthropology* (2004) 33(1):393–418.

2 Benjamin Isaac, 'Proto-racism in Graeco-Roman antiquity', *World Archaeology* (2006) 38(1):32–47, JSTOR, www.jstor.org/stable/40023593.

3 https://www.ons.gov.uk/peoplepopulationandcommunity/birthsdeathsandmarriages/lifeexpectancies/bulletins/trendinlifeexpectancyatbirthandatage65bysocioeconomicpositionbasedonthenationalstatisticssocioeconomicclassificationenglandandwales/2015-10-21.

4 http://tubecreature.com/#/livesontheline/2013.

5 Aaron Antonovsky, 'Social class, life expectancy and overall mortality', *The Milbank Memorial Fund Quarterly* (1967) 45(2):31–73, JSTOR, www.jstor.org/stable/3348839.

6 E. Shils, *A Fragment of Sociological Autobiography*.

7 https://www.economist.com/news/leaders/21731626-case-taxing-inherited-assets-strong-hated-tax-fair-one.

8 Francis Galton, 'Statistical inquiries into the efficacy of prayer', *Fortnightly Review* (1872) 12:125–135.

9   'Statistical Inquiries Into the Efficacy of Prayer', *The Fortnightly Review* (August 1872) LXVIII, p. 127.
10   Ibid., p.127
11   R. G. Wilkinson, 'Income distribution and life expectancy', *BMJ* (1992) 304:165–168.
12   D. A. Redelmeier, S. M. Singh, 'Survival in Academy Award-winning actors and actresses', *Ann Intern Med* (May 2001) 134:955–962, DOI: 10.7326/0003-4819-134-10-200105150-00009.
13   https://visual.ons.gov.uk/how-has-life-expectancy-changed-over-time/.
14   https://visual.ons.gov.uk/how-has-life-expectancy-changed-over-time/.
15   S. Pinker, *The Better Angels of Our Nature: Why Violence Has Declined*, Penguin (2012).
16   https://ourworldindata.org/homicides/.
17   Frederick Burkle Jr, Richard Garfield, 'Civilian mortality after the 2003 invasion of Iraq', *The Lancet* (March 2013) 381(9870):877–879.
18   Ronald and Margaret Bottrall (eds), *Collected English Verse*, Books for Libraries Press (New York, 1969), p. 429.
19   https://www.economist.com/blogs/graphicdetail/2017/11/daily-chart-20.
20   https://www.washingtonpost.com/news/worldviews/wp/2015/07/30/why-the-language-we-use-to-talk-about-refugees-matters-so-much/?utm_term=.4e45bca5a7c1.
21   Francis Galton, *Hereditary Genius*, University Press of the Pacific (Honolulu, HI, 2001), p. 25.
22   E. Schrödinger, *What Is Life?* CUP (Cambridge, 1992), p. 153.
23   Francis Galton, letter to the editor of *The Times*, 5 June 1873.
24   https://www.nature.com/articles/462035c.
25   J. Diamond, *The Rise and Fall of the Third Chimpanzee*, Harper Perennial (2007).
26   C. James, *The Blaze of Obscurity*, Picador (2010), p. 3.

Sleep

1   D. R. Samson, R. W. Shumaker, 'Orangutans (Pongo spp.) have deeper, more efficient sleep than baboons (Papio papio) in captivity', *Am J Phys Anthropol* (Jul 2015) 157(3):421–427, DOI:10.1002/ajpa.22733.
2   M. Montaigne, *On Sleep*.
3   Allan Rechtschaffen, Bernard Bergmann, 'Sleep deprivation in the rat by the disk-over-water method', *Behavioural Brain Research* (1995) 69:55–63.

4   P. Cortelli, P. Gambetti, P. Montagna, et al., 'Fatal familial insomnia: Clinical features and molecular genetics', *J Sleep Res* (Jun 1999) 8(Suppl 1):23–29, PubMed PMID: 10389103.
5   M. Jouvet, *The Paradox of Sleep: The Story of Dreaming*.

Race

1   Steven Rose, 'Darwin, race and gender', *EMBO reports* (2009) 10(4): 297–298.
2   https://www.economist.com/blogs/graphicdetail/2018/02/daily-chart-9, from A. Alesina, S. Stantcheva, E. Teso, *Intergenerational Mobility and Support for Redistribution*, NBER Working Paper no. 23027, issued in Jan 2017, revised in Jun 2017.
3   Matthew Arnold, *Culture and Anarchy*, OUP (Oxford, 2006), p. 104.
4   Elizabeth Carr, *Shura Cherkassky: The Piano's Last Czar*, Scarecrow Press (1996), p. 123.
5   John Stuart Mill, *Principles of Political Economy with some of their Applications to Social Philosophy*, John Parker (London, 1848).
6   M. Marmot, *The Status Syndrome*, Bloomsbury (London, 2015).
7   John Stuart Mill, *Principles of Political Economy with some of their Applications to Social Philosophy*.

Creativity

1   Michael Henry Heim, Simon Karlinsky (transl.), *Anton Chekhov's Life and Thought*, Northwestern University Press (Evanston, IL, 1997), p. 121.
2   https://ebooks.adelaide.edu.au/k/keats/john/letters/letter72.html.
3   N. Roe (ed.), *John Keats and the Medical Imagination*, Palgrave Macmillan (2017).
4   T. Dobzhansky, *Mankind Evolving*, Yale University Press (1962), p. 78.

Eating and drinking

1   Honoré de Balzac, *Le Gastronome français* (1828), Mark Kurlansky (transl.), *Choice Cuts*.
2   Ibid.
3   David Grayson, *Adventures in Contentment*, The Book League of America (1910), p. 143.
4   https://www.nytimes.com/2017/03/17/health/cholesterol-drugs-repatha-amgen-pcsk9-inhibitors.html.

5   Ramón Estruch, Emilio Ros, Jordi Salas-Salvadó, et al., for the PRE-
DIMED Study Investigators*, 'Primary prevention of cardiovascular disease with a Mediterranean diet', N Engl J Med (4 Apr 2013)
368:1279–1290, DOI: 10.1056/NEJMoa1200303.

6   The GBD 2015 Obesity Collaborators, 'Health effects of overweight
and obesity in 195 countries over 25 years', N Engl J Med (6 Jul
2017) 377:13–27, DOI: 10.1056/NEJMoa1614362.

7   The GBD 2015 Obesity Collaborators, 'Health effects of overweight
and obesity in 195 countries over 25 years', N Engl J Med (6 Jul
2017) 377:13–27, DOI: 10.1056/NEJMoa1614362.

8   R. Peto, Harveian Oration 2012, 'Halving premature death', Clin
Med (Lond) (Dec 2014) 14(6):643–657, DOI: 10.7861/clinmedicine.
14-6-643, PubMed PMID: 25468852; PubMed Central PMCID:
PMC4954139.

9   R. Collins, C. Reith, J. Emberson, et al., 'Interpretation of the evidence for the efficacy and safety of statin therapy', The Lancet (19
Nov 2016) 388(10059):2532–2561, DOI: 10.1016/S0140-6736(16)
31357-5, Epub 8 Sep 2016, Review, erratum in The Lancet (11 Feb
2017) 389(10069):602, PubMed PMID: 27616593.

10 S. S. Abumweis, R. Barake, P. J. Jones, 'Plant sterols/stanols as cholesterol lowering agents: A meta-analysis of randomized controlled
trials', Food & Nutrition Research (2008) 52, DOI: 10.3402/fnr.
v52io.1811.

11 C. P. Cannon, M. A. Blazing, R. P. Giugliano, et al., IMPROVE-IT
Investigators, 'Ezetimibe added to statin therapy after acute coronary
syndromes', N Engl J Med (18 Jun 2015) 372(25):2387–2397, DOI:
10.1056/NEJMoa1410489, Epub 3 Jun 2015, PubMed PMID:
26039521.

12 E. D. Kantor, C. D. Rehm, M. Du, et al., 'Trends in dietary supplement
use among US adults from 1999–2012', JAMA (2016) 316(14):-
1464–1474, DOI:10.1001/jama.2016.14403.

13 E. Guallar, S. Stranges, C. Mulrow, et al., 'Enough is enough: Stop
wasting money on vitamin and mineral supplements', Ann Intern
Med (December 2013) 159:850–851, DOI: 10.7326/0003-4819-
159-12-201312170-00011.

14 Myocardial Infarction Genetics Consortium Investigators, N. O.
Stitziel, H. H. Won, et al., 'Inactivating mutations in NPC1L1 and
protection from coronary heart disease', N Engl J Med (27 Nov
2014) 371(22):2072–2082, DOI: 10.1056/NEJMoa1405386, Epub
12 Nov 2014, PubMed PMID: 25390462; PubMed Central PMCID:
PMC4335708.

15 Brian A. Ference, Wonsuk Yoo, Issa Alesh, et al., 'Effect of long-term

exposure to lower low-density lipoprotein cholesterol beginning early in life on the risk of coronary heart disease: A Mendelian randomization analysis', *Journal of the American College of Cardiology* (2012) 60(25)2631–2639.

16 *The Times*, editorial (1842); cited in Peter Medawar, *Limits of Science* (see chapter on Youth).

17 From L. Golding, A. Simon (eds), *We Shall Eat and Drink Again* Hutchinson (1944).

Beauty

1 Hammad Ali, Basil Donovan, Handan Wand, et al., 'Genital warts in young Australians five years into national human papillomavirus vaccination programme: National surveillance data', *BMJ* (2013) 346:f2032.

2 Charles Darwin, *The Descent of Man*, John Murray (London, 1871).

3 Henry James, *Selected Letters*, Leon Edel (ed.), Belknap Press of Harvard University Press (1987).

4 Julia Peakman, *Emma Hamilton: Life and Times*, Haus Publishing (2005), p. 88.

Happiness

1 P. R. Albert, C. Benkelfat, L. Descarries, 'The neurobiology of depression – revisiting the serotonin hypothesis. I. Cellular and molecular mechanisms', *Philosophical transactions of the Royal Society of London. Series B: Biological Sciences* (2012) 367(1601):2378–2381.

2 Joseph J. Schildkraut, 'The catecholamine hypothesis of affective disorders: A review of supporting evidence', *Am J Psychiatry* (1965) 122(5):509–522.

3 I. Kirsch, 'Antidepressants and the placebo effect', *Zeitschrift für Psychologie* (2014) 222(3):128–134.

4 E. H. Turner, A. M. Matthews, E. Linardatos, et al., 'Selective publication of antidepressant trials and its influence on apparent efficacy', *N Engl J Med* (17 Jan 2008) 358(3):252–260, DOI: 10.1056/NEJMsa065779, PubMed PMID: 18199864.

5 J. C. Fournier, R. J. DeRubeis, S. D. Hollon, et al., 'Antidepressant drug effects and depression severity: A patient-level meta-analysis', *JAMA* (2010) 303(1):47–53, DOI:10.1001/jama.2009.1943.

6 I. Kirsch, 'Antidepressants and the placebo effect', *Zeitschrift für Psychologie* (2014) 222(3):128–134.

7 K. P. Hill, J. S. Ross, D. S. Egilman, et al., 'The ADVANTAGE seed-

ing trial: A review of internal documents', *Ann Intern Med* (Aug 2008) 149:251–258, DOI: 10.7326/0003-4819-149-4-200808190-00006.

8   J. G. Rabkin, J. S. Markowitz, J. Stewart, et al., 'How blind is blind? Assessment of patient and doctor medication guesses in a placebo-controlled trial of imipramine and phenelzine', *Psychiatry Res* (Sep 1986) 19(1):75–86, PubMed PMID: 3538107.

9   J. P. Ioannidis, 'Effectiveness of antidepressants: An evidence myth constructed from a thousand randomized trials?' *Philos Ethics Humanit Med* (27 May 2008) 3:14, DOI: 10.1186/1747-5341-3-14, PubMed PMID: 18505564; PubMed Central PMCID: PMC-2412901.

10 E. H. Turner, A. M. Matthews, E. Linardatos, et al., 'Selective publication of antidepressant trials and its influence on apparent efficacy', *N Engl J Med* (2008) 358:252–260.

11 I. Kirsch, B. J. Deacon, T. B. Huedo-Medina, et al., 'Initial severity and antidepressant benefits: A meta-analysis of data submitted to the Food and Drug Administration', *PLoS Medicine* (2008) 5:e45.

12 Andrea Cipriani, Toshi A. Furukawa, Georgia Salanti, et al., 'Comparative efficacy and acceptability of 21 antidepressant drugs for the acute treatment of adults with major depressive disorder: A systematic review and network meta-analysis', *The Lancet* (Feb 2018) 391(10128):1357–1366.

13 Yuval Noah Harari, *Homo Deus*, (see chapter on Death), p. 40.

14 https://www.nobelprize.org/nobel_prizes/medicine/laureates/1949/.

15 https://www.nobelprize.org/nobel_prizes/medicine/laureates/1949/moniz-article.html.

16 V. W. Swayze, 2nd. 'Frontal leukotomy and related psychosurgical procedures in the era before antipsychotics (1935–1954): A historical overview', *Am J Psychiatry* (Apr 1995) 152(4):505–515, PubMed PMID: 7900928.

17 S. Rose, '50 years of neuroscience', *The Lancet* (Feb 2015) 385 (9968):598–599.

18 Cited in Joseph Epstein's essay *Hitting Eighty* – see https://www.weeklystandard.com/joseph-epstein/hitting-eighty-2006085.

19 J. Roger, *Buffon: A Life in Natural History*, Cornell University Press (New York, 1997).

Mind and intellect

1   Emily Dickinson, *Poems*, ed. Mabel Loomis Todd and Thomas Wentworth Higginson, The Floating Press (Auckland, 2009), p. 260.

2   W. V. Harvey, *Mental Disorders in the Classical World*, Brill (Boston, 2013).

3   A. G. Franke, C. Bagusat, P. Dietz, et al., 'Use of illicit and prescription drugs for cognitive or mood enhancement among surgeons', *BMC Med* (9 Apr 2013) 11:102, DOI: 10.1186/1741-7015-11-102, PubMed PMID: 23570256; PubMed Central PMCID: PMC3635891.

4   L. M. Garnier-Dykstra, K. M. Caldeira, K. B. Vincent, et al., 'Non-medical use of prescription stimulants during college: Four-year trends in exposure opportunity, use, motives, and sources', *Journal of American College Health* (2012) 60(3):226–234.

5   B. Sahakian, J. LaBuzetta, *Bad Moves: How Decision Making Goes Wrong, and the Ethics of Smart Drugs*, OUP (2013).

6   A. Chatterjee, 'The promise and predicament of cosmetic neurology', *Journal of Medical Ethics* (2006) 32(2):110–113.

7   D. Repantis, P. Schlattmann, O. Laisney, et al., 'Modafinil and methylphenidate for neuroenhancement in healthy individuals: A systematic review', *Pharmacol Res* (Sep 2010) 62(3):187–206, DOI: 10.1016/j.phrs.2010.04.002, Epub 21 Apr 2010, Review, PubMed PMID: 20416377.

8   R. M. Battleday, A. K. Brem, 'Modafinil for cognitive neuroenhancement in healthy non-sleep-deprived subjects: A systematic review', *Eur Neuropsychopharmacol* (Nov 2015) 25(11):1865–1881, DOI: 10.1016/j.euroneuro.2015.07.028, Epub 20 Aug 2015, Review, PubMed PMID: 26381811.

9   Nigel Hawkes, 'Modafinil does enhance cognition, review finds', *BMJ* (2015) 351:h4573.

10 S. Rose, 'Brainocentrism?' *The Lancet* (March 2017) 389(10072):898.

11 Cornelius A. Rietveld, Tõnu Esko, Gail Davies, et al., 'Common genetic variants and cognitive performance', *Proceedings of the National Academy of Sciences* (Sep 2014) 111(38):13790–13794, DOI: 10.1073/pnas.1404623111.

12 Ewen Callaway, '"Smart genes" prove elusive', *Nature*, News (8 Sep 2014).

13 D. Burch, 'What could computerized brain training learn from evidence-based medicine?' *PLoS Med* (2014) 11(11):e1001758, https://DOI.org/10.1371/journal.pmed.1001758.

14 Charles Darwin, *Origin of Species* (1859).

15 Alfred Russel Wallace, *Contributions to the Theory of Natural Selection* (1871), p. 343, cited here: http://people.wku.edu/charles.smith/wallace/S165.htm.

16 http://charles-darwin.classic-literature.co.uk/more-letters-of-charles-darwin-volume-ii/ebook-page-23.asp.

17 William Hazlitt, *Sketches and Essays*, John Templeman (London, 1839), p. 40.

18 Cited in *The Oxford Handbook of Child Psychological Assessment*, Donald H. Saklofske, Cecil R. Reynolds, Vicki L. Schwean (eds), OUP (2013), p. 9.

19 E. Schrödinger, *What Is Life? The Physical Aspect of the Living Cell*, CUP (1944).

20 S. Rose, '50 years of neuroscience', *The Lancet* (Feb 2015) 385 (9968):598–599.

21 C. Sherrington, *Man on His Nature*, CUP (1940).

22 Erwin Schrödinger, *What Is Life?*, Cambridge University Press (1992), p. 157.

23 Peter Medawar, *The Strange Case of the Spotted Mice*, OUP (1996).

24 https://www.darwinproject.ac.uk/letter/DCP-LETT-8658.xml.

25 As quoted in *New Scientist* (8 March 1979), 777.

26 S. J. Gould, 'Racist Arguments and IQ', *Ever Since Darwin*, W. W. Norton (New York, 1977), pp. 246–247.

27 D. Burch, 'What could computerized brain training learn from evidence-based medicine?' *PLoS Med* (2014) 11(11):e1001758, https://DOI.org/10.1371/journal.pmed.1001758.

28 J. Verghese, R. B. Lipton, M. J. Katz, et al., 'Leisure activities and the risk of dementia in the elderly', *N Engl J Med* (19 Jun 2003) 348(25): 2508–2516, PubMed PMID: 12815136.

29 Robert S. Wilson, Patricia A. Boyle, Lei Yu, et al., 'Life-span cognitive activity, neuropathologic burden, and cognitive aging', *Neurology* (Jul 2013) 81(4):314–321, DOI: 10.1212/WNL.0b013e31829c5e8a.

Biomodification

1 M. J. Dewhurst, N. J. Linker, (2014), 'Current evidence and recommendations for cardiac resynchronisation therapy', *Arrhythmia & Electrophysiology Review* (May 2014) 3(1):9–14.

2 http://www.abstractsonline.com/Plan/ViewAbstract.aspx?sKey= 8aee1902-36d1-4626-9e3b-3fb48ce6bb61&cKey=cbe5d81e-5b06-4de5-9dda-7d7b4c599010&mKey=4393d428-d755-4a34-8a63-26b1b7a349a1.

3 Baron Cuvier, 'Biographical Memoir of M. de Lamarck', *The Edinburgh New Philosophical Journal* (17 July 1835) vol. XX (Edinburgh, 1836), p. 14.

4 S. Hirata, K. Watanabe, K. Masao, '"Sweet-Potato Washing" Revisited', in T. Matsuzawa, (ed.), *Primate Origins of Human Cognition and Behavior*, Springer (Tokyo, 2008).

5   H. F. Harlow, R. O. Dodsworth, M. K. Harlow, 'Total social isolation in monkeys', *Proc Natl Acad Sci USA* (Jul 1965) 54(1):90–97.
6   D. Healey, *The Time of My Life*, Methuen (2015).
7   A. Momigliano, *Annali della Scuola normale superiore di Pisa. Classe di Lettere e Filosofia*, La Scuola (1978), p. 452.
8   S. Rose, '50 years of neuroscience', *The Lancet* (Feb 2015) 385 (9968):598–599.
9   See https://cnp.epfl.ch/page-87258-en.html and http://www.bbc.co.uk/news/health-42430895.
10 See http://www.project-rewalk.com/en/home for a video of the rat and https://cnp.epfl.ch/page-87646-en.html for the group's website.
11 A. B. Ajiboye, F. R. Willett, D. R. Young, et al., 'Restoration of reaching and grasping movements through brain-controlled muscle stimulation in a person with tetraplegia: A proof-of-concept demonstration', *The Lancet* (6 May 2017) 389(10081):1821–1830.
12 Steve I. Perlmutter, 'Reaching again: A glimpse of the future with neuroprosthetics', *The Lancet* (March 2017) 389(10081):1777–1778.
13 J. L. Collinger, B. Wodlinger, J. E. Downey, et al., 'High-performance neuroprosthetic control by an individual with tetraplegia', *The Lancet* (Feb 2013) 381(9866):557–564.
14 O. C. Aszmann, A. D. Roche, S. Salminger, et al., 'Bionic reconstruction to restore hand function after brachial plexus injury: A case series of three patients', *The Lancet* (May 2015) 385(9983):2183–2189.
15 http://www.nytimes.com/2008/07/13/health/13debakey.html.
16 M. Mumme, A. Barbero, S. Miot, et al., 'Nasal chondrocyte-based engineered autologous cartilage tissue for repair of articular cartilage defects: An observational first-in-human trial', *The Lancet* (Oct 2016) 388(10055):1985–1994.
17 Kulwinder S. Dua, Walter J. Hogan, Abdul A. Aadam, et al., 'In-vivo oesophageal regeneration in a human being by use of a non-biological scaffold and extracellular matrix', *The Lancet* (April 2016) 388 (10039):55–61.
18 Atlántida M. Raya-Rivera, Diego Esquiliano, Reyna Fierro-Pastrana, et al., 'Tissue-engineered autologous vaginal organs in patients: A pilot cohort study', *The Lancet* (July 2014) 384(9940):329–336.
19 M. J. Elliott, P. De Coppi, S. Speggiorin, et al., 'Stem-cell-based, tissue engineered tracheal replacement in a child: A 2-year follow-up study', *The Lancet* (July 2012) 380(9846):994–1000.
20 M. Olausson, P. B. Patil, V. K. Kuna, et al., 'Transplantation of an allogeneic vein bioengineered with autologous stem cells: A proof-of-concept study', *The Lancet* (July 2012) 380(9838):230–237.
21 D. Burch, *Digging Up the Dead*, Chatto (2007).

22 Todd N. McAllister, Marcin Maruszewski, Sergio A. Garrido, et al., 'Effectiveness of haemodialysis access with an autologous tissue-engineered vascular graft: A multicentre cohort study', *The Lancet* (April 2009) 373(9673)1440–1446.

Genetics

1   I. Loudon, 'Deaths in childbed from the eighteenth century to 1935', *Med Hist* (Jan 1986) 30(1):1–41, PubMed PMID: 3511335; PubMed Central PMCID: PMC1139579.

2   https://ourworldindata.org/maternal-mortality.

3   Philipp Mitteroecker, Sonja Windhager, Mihaela Pavlicev, 'Cliff-edge model predicts inheritance of Caesarean', *Proceedings of the National Academy of Sciences* (Oct 2017) 114(44):11669–11672, DOI: 10.1073/pnas.1712203114.

4   Philipp Mitteroecker, Sonja Windhager, Mihaela Pavlicev, 'Cliff-edge model predicts inheritance of Caesarean', *Proceedings of the National Academy of Sciences* (Oct 2017) 114(44):11669–11672, DOI: 10.1073/pnas.1712203114.

5   C. R. Gale, F. J. O'Callaghan, M. Bredow, et al., 'Avon Longitudinal Study of Parents and Children Study Team. The influence of head growth in fetal life, infancy, and childhood on intelligence at the ages of 4 and 8 years', *Pediatrics* (Oct 2006) 118(4):1486–1492, PubMed PMID: 17015539.

6   Frederick Hulse's study of height in Switzerland, varying by marriage within a canton or without. Cited in S. Garn, *Human Races*, Charles Thomas (Springfield, 1961).

7   L. Cavalli-Sforza, W. Bodmer, *The Genetics of Human Populations*, Freeman (San Francisco, 1971).

8   Karl Pearson, *The Life, Letters and Labours of Francis Galton*, vol. 3, Cambridge University Press (2011), p. 355.

9   Francis Galton, 'Hereditary Improvement', *Fraser's Magazine* (1873) 7:116–130.

10 *The Scientific Basis of Evolution*, W. W. Norton (New York, 1932), Chapter 10, p. 203.

11 S. L. Chen, 'Economic costs of hemophilia and the impact of prophylactic treatment on patient management', *Am J Manag Care* (Apr 2016) 22(5):S126–S133, Review, PubMed PMID: 27266809. In the USA and for Europe P. Rocha, M. Carvalho, M. Lopes, et al., 'Costs and utilization of treatment in patients with hemophilia', *BMC Health Services Research* (2015) 15:484, DOI:10.1186/s12913-015-1134-3.

12 G. Hütter, D. Nowak, M. Mossner, et al., 'Long-term control of HIV

by CCR5 Delta32/Delta32 stem-cell transplantation', *N Engl J Med* (12 Feb 2009) 360(7):692–698, DOI: 10.1056/NEJMoa0802905. PubMed PMID: 19213682.

13 F. Eichler, C. Duncan, P. L. Musolino, et al., 'Hematopoietic stem-cell gene therapy for cerebral adrenoleukodystrophy', *N Engl J Med* (26 Oct 2017) 377(17):1630–1638, DOI: 10.1056/NEJMoa1700554, Epub 4 Oct 2017, PubMed PMID: 28976817; PubMed Central PMCID: PMC5708849.

14 M. Engelen, 'Optimizing treatment for cerebral adrenoleukodystrophy in the era of gene therapy', *N Engl J Med* (26 Oct 2017) 377(17): 1682–1684, DOI: 10.1056/NEJMe1709253, Epub 4 Oct 2017, PubMed PMID: 28976819.

15 H. Ma, N. Marti-Gutierrez, S. W. Park, et al., 'Correction of a pathogenic gene mutation in human embryos', *Nature* (24 Aug 2017) 548(7668):413–419, DOI: 10.1038/nature23305, Epub 2 Aug 2017, PubMed PMID: 28783728.

16 P. Liang, C. Ding, H. Sun, et al., *Protein Cell* (2017) 8:811, https://DOI.org/10.1007/s13238-017-0475-6.

17 https://www.genome.gov/10001772/all-about-the--human-genome-project-hgp/; accessed 15 Jan 2018.

18 D. Kalladka, J. Sinden, K. Pollock, et al., 'Human neural stem cells in patients with chronic ischaemic stroke (PISCES): A phase 1, first-in-man study', *The Lancet* (Aug 2016) 388(10046):787–796.

19 Cesar V. Borlongan, 'Age of PISCES: Stem-cell clinical trials in stroke', *The Lancet* (Aug 2016) 388(10046):736–738.

20 Konstantinos Malliaras, Eduardo Marbán, 'Cardiac cell therapy: Where we've been, where we are, and where we should be headed', *British Medical Bulletin* (1 Jun 2011) 98(1):161–185, https://DOI.org/10.1093/bmb/ldr018.

21 https://www.genome.gov/12011238/an-overview-of-the-human-genome-project/; accessed 15 Jan 2018.

22 S. Levy, G. Sutton, P. C. Ng, et al., 'The diploid genome sequence of an individual human', *PLoS Biol* (2007) 5(10):e254, https://DOI.org/10.1371/journal.pbio.0050254.

23 M. Wadman, 'James Watson's genome sequenced at high speed', *Nature* (17 Apr 2008) 452(7189):788, DOI: 10.1038/452788b, PubMed PMID: 18431822.

24 https://www.huffingtonpost.com/peter-diamandis/outpaced-by-innovation-ca_b_3795710.html; accessed 15 Jan 2018.

25 https://www.forbes.com/sites/matthewherper/2017/01/09/illumina-promises-to-sequence-human-genome-for-100-but-not-quite-yet/#4987f3f3386d; accessed 15 Jan 2018.

26 https://report.nih.gov/NIHfactsheets/ViewFactSheet.aspx?csid=45.

27 P. K. Hatemi, S. E. Medland, R. Klemmensen, et al., 'Genetic influences on political ideologies: Twin analyses of 19 measures of political ideologies from five democracies and genome-wide findings from three populations', *Behavior Genetics* (2014) 44(3):282–294.

28 K. K. Ray, U. Landmesser, L. A. Leiter, et al., Inclisiran in patients at high cardiovascular risk with elevated LDL cholesterol', *N Engl J Med* (13 Apr 2017) 376(15):1430–1440, DOI: 10.1056/NEJMoa 1615758, Epub 17 Mar 2017, PubMed PMID: 28306389.

29 Y. Guan, Y. Ma, Q. Li, et al., 'CRISPR/Cas9-mediated somatic correction of a novel coagulator factor IX gene mutation ameliorates hemophilia in mouse', *EMBO Mol Med* (2 May 2016) 8(5):477–488, DOI: 10.15252/emmm.201506039, Print May 2016, PubMed PMID: 26964564; PubMed Central PMCID: PMC5125832.

30 S. Rangarajan, L. Walsh, W. Lester, et al., 'AAV5-factor VIII gene transfer in severe hemophilia A', *N Engl J Med* (28 Dec 2017) 377(26):2519–2530, DOI:10.1056/NEJMoa1708483, Epub 9 Dec 2017, PubMed PMID: 29224506.

31 L. A. George, S. K. Sullivan, A. Giermasz, et al., 'Hemophilia B gene therapy with a high-specific-activity factor IX variant', *N Engl J Med* (7 Dec 2017) 377(23):2215–2227, DOI: 10.1056/NEJMoa1708538, PubMed PMID: 29211678; PubMed Central PMCID: PMC6029626.

32 'Successful correction of hemophilia by CRISPR/Cas9 genome editing in vivo: Delivery vector and immune responses are the key to success', *EMBO Mol Med* (4 Apr 2016) 8(5):439–441, DOI:10.15252/ emmm.201606325.

33 G. Church, 'Compelling reasons for repairing human germlines', *N Engl J Med* (16 Nov 2017) 377(20):1909–1911, DOI: 10.1056/ NEJMp1710370, PubMed PMID: 29141159.

The book of life

1 https://jamanetwork.com/journals/jama/fullarticle/2.528216.

2 A. Verghese, N. H. Shah, R. A. Harrington, 'What this computer needs is a physician: Humanism and artificial intelligence', *JAMA* (2018) 319(1):19–20, DOI:10.1001/jama.2017.19198.

3 D. Burch, *Taking the Medicine*, Chatto & Windus (2009).

4 J. Watson, *Avoid Boring People*, OUP (Oxford, 2007), p. 34.

5 L. Thomas, *The Fragile Species*, Touchstone (1996).

6 G. Chapman, N. Talbot, D. McCartney, et al., 'Evidence based medicine – older, but no better educated?' *The Lancet* (2013) 382(9903): 1484.

7   http://edition.cnn.com/HEALTH/9511/conquer_cancer/cancer25/
    index.html; accessed18 Jan 2018.
8   A. Kumar, H. Soares, R. Wells, et al., 'Are experimental treatments
    for cancer in children superior to established treatments? Observa-
    tional study of randomised controlled trials by the Children's Oncol-
    ogy Group', *BMJ* (Clinical research ed.) (2005) 331(7528):1295.
9   Alfred Russel Wallace, *The Wonderful Century*, Swan Sonneschen
    & Company (London, 1899), p. 343.
10 J. A. Wheeler, K. Ford, *From Geons, Black Holes and Quantum
    Foam: A Life in Physics*, Dodd, Mead & Co. (New York, 1899).
11 S. J. Gould, *The Lying Stones of Marrakech* (see chapter on Culture).
12 S. Rose, 'Routes to a biology of the spirit', *New Scientist* (2 Aug
    1984), p. 42.
13 *The Collected Works of William Hazlitt: Fugitive Writings*, volume
    12 of the *Collected Works of William Hazlitt*, edited by Alfred
    Rayney Waller and Arnold Glover, J. M. Dent (publisher), the Uni-
    versity of Michigan (1904), p. 172.
14 Ed. Dov Gabbay and John Woods, *British Logic in the Nineteenth
    Century* volume IV, Elsevier (2008), p. 183.
15 C. James, *Cultural Amnesia*, essay on Charles Chaplin, Picador
    (2012), p. 117.
16 Percy Bysshe Shelley, *A Defence of Poetry* (1821).
17 G. Santayana, *The Life of Reason: The Phases of Human Progress*,
    Project Gutenberg / Dover Publications (New York, 2005).
18 Samuel Johnson, from his *Rambler* essay on procrastination.
19 Norman Maclean, *A River Runs Through It*. Although among the
    good things, Maclean specifically mentioned only eternal salvation
    and trout.
20 W. R. Bion, *The Long Week-end*, 1897–1919, Routledge (1982),
    p. 128.
21 https://en.wikisource.org/wiki/The_Code_of_Hammurabi_(Harper_
    translation); see entry 108.
22 http://etcsl.orinst.ox.ac.uk/cgi-bin/etcsl.cgi?text=t.2.1.5&display=
    Crit&charenc=gcirc&lineid=t215.p16#t215.p16.
23 http://etcsl.orinst.ox.ac.uk/cgi-bin/etcsl.cgi?text=t.5.1.3#.
24 W. A. Murphy Jr, Dz Dz Nedden, P. Gostner, et al., 'The iceman: Dis-
    covery and imaging', *Radiology* (Mar 2003) 226(3):614–629, Epub
    24 Jan 2003, PubMed PMID: 12601185.
25 P. W. Anderson, 'More is different', *Science* (4 Aug 1972) 393–396.
26 Immanuel Kant, *Idea for a General History with a Cosmopolitan
    Purpose* (1784). Published in English in *The London Magazine* 10:
    385–393.

27 Cited in J. Epstein, F. Raphael, *Distinct Intimacy*, Yale University Press (2013).

28 H. L. Mencken, *Minority Report* (1956), John Hopkins University Press (2006).

29 William Whewell, *The Philosophy of the Inductive Sciences Founded Upon Their History*, vol. 1, John Parker (London, 1847), p. 42.

30 Cited in P. Ward, J. Arac (eds), *The American Novel 1870–1940*, vol. 6, OUP (2014), p. 378.

31 Walt Whitman, *One's-Self I Sing* (1871).

32 http://www.bartleby.com/229/1102.html.

Image credits

Fig. 1   Percentage survival at period rates for males in England and Wales. Reproduced by permission of the Clinical Trial Service Unit, University of Oxford.

Fig. 2   Luke Fildes, *The Doctor*, Public domain.

Fig. 3   Use of the terms 'evils of the modern world' and 'blessings of the modern world', in Google's record of English language literature, Google Books Ngram Viewer.

Fig. 4   Global Health Estimates 2016: Deaths by Cause, Age, Sex by Country and by Region, 2000–2016, Geneva, World Health Organisation, 2018.

Fig. 5   Life expectancy at birth, England and Wales, 1841 to 2011, ONS digital.

Acknowledgements

The iniquity of oblivion blindly scattereth her poppies but in the fields of remembrance some also blow. To Joseph Epstein I owe a strengthening of my inclination to be quotatious, and to George Saintsbury a warrant for refusing to accompany every borrowing with a reference. ("Nothing pleases me so much as an allusion that I understand – except one that I don't and have to hunt up.") Debts to people one has never met are pleasing to owe.

Pleasing too are those to figures from one's external life. Peter Buckman, my agent, prompted the idea for this book and has correctly suggested I owe him a non-pecuniary debt payable in bottles of Chateau Lynch-Bages; Saintsbury would have approved. Neil Belton, Florence Hare and Christian Duck have kindly provided their professional help and Greg Wagland is due to add his in the form of audio narration; the fact his homepage centres on a sample of the wonderful J. L. Carr shows life can quote back.

David Roberts, whose state school visits encouraging applicants to Oxford led to my admission, has generously pointed out where his efforts were wasted. His corrections to my knowledge of genetics, now and thirty years ago, have been gratefully received, and in this electronic age I can even read his writing.

Roger Barbee's advice has been much appreciated, as has the encouragement of Richard Holmes (manifest years before his 2003 seminars in the vitalising form of his Coleridge). Sebastian Thomas and Jonathan Points have provided direct help, some of it in a non-vinous form. Marion Mafham and Theo & Rachel Burch all helped too but only Marion's help involved annotations.

My mother died between the writing of the text and of these acknowledgements. I should have given her a copy early, as she'd asked.

Index

Page numbers for illustrations are in *italics*.